TECHNOLOGY IN MENTAL HEALTH

ABOUT THE EDITORS

Stephen Goss, PhD, MBACP, is an independent consultant in counselling technology, research and evaluation and a counselling practitioner and online supervisor. He coedited *Technology in Counselling and Psychotherapy: A Practitioner's Guide* with Kate Anthony and coauthored the first and third editions of the British Association for Counselling and Psychotherapy's *Guidelines for Online Counselling and Psychotherapy*. He is coeditor (counselling) of the *British Journal of Guidance and Counselling* and is Principal Lecturer on the DPsych by Professional Studies at the Metanoia Institute in London. Among his other books are *Making Research Matter* in 2016 and *Evidence Based Practice for Counselling and Psychotherapy* in 2000. He is the author of over 100 other reports and publications.

Kate Anthony, DPsych, FBACP, is a psychotherapist, consultant and international expert regarding online therapy and coaching. She is cofounder of the Online Therapy Institute, and has trained thousands of practitioners in adding online services to their practice. She is widely published on such topics as the use of email, bulletin boards, IRC, videoconferencing, stand-alone software and virtual reality – and the omnichannelling of such tools. She coedited *Technology in Counselling and Psychotherapy: A Practitioner's Guide* with Stephen Goss in 2003, coauthored *Therapy Online [a practical guide]* with DeeAnna Merz Nagel in 2010, and coauthored all three editions of the British Association for Counselling and Psychotherapy's *Guidelines for Online Counselling and Psychotherapy* and the most recent BACP Good Practice Guidance for working online.

LoriAnn Sykes Stretch, PhD, LPC-S, NCC, ACS, is a psychotherapist and consultant for online counseling and supervision. She is the Program Director/Department Chair for the Clinical Mental Health Counseling Program for The Chicago School of Professional Psychology – Online Campus and has a fully online clinical practice through Breakthrough. She has presented at state, regional, national and international conferences on distance counseling and supervision. Her specialty is training and advising clinical professionals on the legal and ethical considerations of online counseling and supervision. She helped draft legislation and the administrative code in the State of North Carolina in the U.S. legalizing and regulating distance supervision.

DeeAnna Merz Nagel, M.Ed., LMHC, BCC, is an international expert regarding online therapy and online coaching. She instructs helping professionals about the use and impact of technology, ethical practice and service delivery. She is cofounder of the Online Therapy Institute and has written several publications representing the counseling and coaching professions. She maintains her Licensed Mental Health Counselor credential and she is a Board Certified Coach. These days you can find DeeAnna online and at her Havana Wellness Studio in Florida.

Second Edition

TECHNOLOGY IN MENTAL HEALTH

Applications in Practice, Supervision and Training

Edited by

STEPHEN GOSS, PH.D., MBACP
Metanoia Institute

KATE ANTHONY, D.PSYCH., FBACP
Online Therapy Institute

LORIANN SYKES STRETCH, PH.D., LPC-S
The Chicago School of Professional Psychology

DEEANNA MERZ NAGEL, M.ED., LMHC, BCC
Havana Wellness Studio

(With 52 Other Contributors)

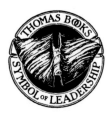

CHARLES C THOMAS • PUBLISHER, LTD.
Springfield • Illinois • U.S.A.

Published and Distributed Throughout the World by

CHARLES C THOMAS • PUBLISHER, LTD.
2600 South First Street
Springfield, Illinois 62704

© 2016 by CHARLES C THOMAS • PUBLISHER, LTD.

ISBN 978-0-398-09105-7 (paper)
ISBN 978-0-398-09106-4 (ebook)

First Edition, 2010

Second Edition, 2016

With THOMAS BOOKS *careful attention is given to all details of manufacturing
and design. It is the Publisher's desire to present books that are satisfactory as to their
physical qualities and artistic possibilities and appropriate for their particular use.*
THOMAS BOOKS *will be true to those laws of quality that assure a good name
and good will.*

Printed in the United States of America
UBC-R-3

Library of Congress Cataloging-in-Publication Data

Names: Goss, Stephen, 1966- editor. | Anthony, Kate, editor. | Stretch,
    Loriann Sykes, editor. | Nagel, DeeAnna Merz, editor.
Title: Technology in mental health : applications in practice, supervision
    and training / edited by Stephen Goss, PH.D., MBACP, Metanoia Institute,
    Kate Anthony, D.PSYCH., FBACP, Online Therapy Institute, Loriann Sykes
    Stretch, PH.D., LPC-S, The Chicago School of Professional Psychology,
    DeeAnna Merz Nagel, M.ED., LMHC, BCC, Havana Wellness Studio,
    (with 52 other contributors).
Other titles: Use of technology in mental health.
Description: Second edition. | Springfield, Illinois : Charles C. Thomas
    Publisher, LTD., [2016] | Revision of: The use of technology in mental
    health. c2010. | Includes bibliographical references and index. |
    Description based on print version record and CIP data provided by
    publisher; resource not viewed.
Identifiers: LCCN 2016000974 (print) | LCCN 2016000022 (ebook)
    ISBN 9780398091064 (ebook) | ISBN 9780398091057 (pbk.)
Subjects: LCSH: Mental health services. | Communication in medicine. |
    Medical informatics.
Classification: LCC RA790.5 (print) | LCC RA790.5 .U84 2016 (ebook) | DDC
    610.285--dc23
LC record available at http://lccn.loc.gov/2016000974

CONTRIBUTORS

Meyran Boniel-Nissim, PhD, is a senior lecturer and researcher at the School of Social Sciences and Humanities, Kinneret Academic College, Sea of Galilee, Israel; and at the Faculty of Education, University of Haifa, Haifa, Israel. Her research interests are in the psychology of the Internet, including online writing therapy, teenagers' blogs, virtual communities, online support groups, electronic media communication, and online risk behavior such as Pro-Ana communities.

Dr. Andrew M. Burck, LPC (CO), PC (OH), is an Associate Professor at Marshall University. Dr. Burck has published articles in the field of assessment, wellness and addictions. He has presented at a variety of state, regional and national conferences. Dr. Burck is a faculty advisor the Marshall University chapter of CSI. Dr. Burck is the current Member at Large (Publications) for AARC (a division of ACA).

Jennifer Askew Buxton, BS, PharmD, CPP, FASHP, is the Director of Pharmacy and Co-Director of Mental Health at Cape Fear Clinic, Inc. in Wilmington, North Carolina. Dr. Buxton, a North Carolina native, received her Doctorate of Pharmacy from the University of North Carolina at Chapel Hill and completed a Primary Care Residency with Coastal Area Health Education Center and New Hanover Regional Medical Center. Dr. Buxton has held local, state, and national leadership positions with the American Society of Health-Systems Pharmacists (ASHP), the North Carolina Association of Pharmacists (NCAP), the International Pharmaceutical Federation (FIP), the American College of Clinical Pharmacy (ACCP), and the American Pharmacists Association (APhA). She is also a preceptor of students and residents and is the author of a book entitled *From Student to Pharmacist: Making the Transition.*

KaRae' N. Carey, PhD, LPC-S, NCC, ACS, DCC, LCAS, BC-HSP, is a psychotherapist and clinical addictions specialist serving clients in both traditional and online format. She also works full-time as a professor in a CACREP accredited University. KaRae' enjoys teaching counseling students new to the field as well as providing training for veteran counselors via presentations at regional and national conferences. She resides and practices in Cary, North Carolina.

Linnea Carlson-Sabelli, PhD, is Professor Emeritus of Psychiatric Nursing at Rush University College of Nursing, Chicago, Illinois, where she has been a faculty member since 1978. She has received grants in excess of one million dollars from the U.S. Department of Health and Human Services to develop creative online methods for clinical psychiatric nurse supervision.

Kate Cavanagh is a Senior Clinical Lecturer in the School of Psychology at the University of Sussex and Honorary Clinical Psychologist in Sussex Partnership NHS Trust. Her research interests include increasing access to evidence-based psychological therapies for common mental health problems and she has been involved in the research, development, and implementation computerised mental health interventions over the past 15 years.

Ginger Clark is a Professor of Clinical Education in the Marriage and Family Therapy program at the University of Southern California. She is also serving as President of the Academic Senate for the 2015–2016 academic year. In addition to her academic position, she is a licensed psychologist and part of a group practice in Long Beach, California. Ginger infuses technology into her academic work, requiring students to utilize online platforms and websites to further enhance their learning process.

Diane H. Coursol, PhD, is currently Co-Chair of the Technology Interest Network for the American Association of Counselor Education and Supervision. She is a Professor of Counselor Education at Minnesota State University, Mankato. She teaches Technology in Counseling, Assessment, Treatment Planning, Counseling Procedures and Skills, Practicum, and Internship. Research interests include technology in counseling and supervision, counseling process and outcome, career and workplace issues, mindfulness and the therapeutic process, diagnosis and treatment planning.

David Coyle, PhD, is a Lecturer in Computer Science at University College Dublin. His research focuses on the design of new technologies to support mental health and emotional wellbeing. Recent interests include the investigation of sustainable approaches to improving mental health services for children and adolescents.

Kathleene Derrig-Palumbo, PhD, is a leading figure and international speaker in the world of online mental health services. She is a lead consultant and expert for the Dr. Phil Show. She is a recent recipient of a Stevie Award for "Best Woman Entrepreneur – Service Business." In addition to many published articles in magazines and journals as well as authored chapters in books, she is well-known for her book, *Online Therapy: A Therapist's Guide to Expanding Your Practice*.

John Devaney, Executive Director of Cape Fear Clinic, has more than 20 years of progressive experience leading nonprofits, with almost 18 years in healthcare. He has held the positions of Vice-President of a national healthcare consulting firm, Director of the largest HIV/AIDS clinic in Virginia, and Director of Operations of one of the oldest pro-bono legal providers in the U.S. He holds a BS in Sociology from Longwood University in Farmville, Virginia.

Vanessa Dodd is a researcher at the International Centre for Guidance Studies at the University of Derby. She received her Master's in Applied Sociology at Clemson University. She has research interests in both quantitative and qualitative methods particularly as it applies to digital contexts. She has managed various projects for governmental and non-profit organizations at local, national and international levels.

Mark Dombeck, PhD, is a licensed psychologist in private practice (https://psychtools. com) near Oakland, California. He is a former director of Mental Help Net (https:// www.mentalhelp.net), one of the first consumer mental health education websites, and presently directs Sift.Care (https://sift.care), a referral sharing resource for mental health professionals.

Glenn Duncan, LPC, LCADC, CCS, ACS, has been working in the behavioral healthcare field for over twenty years. He has lectured nationally in the USA on many topics including the *Diagnostic and Statistical Manual of Mental Disorders*, clinical supervision and emerging drugs of abuse. Glenn is a Licensed Professional Counselor, a Licensed Clinical Alcohol/Drug Counselor, a Certified Clinical Supervisor, and an

Approved Clinical Supervisor. Glenn has a Master's in Clinical Psychology from Western Carolina University. Glenn is currently at Hunterdon Drug Awareness Program, Inc. as Executive Director since 2003. Glenn specializes in working with clients who have co-occurring substance use disorders, depressive disorders, and anxiety disorders.

Joe Ferns is UK Knowledge and Portfolio Director for the Big Lottery Fund. He was previously Deputy Director of Policy and Projects at Samaritans. He is a media spokesperson and has worked on several national and international advisory groups on suicide prevention. Prior to Samaritans, he worked for the Institute of Psychiatry on a project running psychoeducational workshops for people with depression and anxiety problems. Joe has over 19 years experience in mental health in settings including residential services, community outreach, day services, advocacy and 1:1 support work.

Rebecca Grist is a Research Fellow for the LifeGuide Project based in the Centre for Applications of Health Psychology (CAHP) at the University of Southampton, where she is involved in exploring perceptions of Internet interventions built using the Life-Guide software. She completed her PhD in Psychology at the University of Sussex in 2014 under the supervision of Dr Kate Cavanagh and Professor Graham Davey.

John M. Grohol, PsyD, has been writing, researching, and publishing in the area of online mental health, psychology and human behavior since 1992. He sits on the editorial board of *Computers in Human Behaviour* and is a founding member of the Society for Participatory Medicine. Since 1995, he has been overseeing the leading mental health network online today, PsychCentral.com, named one of the 50 Best Websites in 2008 by *TIME*.

Melissa Groman is a Licensed Clinical Social Worker with a private practice in Nutley, New Jersey. She is the founder and director of the Good Practice Institute for Professional Psychotherapists (www.goodpracticeinstitute.com), a clinical resource and learning center for psychotherapists. The Good Practice Institute offers individual and group clinical supervision and consultation and classes via telephone, bringing together clinicians from around the world to consult, learn, study and advance their practice.

Samara (Rainey) Harms is a freelance research consultant based in the northeast United States. Published in the areas of mental health, technology and the law, she frequently collaborates with Dr. Patricia Recupero and her colleagues at Butler Hospital. A major research and teaching psychiatric hospital in Providence, Rhode Island, Butler is affiliated with The Warren Alpert Medical School of Brown University.

Tristram Hooley is Professor of Career Education at the International Centre for Guidance Studies at the University of Derby. His research interests include career education and guidance, the interface between policy and practice and the social and educational role of Internet technologies. He also writes the Adventures in Career Development blog at https://adventuresincareerdevelopment.wordpress.com/.

Roy Huggins, MS, LPC, NCC, is a counselor in private practice in Portland, Oregon, who also directs Person-Centered Tech. Roy worked as a professional Web developer for 7 years before changing paths to counseling. He is an adjunct instructor at the Portland State University Counseling program where he teaches Ethics, is a member of the Zur Institute advisory board and routinely consults for colleagues on issues of tech in clinical practice.

Audrey Jung, a Licensed Professional Counselor and National Certified Counselor, is the owner of Affiliated Psych Services in Chandler, Arizona. Audrey earned her B.A. at the University of Maryland College Park, in Psychology, and her M.A. in Counseling at Gallaudet University. Audrey is a former Executive Board Member for the International Society of Mental Health Online. Audrey offers a variety of experience including, but not limited to, marital counseling, stress reduction and pregnancy/post-partum issues.

Eva Kaltenthaler, PhD, is a Professor of Health Technology Assessment at the School of Health and Related Research at the University of Sheffield. She has a special interest in mental health issues, especially patient acceptability of technologies. She has completed comprehensive systematic reviews of Computerised Cognitive Behaviour Therapy for the National Institute for Health and Care Excellence. She has also completed systematic reviews of group cognitive behaviour therapy for postnatal depression, art therapy to treat mental health disorders and sexual health interventions for people with severe mental illness.

Thomas J. Kim, MD, received his BA in Philosophy from Georgetown University and MD, MPH from Tulane University. He continued at Tulane to complete a combined residency in Internal Medicine and Psychiatry and a General Medicine fellowship in health services research. At present, he serves as Physician Advisor for Government Affairs at Athenahealth, an integrated web-based practice management company.

Reid Klion, PhD, is the Chief Science Officer of pan-A TALX Company (www.panpowered.com). He is an expert in web-based assessment and is actively involved in scientific, regulatory and industry issues related to testing. He has published extensively and presents regularly at international professional conferences. A licensed psychologist, he is a graduate of Hobart College and received his doctorate in Clinical Psychology from Miami University.

Jonathan Lent, PhD, PC, Certified School Counselor is a full-time Counselor Educator at Marshall University in Huntington, West Virginia. He is also works directly with local schools in providing workshops and consultation regularly. He has presented at national conferences and published on many topics, specifically technology in Counselor Education, burnout, wellness and career issues.

Jacqueline Lewis is a Professor in the Department of Counseling and Student Personnel at Minnesota State University, Mankato. She currently serves as Co-Chair of the Technology Interest Network for the American Association of Counselor Education and Supervision. Her research areas include technology in counseling and student affairs, career development and diversity in counseling and student affairs.

Michèle Mani, MEd, is a Registered Psychotherapist with over 13 years experience in the field of Employee and Family Assistance Programs (EFAP). As a Clinical Supervisor, Michèle has provided training and supervision to crisis counsellors, tele-counsellors and online counsellors practicing E-Counselling and Online Group Counselling for Morneau Shepell. Michèle draws upon a variety of clinical methods and applies narrative, solution-focused and CBT approaches online.

Dr. Mark Matthews is a Research Associate at Cornell University. His research focuses on developing low-cost technologies for people experiencing mental illness with a focus on solutions with real world applicability. He has been working for over 10 years to create innovative technologies to support mental wellness, including the award-winning Personal Investigator and MoodRhythm, an award-winning app designed to help people with bipolar disorder stabilize their sleep and social patterns. He is passionate about using play to both diagnose and treat a wide range of mental illnesses.

Paul McCrone, PhD, is Professor in Health Economics at the Institute of Psychiatry, Psychology and Neuroscience (King's College London), where he has worked for 23 years after having previously worked at the University of Kent. He has worked on a large number of economic studies in health and social care. Currently he is involved in evaluations in psychiatry, neurology, cancer, HIV and palliative care. He teaches health economics to Masters-level students and has published widely in peer-reviewed journals.

Siobhan Neary, EdD, is the Deputy Head of the International Centre for Guidance Studies (iCeGS), University of Derby. She is a career guidance professional who has worked in the sector as a practitioner, trainer, manager, lecturer and researcher for over twenty-five years. Siobhan's research interests focus on the continuing professional development, workforce development and professional identity of career development practitioners.

Deb Osborn, PhD, is an Associate Professor in the Educational Psychology and Learning Systems Department at Florida State University, a Nationally Certified Counselor and Fellow of the National Career Development Association and American Counseling Association. She is Past President of NCDA, and currently serves on the NCDA and ACA boards as a governing council representative. She has multiple publications and presentations on the design and use of technology in counseling.

Gregory Palumbo is a pioneer in online mental health services technology. He has overseen the project management of enterprise-level software systems designed for use by mental healthcare providers. He is currently overseeing the development of a suite of Web 2.0 solutions adapted for use by mental healthcare providers. Previous to this work, he served as CEO of Galilay Entertainment, COO of Innerlight Entertainment and CTO for Magic Image Films, a subsidiary of Digital Magic, now Todd AO West.

Daniel M. Paredes, PhD, is a clinical counselor in the North Carolina Agricultural and Technical State University's Counseling Service. A member of national and state professional associations, he has been inducted into the Chi Sigma Iota Counseling Academic and Professional Honor Society. He is a graduate of the University of California at San Diego and of the University of North Carolina at Greensboro.

Marcos A. Quinones is a Spanish-bilingual psychotherapist treating patients in New York City. As a member of the Association for Contextual and Behavioral Sciences, he focuses on behavioral and cognitive therapies with a clinical interest in interpersonal relationships. Marcos is completing a masters degree in social neuroscience at Columbia University and works as an adjunct professor of social work at New York University, where he teaches dialectical behavioral therapy and at Hunter College where he teaches Cognitive Behavioral Therapy.

Patricia Ryan Recupero, JD, MD, is the SVP of Education and Training for Care New England Health System and past President and CEO of Butler Hospital. She serves as Clinical Professor of Psychiatry in the Department of Psychiatry and Human

Behavior at the Warren Alpert Medical School of Brown University. She holds board certification in Forensic Psychiatry and Addiction Psychiatry and writes on technology in medical practice.

Dr. Corinne Reid is a clinical psychologist and Associate Professor leading the post-graduate program at Murdoch University in Western Australia. She uses video therapy in her work with élite athletes as they compete around the world and also in working with other clients and professionals working in rural and remote settings across the vast geographical expanse of Australia. Her particular interest is in person-centred approaches and how the therapeutic relationship can best translate in a technological setting.

Claudia Repetto PhD, PsyD, is a Research Fellow in Neuropsychology at the Catholic University of the Sacred Heart, Milan. Her research combines neuroscience and new technology frontiers to build powerful tools for improving language abilities.

Dr Lisa K. Richardson is a Clinical Psychologist from Perth, Western Australia. She works for the Statewide Community Forensic Mental Health Service and Joondalup Older Adult Mental Health Service in WA and is an adjunct lecturer at Murdoch University in Perth. She wrote her doctoral research in the use of telepsychology to provide community mental health clinic-based clinical psychology interventions to regional WA centres and was awarded a Fulbright Research Scholars award to study in the USA to complete this work.

Giuseppe Riva, PhD, is Full Professor of Communication Psychology and Director of the Communication and Ergonomics of New Technologies Lab. – ICE NET Lab. – at the Catholic University of Milan, Italy. He also serves as Head Researcher at the Applied Technology for Neuro-Psychology Laboratory – ATN-P Lab., Istituto Auxologico Italiano, Milan, Italy. Currently he is Editor in Chief for the *Emerging Communication* book series and for the online journals *Annual Review of Cybertherapy and Telemedicine and Psychology*. More, he is European Editor for the *CyberPsychology & Behavior* journal.

Denise E. Saunders, PhD, maintains a private practice in Chapel Hill, North Carolina, providing psychotherapy, counseling and consultation services to her clients. In addition to work with individual clients, she consults with higher educational institutions, for-profit organizations, community groups and government agencies. She has served as counselor and trainer for a provider of distance career counseling services. She is a Licensed Psychologist in the state of North Carolina, a National Certified Counselor and a Distanced Credentialed Counselor.

John W. Seymour, PhD, LMFT, is a Professor in Counseling at Minnesota State University, Mankato. He is an Approved Supervisor with the American Association of Marriage and Family and a Registered Play Therapist-Supervisor with the Association for Play Therapy. Prior to teaching graduate supervision, family therapy and play therapy courses at the University, he worked in a variety of settings, including hospital, agency and residential treatment.

Susan Simpson is senior lecturer and Psychology Clinic Director on the postgraduate training program for clinical psychology at the University of South Australia, where she teaches and supervises videoconferencing-based psychotherapy. She previously ran a telepsychology service between Aberdeen and Shetland within NHS Grampian for many years, and has carried out research into the effectiveness and acceptability of videoconferencing-based psychotherapy for a range of clinical problems. She is particularly interested in the way in which the technologies can influence therapeutic rapport.

Cedric Speyer is Clinical Supervisor, E-Counselling, for Morneau Shepell, Toronto, Canada and Director, InnerView Guidance International (IGI). He holds Master degrees in Creative Writing, Counseling Psychology and Education. As founder and pioneer of the Shepell E-Counselling service, he developed and implemented a short-term counselling model for online practitioners, edited a textbook on the subject, and continues to engage in related writing and publishing, while serving as an e-therapy mentor.

Anne Stokes is a senior accredited BACP counsellor and trainer and also has a large supervision practice. She is a Director of Online Training Ltd., founding the OCTIA Conferences (Online Counselling and Therapy In Action) with her co-director, Gill Jones, some six years ago, and was instrumental in setting up ACTO (The Association for Counselling and Therapy Online). Currently she divides her time between her home in the UK and her home in France, working with clients, supervisees and students online.

Jean-Anne Sutherland, PhD, is Associate Professor of sociology at University of North Carolina, Wilmington, and focuses on two areas of research: the sociology of mothering, guilt, and shame and sociology through film. Her chapter, entitled "Ideal Mama, Ideal Worker: Negotiating Guilt and Shame in Academe" appears in, *Women Write About Motherhood and the Academy*. Her textbook, edited with Kathryn Feltey, is entitled *Cinematic Sociology: Social Life in Film.*

Leon Tan (PhD, *Auck*) is an art and culture historian, critic, artist, educator and registered psychotherapist. He publishes on contemporary art, public art, globalization, digital culture and social activism; advises artists and arts organizations and is a member of the International Association of Art Critics. He is a senior lecturer and MDes programme leader at Unitec's Department of Design and Contemporary Arts, and a member of Auckland Council's newly established Advisory Panel on Art in Public Places (New Zealand).

Allison Thompson is a Counselor for St. Aloysius Orphanage where she works with children, adolescents and families. She is a graduate from Xavier University's Master of Arts program in Counseling (2008) and earned a Bachelor of Science from Ohio University (2004). She was published in the August 2008 issue of *Counseling Today* and in *The Use of Technology in Mental Health: Applications, Ethics and Practice* (1st edition).

Karen Turner runs www.elderwisdom.com, helping clients to expand their self-knowledge and to access and learn to trust the authentic self within them. Utilizing the tools and techniques used from the Online Therapy Institute course, plus the experience of a long career in integrating tools of Eastern and Western psychology, she works both in-person and online in private practice.

Barb Veder, Vice President Clinical Services and Research Lead, has spent over 20 years as clinical leader with Morneau Shepell. Barb has extensive clinical experience and is deeply involved with clinical research and counsellor education. She is committed to the development of clinical best practices, resources and support for individuals struggling with depression, anxiety and other mental health issues. She is actively involved with EASNA, EAPA, and EARF (Employee Assistance Research Foundation).

Kristin Ann Vincenzes, PhD, LPC, NCC, ACS, is a psychotherapist and clinical supervisor. She is the Program Director for the Online Clinical Mental Health Counseling Program for Lock Haven University. She has presented at state and national conferences and her professional specialties include: online learning and clinical supervision as well as counseling children, adolescents and the military/veteran population.

John Yaphe, MD, CM (McGill University), **MClSc** (Western Ontario), is a family physician and Associate Professor in community health at the School of Medicine, University of Minho, Braga, Portugal. He has been an active online counsellor with the Morneau Shepell Employee and Family Assistance Program (EFAP) since 2004. Dr. Yaphe has contributed to the theory and practice of online counselling by publishing articles, conducting seminars and presenting related papers worldwide.

For Catriona, Andrew and for E
for the best motivations I will ever know.

For my nephew Azza Kemp (SuperStar) and as ever for P
for keeping my warmest dreams afloat.

To my two beautiful children, countless students, mentors and peers
who inspire me to be my best.

To Stephen and Kate for your dedication and commitment
to this project while supporting my career at the crossroads.
I have landed in a very different yet familiar place
with our collective experience to guide my work
with coaches and healers. XO!

INTRODUCTION

Kate Anthony

It was with excitement and also trepidation that we received the invitation from our publisher to produce a second edition of this textbook. Excitement at the opportunity to refresh and update the valuable work from the extensive list of colleagues who contributed to the first edition, but also trepidation in considering the task of assessing what to include this time around and deciding what information needed to be assigned to the history of using technology in mental health. In addition, it was an opportunity to include a whole new section on the use of technologies in the field of supervision, both clinical and peer, and to ensure that this vital strand of input into the professions of counselling, psychotherapy and coaching got the attention it deserves.

In the half-decade since the publication of the first edition, we have seen changes in society brought about by the rise of technology in our everyday lives that also have a distinct impact on our mental health. The most important of these has been the shift in the way human interaction itself is conducted, with electronic text-based exchanges becoming more normal than the picking up of the telephone to use our voices and the ubiquity of social media leading us to consider even the core nature of privacy itself. The large consumer organisations have become verbs themselves – we are likely to Google a mental health problem before making an appointment at the doctors, or Facebook a friend before dialling their number. We tweet information we want to disseminate, and we YouTube how-to videos rather than consulting a manual. Even the early formation of human relationship making is changing – we swipe until we find a potential match or, conversely, may not wish to meet a stranger unless we have searched all the information the Internet has to offer us about them.

Alongside these shifts, the mental health field has rushed to keep up. Amongst the following pages, you will see the theoretical development about human behaviour as we witness it playing out in Cyberspace; the ethical development as each new technology brings its own concerns about how it is affecting the client and the practitioner (and the therapeutic process itself); and the exciting application of those technologies in delivering innovative and robust ways of improving the mental health of human beings in a world where our connections are available 24 hours a day and our electronic devices have (for many) become our constant companions.

Perhaps the most fundamental shift in our thinking since the last edition is in the attitude to how we approach it. From the caution employed (rightly) in the first decade of this century in the application of technology within counselling, psychotherapy and its associated professions such as coaching, we have matured into no longer being surprised by its existence. Text-messaging is used to make, remind and cancel appointments as standard. Our medical records, including those about our mental health, are electronically stored in "the cloud." We use videoconferencing to conduct sessions with clients and create whole virtual worlds to explore the inner workings of our psyches. We are no longer restricted by geographical boundaries to communicate, or beholden to time zones in choosing when to do so. The global environment of society and how we relate to each other has changed fundamentally. It has been an incredibly exciting time to be a professional in the field of mental health.

So where did we start in producing a second edition of such a potentially vast area of study? We decided early on to cover better the area of supervision, and brought a fourth editor on board, LoriAnn Sykes Stretch, to add her expertise to the core of the original editors in myself, Stephen, and DeeAnna. We then approached our original authors to revisit and revise their specialist topic, or to suggest a new author where their own careers had taken a different turn, and invited new specialists in the field of cybersupervision to add their voices. As with the first edition of the book, its creation and development had taken time, but we hope you agree it has been worth waiting for. We have included the new technologies that we were looking forward to in our last edition, and now eagerly anticipate the technologies of the future for our next edition!

OVERVIEW

As before, the book is designed to be both useful to the reader wishing to dip into information on a certain technology and its application to their service provision, or for the reader looking for a comprehensive overview of the state of the art as a whole at the time of writing. It should be noted that each author may have a different view of how these technologies are best implemented. As example, the editors conclude that the use of encryption is paramount and nonnegotiable, but the legal implications of what service, product or platform to utilise is not within the purview of this book. The editors advise practitioners to seek legal counsel regarding such matters, particularly concerning terms of use and privacy issues.

What you will also again find in the book is a wide range of styles, from the individual practitioner exploring a new technology and writing anecdotally about their personal experience, to medical practitioners writing an academic overview of a technology and its uses in the profession. Within each chapter, you will find reference to definitions of the technology, application to the therapeutic intervention being discussed, case material and illustrations, ethical examination and concluding thoughts on the future impact of the technology on the profession. All case illustrations are fictionalized, although all are based on authors' direct, practical experience. This book is an extensive body of work on the topic and we hope you find it of use professionally and personally in your online and offline life.

Finally, the book is now in two clear sections, the first addressing the technologies as they apply to being used in counselling and psychotherapy itself and second section applying to training and supervision.

PART ONE: THE USE OF TECHNOLOGY IN MENTAL HEALTH

In Chapter 1, "Using Email to Conduct a Therapeutic Relationship," Patricia Ryan Recupero and Samara Harms revisit the impact of the use of email for therapeutic use, its application and ethical issues such as risks to confidentiality, appropriateness for client work, standards of care and administrative issues before turning to the cases of clients "Sheila" and "John" by way of short illustration. They conclude, as do many other authors in the book, that even now further research is still needed to be able to provide an ethical, practical, and beneficial service via the technology discussed in the chapter.

In Chapter 2, "Using Chat and Instant Messaging (IM) to Conduct a Therapeutic Relationship," Kathleene Derrig-Palumbo considers how to conduct a therapeutic relationship via chat rooms and instant messaging. She discusses issues such as identity, how the therapeutic relationship is formulated and maintained, practical strategies for encouraging progress of the work via text, and some theoretical orientations that successfully underpin. She then gives a chat room session with a client "Joshua," who was unable to communicate face-to-face, but through chat rooms developed an ability to open up and therefore communicate better with his parents. She concludes that in the future, online therapy may well be regarded as no different than in-person therapy.

In Chapter 3, "Using Mobile Phone Communication for Therapeutic Intervention," Roy Huggins looks at the use of mobile phone texting (SMS or "Short Message Service") and how we as humans connect in the modern world. Such modern use of text to communicate with each other has shifted our expectations of being in demand and also our definitions of what is private and what is not. In a therapeutic context, this "asynchronous yet semi-interruptive" technology has meant that many clients perceive their mental health practitioner to be available all of the time, creating boundary issues that didn't exist pre-smartphones. Keeping up with the new rules for keeping in touch with our clients, and how we do this, is fast becoming essential within the modern practitioner's service provision, alongside a close consideration of how such convenient communicative tools can be ethically used.

Chapter 4, "The Rise of Social Networks and the Benefits and Risks to the Mental Health Profession," is by Allison Thompson and studies the impact of online communities and their role in impacting on mental health. She examines the dangers of dual relationships and the importance of boundaries and gives two clear examples of when this can impact negatively on therapeutic or professional work. She concludes with the need for research in this topic, and also points out that social media may influence on how organizations around the world may monitor the private lives of counselors who belong to online communities.

In Chapter 5, "Using Forums to Enhance Client Peer Support," the book shifts towards looking at technologies for peer support with an updated chapter on the topic from Meyran Boniel-Nissim. She describes and defines online support groups, looks at both the positive and negative aspects within them, and points out the differences between them and conducting therapy online. She discusses the research into the field and concludes that the advent of online support groups has significantly positively changed the mental condition of many people suffering from various types of personal distress. Future research into how peer communities are flourishing on social networking sites is rightly identified as being essential.

Chapter 6, "Using Cell/Mobile Phone SMS to Enhance Client Crisis and Peer Support," by Stephen Goss and Joe Ferns, examines SMS Crisis Support and Peer Support, based on a presentation given at the first Online Counselling and Therapy In Action (OCTIA) conference in the UK in 2009. They explore the development process and use of SMS text messaging systems in support services, in particular The Samaritans in the UK. They include case material – text messages sent and responded to – to illustrate the chapter and conclude that as in the case of many of the technologies examined in this book, the initial fears and doubts about the use of SMS in mental health services are steadily being dispelled.

Chapter 7, "Using Websites, Blogs, and Wikis in Mental Health," is reviewed and updated by John M. Grohol, who offers an examination of websites, blogs, and wikis. He discusses the application of these technologies and also the ethical implications and issues that are inherent in them. For example, wikis can be a huge source of *mis*information as well as information and blogs "can provide people with all sorts of potentially harmful (or at the very least, useless) personal opinions that carry some legitimacy if the blog is popular." The case example of "Jane" describes her journey in exploring options to treat her depression via websites and blogs on the topic, before finally taking the plunge to seek professional help from an individual. He concludes with thoughts on the role of the Internet in lessening isolation and the stigma around seeking help for mental health issues.

In Chapter 8, "The Role of Blogging in Mental Health," DeeAnna Merz Nagel and Gregory Palumbo take a look at blogging in detail, noting how the Internet brought change not only to how people could distribute their writings, but also to how those writings could remain dynamic and alive. The most popular example of technologies that support this interactivity is blogging. The authors examine the business applications of blogging as well as the use of blogs in mental health for disseminating information and education and also as a form of journaling for clients, all with examples. They also visit micro-blogging sites such as Twitter. They conclude that "whether for professional or personal pursuits, when used responsibly, blogging can make a substantial and positive impact on the counseling profession and the world at large."

At Chapter 9, "Using the Telephone for Conducting a Therapeutic Relationship," the book again shifts towards non-text-based technological interventions with an updated chapter on using the telephone for mental health services from Denise Saunders and Debra Osborn. They define "telephone counseling," examine the state of it in practice via evidence-based findings, the benefits and limitations, the ethical considerations of telephone use such as security and confidentiality and the practical applications. They offer the case examples of "May" and "Jonathan," describing their experience working by telephone. They conclude with thoughts on the possibility that "one day it will be commonplace for counselors to provide distance services to clients exclusively" and state the prominent role the telephone will have in this.

Continuing the theme of voice-based interactions, Chapter 10, "Therapeutic Alliance in Videoconferencing-Based Psychotherapy," is by Susan Simpson, Lisa Richardson, and Corinne Reid, who look at the role of videoconferencing. This particular technology has seen an increase in its use since the first edition of this book and this valuable chapter is updated accordingly. As well as examining what we already know about videoconference use in mental health services, the authors examine the factors associated with the quality of the therapeutic alliance and give extensive recommendations for enhancing the quality of the interaction. They also examine what videoconferencing platforms are suitable for professional mental health services and, perhaps more importantly, which aren't (and why).

In Chapter 11, "Using Virtual Reality Immersion Therapeutically," Guiseppe Riva and Claudia Repetto re-examine immersion in four virtual environments: full, CAVE, augmented, and desktop. They give an examination of the role of virtual reality (VR) in clinical psychology in relation to conditions such as phobias, posttraumatic stress and anxiety disorders. They also note, however, that VR has further implications for treatment beyond desensitisation and exposure therapy, such as being immersed in the environment with the practitioner in such a way that is indistinguishable from the non-virtual world via the role of "presence." Riva and Repetto identify four major issues that limit the use of VR in practice and discuss how they and colleagues have addressed this.

In Chapter 12, "The Use of Computer-Aided Cognitive Behavioural Therapy (CCBT) in Therapeutic Settings," Kate Cavanagh and Rebecca Grist give a history of the evolution of cognitive behavioural theories into providing these interventions via Computerised Cognitive Behavioural Therapy (CCBT). They revisit various software packages before focusing down on Beating the Blues and FearFighter and the evidence of outcomes for such programmes. Ethical consideration is given to their use and the importance of balancing this with in-person intervention. The authors conclude with showing how CCBT is important as a hands-on early option for effective self-help in a growing number of mental health problems.

Chapter 13, "The Role of Gaming in Mental Health," by Mark Matthews and David Coyle, revisits and updates us on the use of games to engage adolescents – a client group notoriously reluctant to access counselling – in the therapeutic process. They show how appropriately designed games (in contrast to the other types that receive so much negative media coverage) can be used for this purpose and to help adolescents get the mental health assistance they need. Matthews and Coyle start with ethical discussion before giving a history of the limited previous research and noting some of the benefits defined by such research, advocating caution in trusting results without further examination. He describes *Personal Investigator*, a 3-D computer game based on Solution-Focused Therapy, and SPARX, a self-help, stand-alone fantasy game to battle depression literally. The authors conclude by looking to the future of gaming for mental health treatment services.

In Chapter 14, "Web-based Clinical Assessment," Reid Klion considers web-based clinical assessment, including its history, application in relation to therapeutic intervention and ethics. He goes on to discuss the case of "Robert," before concluding with a look to the future, where he postulates that tests will be developed specifically for Internet-based delivery and that we are at the edge of the revolution when it comes to web-based assessment.

In Chapter 15, "The Role of Behavioral Telehealth in Mental Health," Thomas J. Kim discusses behavioural telehealth, showing how technology has transformed healthcare and defines its role through historic examination, looking at the current landscape and offering opinions based on clinical and program development experience. Kim starts with a case study to illustrate post-disaster intervention via psychiatric telehealth, before offering a telehealth model. He goes on to show the challenges the profession faces in this field such as licensure and malpractice suits, some future directions and a call for meaningful healthcare reform.

In Chapter 16, "The Use of Virtual Reality for Peer Support," Leon Tan takes a look at the use of Virtual Reality for this purpose. He describes both in-vivo exposure therapy (IVET) and Virtual Reality exposure therapy (VRET) before discussing mental health affordances, defined as the "opportunities and risks provided by a social environment to affect the mental health of individuals" and its application to VR, in this case Second Life (SL). He illustrates his chapter with reports from CBS news about a woman, "Patricia," who suffered from agoraphobia but overcame her difficulties through SL. Tan discusses some of the psychological processes a client can undergo in such environments and in which peers can assist. He concludes with pointing out the powerful impact such environments can have on an individual's mental health.

In Chapter 17, "The Use of Podcasting in Mental Health," Marcos A. Quinones describes his work with podcasting in helping clients improving their mental and physical health by downloading audio or video files on various topics. He also defines best practice for testing in Mental Health and gives anecdotal evidence to support the success this method of communicating to clients. He recommends structures for content and the hardware and software required, before examining the ethical considerations needed when planning to podcast.

Chapter 18, "The Use of Online Psychological Testing for Self-Help," is a study of online psychological testing, by Mark Dombeck, as it applies to self-help. Dombeck reviews how online testing supports mental health self-help efforts, discusses problems and concerns associated with online testing and self-help practices and offers informed speculation concerning the ways in which online psychological testing and self-help technologies are likely to develop in the future. He also examines in detail the downsides of this technology.

In Chapter 19, "Text-Based Credentialing in Mental Health," Daniel M. Paredes examines how text-based continuing education (CE) in the USA and continuing professional development (CPD) in the UK can meet the requirements imposed by credentialing bodies for the profession. He defines what text-based CE/CPD is and examines some of the issues inherent in it. He also examines the ethical considerations needed and a framework to classify CE activities according to general content area, including research into the topic to illustrate it.

Chapter 20 is about "Online Research Methods for Mental Health," by Tristram Hooley and Vanessa Dodd. The chapter focuses on online methods for counselling and psychotherapy research, including a brief history and considering the ethical issues inherent in conducting research in this way. They conclude that although online research should not be seen as a replacement for traditional onsite methods, they will continue to be an essential part of the researchers' toolkit.

Chapter 21, "Evaluating the Role of Electronic and Web-Based (e-CBT) CBT in Mental Health," returns to the updated subject of Computerised CBT (CCBT) from Eva Kaltenthaler, Kate Cavanagh and Paul McCrone. They give an evaluation of stand-alone computer software programs for depression and anxiety, with attention to issues of trial design and the components of CCBT packages. Program and client considerations are taken into account, as well as logistical and ethical balances.

In Chapter 22, "The Role of Film and Media in Mental Health," Jean-Anne Sutherland turns the reader's attention to the use of films and media in educating counselors and supervisors by noting how they provide an opportunity for clients in a therapeutic setting to recognize and potentially identify and struggle with deep-seated conflicts. She reviews the literature and notes cautions and considerations before concluding that films can be an ideal tool for illustrating life and how it is the work of the therapist to frame those representations in such as way as to provide meaningful analysis for the client.

PART TWO: THE USE OF TECHNOLOGY IN TRAINING AND SUPERVISION

In Chapter 23, "An Approach to the Training and Supervision of Online Counsellors," the authors Cedric Speyer and John Yaphe offer us one model of online supervision as it applies to asynchronous communication, as well as reviewing practices that have emerged within the framework of an established e-counselling service. They present the principles of online supervision used in their service, discuss common challenges faced by counsellors and present some online supervisory interventions using composite case excerpts. The authors conclude with reflections on future developments for Internet supervision of distance counselling.

In Chapter 24, "Using Chat and Instant Messaging (IM) to Enrich Counselor Training and Supervision," DeeAnna Merz Nagel and I discuss the use of chat and instant messaging for online supervision and illustrate this with the experience of the authors of the first edition of the chapter working together in an agency setting that offered in-home counseling and evaluation services to clients in rural locations. We define chat, clinical supervision, peer supervision, and field supervision and conclude that chat supervision can be used as a stand-alone method of delivery or it can be combined with other technology and face-to-face supervision, enriching any supervisory experience.

Chapter 25, "Using Forums to Enrich Counselor Training and Supervision," is by Linnea Carlson-Sabelli. Her goals are to provide definitions, applications, ethical considerations, illustrations of supervision techniques and speculation on the future of online text-based clinical supervision based on extensive experience supervising graduate-level Psychiatric Mental Health Nurse Practitioner students at a major medical university located in the Midwest United States. She also looks at future applications of technologies using virtual reality environments and how they may best be implemented in the future to enrich counsellor training and supervision.

In Chapter 26, "Traditional Uses of Technology in Counseling Education and Supervision," Ginger Clark gives an overview of the traditional use of technology in counseling education and supervision. She defines various types of technologies used for this purpose and examines the ethical issues in each, the effect on the trainee practitioner, the client and the therapeutic process itself, illustrated with case vignettes. She concludes that it is unlikely that any of these technologies will disappear in the near future but that their implementation will change and develop – as it already has in the years since our first edition.

In Chapter 27, "The Use of Telephone to Enrich Counselor Training and Supervision," Mellissa Groman gives an analysis of the use of the telephone for supervision and consultation. Among the questions she considers are how the relationship between consultant and therapist gets established and develops, whether the benefits of clinical consultation and supervision can apply across the airways and whether the goals of supervision can be met without visual cues and sight induced transferences. She concludes that "phone supervision's appeal will likely continue to grow as technology continues to dissolve geographic limitations."

Chapter 28, "CyberSupervision: Supervision in a Technological Age," by Diane Coursol, Jacqueline Lewis, and John Seymour, considers the same field but in relation to the use of videoconferencing software and hardware. They discuss the concept of what they name "cybersupervision," its implementation and the process, illustrating these with case examples. They give an overview of the ethical implications of cybersupervision, before concluding that there is increasing evidence for its viability and the likelihood of this perception growing.

In Chapter 29, "Mentoring Therapists to Work Online Effectively," I team up with DeeAnna and also our respected colleague Audrey Jung and one of our graduates, Karen Turner. We examine the history of how training has been provided – both face-to-face and online – and conclude that the future of training therapists to be effective when working online seems to invite blended technologies – including face-to-face work where appropriate – to provide a suite of trainings in the use of technology for mental health that reflect the increasing blending of online and offline aspects of day-to-day living.

Chapter 30 presents "An Updated Ethical Framework for the Use of Technology in Supervision," which was written originally in 2012 by three of this book's editors – LoriAnn Sykes Stretch, DeeAnna Merz Nagel, and I. Presented as part of the suite of Ethical Frameworks by the Online Therapy Institute, the Supervision Framework covers such areas as: ethical and statutory considerations; informed consent; appropriate qualifications; screening; the types of modality used; contracting and record keeping; security; gatekeeping; and research.

In Chapter 31, Michèle Mani and Barbara Veder look at "Supervising the Delivery of Online Counselling Services in an Employee and Family Assistance Program (EFAP) Setting." The chapter looks at Employee Assistance Programs (EAPs): employer or group-sponsored programs that are designed to alleviate workplace problems due to a variety of issues including mental health, substance abuse, personal problems and workplace difficulties. They look at the specific EAP resources, structure and supervisory practices at Morneau Shepell, a Canadian EFAP provider, that works within a short-term counselling framework.

Chapter 32, "The Use of Technology in Clinical Supervision: A Case Report from Cape Fear Clinic," looks at a specific case study by Jennifer Askew Buxton and John Devaney. The Cape Fear Clinic is a nonprofit clinic that has served low-income and uninsured patients in southeastern North Carolina for 22 years. The clinic's mission is "to provide compassionate and affordable patient-centered health care to low income individuals and families in the Cape Fear region, regardless of ability to pay." The authors describe their journey in turning to technology to address the operations of the clinic, which they describe as tedious and time-consuming in the early days. They conclude by looking to the future of how technology can assist them becoming even more efficient in meeting the needs of their client population.

Chapter 33, considers is given to supervision *in* private practice, rather than *of* private practice and is authored by Anne Stokes. Ways of conducting online supervision are discussed, including advantages and disadvantages. Anne includes the pros and cons of a private online supervision practice itself and concludes by noting that an important area for the online supervisor to consider is the value of undertaking a specific training in online supervision. She notes that "in the same way as it is now considered sound ethical practice to undertake post initial F2F training to work as an online counsellor, there is a growing recognition of importance of online supervision training to adapt to the particulars of online supervision."

In Chapter 34, one of this book's editors, LoriAnn Sykes Stretch, and her colleague Kristin Vincenzes visit the interesting topic of "Distance Group Supervision for Play Therapy," noting that one client population that requires a unique skill-set is children. The authors offer us a model for distance supervision based on the work in a small private practice in a rural portion of North Carolina, which had four mental health practitioners seeking supervision for play therapy. The authors conclude by noting the needs of future distance group supervision models, where facilitators will be encouraged to utilize more secure videoconferencing software. They note that professional associations, such as the ACA, NBCC, and APT, are providing more guidance regarding the use of distance technologies in both clinical practice and supervision. Finally, as with many of the authors in this book, they note that more research needs to be conducted to better understand best practices for distance supervision.

Chapter 35, by Jonathan Lent, Andrew Burck and LoriAnn Sykes Stretch, is an overview of "Practica and Internship Field Placements Using Cybersupervision". Their work in this case study drew them to identify some important lessons to consider when implementing a cybersupervision program, including: "factor in time to work out technical glitches, provide training for new technologies, assess readiness for technology-assisted supervision, understand legal and ethical requirements, review raw clinical data, provide ongoing evaluation of supervisee skills, ensure a secure transmission of information and engage in a continuous program evaluation process."

In Chapter 36, KaRae' Carey and LoriAnn Sykes Stretch examine the topic of "Teaching Counseling Techniques Using Technology" and note that in the modern world, "students are being taught professional counseling techniques in both land-based and hybrid (combined online/land-based) classroom environments." They also note that research supports both land-based and online methods of learning as effective tools for teaching and learning counseling techniques. They identify that the challenge now is for programs to focus less on justifying the use of technology and moving more toward maximizing the use of technology for counselor educator training.

Chapter 37 is by Tristram Hooley and Siobhan Neary, who visit the strongly documented relationship between positive career building and good mental health and, specifically, "The Role of Online Careers Work in Supporting Mental Health." The growth of online recruitment, e-learning and online career support has transformed the lived experience of those in work and learning and the authors examine the growing range of career guidance practice taking place in online spaces in recent years. The chapter demonstrates how the development of such practice is rapidly outpacing evidence and research, meaning that the efficacy and appropriate use of such technologies is often poorly understood. The authors identify "a clear need for a concerted research effort in this space in order to highlight the opportunities that new technologies offer."

Chapter 38 of the book is by Ginger Clark, "Using Technology to Enhance Supervision at The University of Southern California." She notes how USC believe technology has made their program more agile and "has allowed us to more easily stay current and relevant as the field changes, because we have easy access to new information and tools."

The final chapter is by Glenn Duncan, "The Use of Supervision in a Community-Based Treatment Program" using Hunterdon Drug Awareness Program as an example. Duncan notes that live supervision using technology "enhances... functioning as a supervisor while helping to deliver the best array of services to the client and... an ethical fidelity to consumer protection" which is a fitting end to part 2 of the book.

The book concludes with the editors' thinking about the future directions of technology in Mental Health. We note how the question is no longer, as it once was, whether we *should* use technology in the delivery of mental health services, counsellor training, or clinical supervision. Instead the question now is *how to best use technology, with whom, and when.*

NOTE ON THE SCOPE OF THE TEXT AND THE LANGUAGE USED

The collaboration of the editors from both sides of the Atlantic is deliberate, as addressing an audience that is international is appropriate when discussing a topic that provides therapeutic, peer support and education services globally, regardless of geographical limitations. Our range of authors reflects that international spread.

The scope and language of the book has been kept as internationally applicable as possible, while US and non-US spellings (e.g., of "counselor" or "counsellor") have generally been retained to reflect each author's original use in their own country. However, some language has been edited for the sake of consistency, such as using "therapy" to indicate counselling/counseling and psychotherapy, which are also used interchangeably (McLeod, 1994) only using the more specific terms where they are clearly applicable. Also, we have adopted "therapists" or "practitioners" in a similar vein and used the term "mental health" to indicate that much of the material here is applicable to different tiers of the profession. Although sometimes the term "patient" may be applicable to the person seeking therapeutic help, the authors, for the most part, use the term "client" throughout. The editors recognise that many of the technologies and their applications from chapter to chapter may overlap and be applicable to other technologies. Duplication of some basic information in chapters is deliberate to allow for each chapter to be read in isolation if preferred.

We hope you enjoy this collection of chapters on technology and mental health, supervision, and training.

REFERENCE

McLeod, J. (1994). The research agenda for counselling. *Counselling*, 5(1), 41–3.

ACKNOWLEDGMENTS

We would like to thank the authors who have contributed to this volume for their wide-ranging expertise and their patience, the team at Charles C Thomas, and our friends, family, and the many colleagues from the online and offline world, too numerous to mention and, particularly, the students of the Online Therapy Institute.

CONTENTS

PART TWO:
THE USE OF TECHNOLOGY
IN TRAINING AND SUPERVISION

TECHNOLOGY IN MENTAL HEALTH

Part One

THE USE OF TECHNOLOGY IN MENTAL HEALTH

Chapter 1

USING EMAIL TO CONDUCT A THERAPEUTIC RELATIONSHIP

Patricia Ryan Recupero and Samara Harms

INTRODUCTION

Written communication between therapists and clients dates back to the origins of psychotherapy when Sigmund Freud corresponded with his patients (Pergament, 1998). Today, such communication often takes the form of electronic mail (email). Although email has been available for well over two decades, unfortunately there are relatively few studies evaluating its use in psychotherapy. This chapter defines email as asynchronous written electronic communication and excludes short-form texting and instant messaging. Email is poised to become more popular as a means of electronic communication between clinicians and clients, as it can offer more data security than text messaging (Cohall, Hutchinson, & Nye, 2007).

Email may be conducted in several formats: directly through a server to recipients within that server; from a server and routed to a recipient through another server; or through a password-protected connection on a secure website (secure, web-based messaging, sometimes referred to as a web board). Emails sent through servers rather than directly through a secure website may be composed and directed online in an Internet browser window, or they may be sent through an email client such as

Microsoft Outlook. Emails may also be sent through smartphones and mobile phones, via the phone's web browser or through an email application on the phone. However, it should be noted that not all of these would be suitable for exchanging emails as part of therapy, given the need to ensure adequate levels of privacy and data security.

In the clinical practice of psychotherapy and mental health counseling, the use of email ranges from incidental emails for prescription refills and appointment setting to therapeutic emails (Anthony, 2004). Incidental emails may be analogous to routine telephone calls. Therapeutic emails range from brief follow-up messages (e.g., brief motivational tips for exercise or quitting smoking, food diaries for eating disorders, etc.) to therapy or treatment conducted, at least in part, via email. Risks associated with the use of email tend to increase as the communication moves away from incidental matters and toward therapeutic uses, just as providing psychotherapy in one's office arguably involves greater risks than confirming or rescheduling a client's appointment.

Email has numerous potential therapeutic uses and in some situations may be especially helpful to clients. Email has been shown to improve communication between clinicians and patients and to improve patient satisfaction (Leong et al., 2005). Although physicians have been slow to adopt regular email contact with patients (Brooks & Menachemi, 2006), client demand is high (Stanfill et al., 2014), and recent years have seen significant growth in doctor-patient electronic communication (Ye et al., 2010; Yellowlees & Nafiz, 2010). Therapists and mental health professionals seem to have been earlier adopters of the technology.

Some psychotherapy clients may be even more receptive to communicating with providers via email, particularly for issues that may be difficult to discuss in person. Women are more likely to seek support through email than via face-to-face (F2F) contact (Lim et al., 2013) and people with low self-esteem often prefer email over F2F communications, particularly when communications involve an element of risk (Joinson, 2004). Persons in the armed forces have also found email follow-up with mental health clinicians helpful, especially for sharing links to informative websites (Stanfill et al., 2014). Furthermore, there is some indication that email communication may facilitate engagement with treatment among clients with particularly challenging case presentations (Roy & Gillett, 2008).

This chapter discusses some relevant applications of the use of email as well as some important ethical considerations.

APPLICATIONS

The use of email by psychotherapists and counselors varies considerably. Even providers who do not communicate with clients through email may address email-related concerns in therapy. Malater writes of clients for whom email becomes an important element of issues explored in therapy (2007). Email may occupy such an important part of the client's life that he or she may bring in copies of emails with third parties, such as family members, to discuss in therapy. Therapists should be aware of the role of email in a client's life and should be aware of the client's use of email as a potential area to explore during sessions. The clinical use of email may be adjunctive (Peterson & Beck, 2003) or offered as a sole form of treatment. Therapists should have a well-thought-out email policy that should be communicated to clients, just as one has a policy for telephone calls. The policy should clarify expectations about the use of email, reasonable expectations for turnaround time for clinician response to client messages (Mattison, 2012), when it is and when it is not appropriate to use email, as well as the various risks associated with email and the available safeguards; this chapter details additional suggestions for email policies in the section on Ethical Considerations.

Adjunctive applications of email may be among the most common. Yager, an early adopter of the technology, uses email with his clients for both administrative and clinical purposes. He has written extensively about his experience using email with adolescents in treatment for eating disorders (Yager, 2003), and his observations and recommendations will be helpful to many clinicians who use email or who are contemplating it. He notes the utility of email for encouraging clients to report daily symptom and behavior diaries, which enhances accountability and self-awareness. Adjunctive email (e.g., for medication reminders and personalized case management) has also been found helpful in the treatment of depression (Watkins et al., 2011; Vernmark et al., 2010; Robertson et al., 2006) and substance use disorders (Collins et al., 2007).

Eating disorders are among the most studied indications for the clinical use of email (Sánchez-Ortiz et al., 2011; Robinson & Serfaty, 2007; Yager, 2003). There is some evidence that automated email messaging may help to improve outcomes in smoking cessation (Lenert et al., 2004) and, interestingly, that email CBT with minimal therapist contact may be helpful for social phobia (Carlbring et al., 2006). Email has shown some potential for helping abuse victims by increasing rates of abuse disclosure and facilitating communication among parents, children and treatment providers; these applications were originally suggested by women in domestic violence shelters (Constantino et al., 2007). Self-directed writing exercises with therapist email were found to be helpful for posttraumatic stress and grief (Lange et al., 2001). Conditions for which email may be helpful range from clinical disorders such as depression to subclinical, "worried well" difficulties, such as work stress (Ruwaard et al., 2007). Email has been proven effective for weight-loss counseling, even when using automated, computer-tailored feedback instead of email counseling by a therapist (Tate et al., 2006).

Email may elicit more honest information about a client's conditions. The Samaritans, a UK-based charity best known for its work with suicide hotlines, noted that their email contacts describe suicidal feelings more frequently than phone contacts (Armson, 1997). Turkle (1999, p. 643) notes: "The relative anonymity of life on the screen . . . gives people the chance to express often unexplored aspects of the self. Additionally, multiple aspects of self can be explored in parallel." The act of writing and thoughtfully composing emails may encourage deeper self-reflection and insight into a client's problems (Mattison, 2012). As email communication between therapist and client delves more deeply into clinical matters and psychological difficulties, ethical considerations abound.

Practically speaking, email offers numerous benefits, including the ability to compose and send communications at any time and from numerous locations. Many consider email's automatic documentation a benefit, although having a complete and literal record carries some risks as well (Recupero, 2005). Email can be used in conjunction with other forms of electronic technology for therapeutic purposes.

Tate and Zabinski (2004) provide a helpful review of technological applications that may be useful adjuncts to therapy, such as online support groups.

ETHICAL CONSIDERATIONS

Most of the important ethical considerations for email are merely extensions of existing ethical standards and problems in the practice of psychotherapy. Among the central ethical concerns for the use of email are:

- confidentiality and privacy;
- the appropriateness of email communication in a particular clinical situation;
- the implications of email for professionalism and the standard of care; and
- administrative issues, such as licensure and reimbursement.

Because clinical scenarios vary significantly among different clients, it is impossible to address every potential ethical concern that may confront the therapist who uses email. This chapter aims, instead, to offer some starting points for reflection and to encourage the reader to seek out additional resources, such as existing ethical guidelines and competencies for therapists and counselors on the use of email (e.g., Anthony & Goss, 2009; Nagel & Anthony, 2009; Hill & Roth, 2014).

Confidentiality and Privacy

Client confidentiality and privacy concerns arise frequently in connection with Internet-based communications, including email. In some countries, communications between therapists and clients are normally subject to therapist-client privilege, a legal principle that protects confidentiality, with some exceptions. Therapists everywhere, in any case, also have an ethical duty to protect clients' confidentiality that arguably transcends legal obligations.

Psychotherapists can be held liable for breach of confidentiality even where no law was broken (Grabois, 1997). Because email carries risks to client confidentiality and privacy, the decision to communicate with clients via email should not be made without involving the patient in a full discussion of the risks and available safeguards.

Emails may be analogous to recorded therapy sessions. They both contain a literal transcript of the client's and therapist's words, unlike summaries in chart notes or even process notes. Even emails deleted by both parties are often retained in storage by third parties such as Internet service providers (ISPs) or on individual parties' hard drives and are typically recoverable by information technology (IT) professionals (Fitzgerald, 2005). The exact words of therapist and client are preserved in email communications, so it is important to be mindful of potential future readers when writing (Recupero, 2008). Clients should be fully informed about this risk and the therapist should make sure that the client has understood before agreeing to communicate by email.

Laws that apply to medical records generally apply to emails as well. In the USA, emails are covered by the Health Insurance Portability and Accountability Act (HIPAA), as well as more restrictive state laws regarding the privacy of protected health information (PHI). Like any medical record, emails are subject to subpoena. Although in most cases therapists should decline to release client emails without the client's consent, courts and legal professionals may still be able to obtain the emails from third parties, such as ISPs, who often retain emails on their servers for a specified period of time. HIPAA requires providers to develop a security policy and to notify clients of privacy practices. An established security policy and open discussion of privacy practices are good risk management practices to help protect clients and therapists. HIPAA requires that all

providers subject to its rules provide patients annually with copies of a privacy statement. Among the things to consider including in that privacy statement would be who has access to emails and what your email retention policy is.

Security issues are an important consideration. While many have expressed concern about risks posed by hackers and high-tech threats, Sands (2004) notes that "the biggest threats to security are low-tech ones: failure to log off or use a screen saver, misaddressing email messages, sharing email accounts and using employer-owned email systems" (p. 268). Although not all possible security-enhancing measures will be addressed in this chapter, the following list offers some suggestions:

- Use secure, web-based messaging systems instead of sending emails through multiple servers; these systems can be configured so that clients only receive a notification email alerting them to log in to the website in order to retrieve your message. These sites are secure and password-protected and they may offer the strongest (although not perfect) security protection for therapist-client email.
- If you work in a multi-provider facility or if you have office staff, additional security measures may be appropriate. Some technological tools to increase security are encryption, authentication, electronic signatures, password-protected screen savers, automatic log-outs, audit trails, return receipts for email, password protection for email accounts, firewalls and virus protection.
- If you have staff, or if you work with others, develop a policy regarding staff/others' access to client emails; be sure that clients are fully informed of these practices.
- If it is necessary to use traditional email (as opposed to secure, web-based

messaging), keep track of clients' email addresses so that you do not confuse two clients' email addresses and send confidential communications to the wrong person. Furthermore, educate yourself about the evolving security threats associated with email, such as malware, spam, phishing, hacking, and social engineering such as spoofing (Stine & Scholl, 2010). Storing clients' personal information and email addresses in an electronic address book (such as the "Contacts" tool) can make them more vulnerable to security threats if the storage method is not secure.

- Instruct clients not to compose or send emails through workplace computers or networks. Many employers routinely screen and monitor emails sent or received by employees. Warn clients about the risk of others reading their emails, particularly if they will be using a shared computer or shared mobile phone. If clients are not technology-aware, it is appropriate to help them learn how to protect their emails from family members who may have a vested interest – or just curiosity – in accessing the sessions.
- An email retention and confidentiality policy will help to clarify client and therapist expectations of email confidentiality (or lack thereof). The policy may address, for example, which ISP the therapist will use, whether the therapist will save or delete emails, how long emails may be retained after therapy has concluded and policies for protecting the security of email communications. There are several questions to address when formulating such a policy. Will you retain all emails in the client's medical record? If so, the client should be aware of this. Will you retain no emails, but instead keep just a record of the content of sessions? If so, what will be your

policy for deleting emails? Some commentators (Sands, 2004) believe that deleting or destroying entire or portions of emails "is tantamount to destroying or altering medical records." If you do delete emails, be sure to keep at least a record of what was communicated, in essence. Even if you will delete emails and keep session notes instead, clients may decide to keep emails, so it may not be possible to guarantee that no permanent record is maintained. There are software packages that help to completely delete emails from hard drives, but clients may not be able to afford these programs and, furthermore, ISPs and other networks may retain emails; clients should be forewarned that even if you delete emails, it is no guarantee that they will be completely erased. Articles and reports from technology news can be helpful sources for tips on increasing data security, software to help remove old files and so forth (Fitzgerald, 2005).

- Concerns about email privacy should not defeat otherwise sound plans to communicate with clients online. In the US, in the case of Warshak v. United States, the Sixth Circuit upheld a district court's opinion that emails should not be subjected to search and seizure without a valid warrant.

Therapists who are interested in learning more about encryption and conducting a risk-benefit analysis to decide which form of encryption to use for email with clients are encouraged to review Caffery and Smith's helpful discussion on the topic (Caffery & Smith, 2010); they provide a decision-support flowchart to help practitioners determine which form of email and encryption pairing will best meet their needs as well as those of their clients. The American Health Information Management Association (AHIMA) has also published a number of helpful practice briefs regarding best practices for security and documentation with email.

Appropriateness of Email for the Clinical Situation

There is an almost infinite variation in clinical situations. In some cases, email will not be an appropriate medium for therapist-client communication. Therapists must consider the needs of the particular client. Demographic and clinical factors alike can affect the advisability of using email. When treating children and adolescents, an email record could be problematic for the young client if the parent requests access to the emails. Generally speaking, parents often have the legal right to view their children's medical records until the child has reached the age of majority. Since courts may consider emails part of the medical record, parents could demand to view the young person's emails, which could have a detrimental effect on the client's progress as well as the therapeutic relationship. Furthermore, parents may own the account and the hardware through which the emails were composed; this risk should be recognized and discussed. Numerous legal and ethical issues related to documents and records must be considered when treating children and adolescents (Recupero, 2008).

The therapist should also consider questions of accessibility. People unfamiliar with technology may need help ensuring they know how to hide messages from family members on shared computers or phones and those who do not have Internet access at home might not have appropriate locations to compose or read therapeutic emails. If the patient must use a public terminal (e.g., a library or Internet café) or a shared mobile phone for email, his or her privacy may be compromised and he or she may not be able to openly discuss important, but sensitive, issues. As previously mentioned, clients should be strongly discouraged from using workplace computers or email addresses/networks for therapy-related emails. Therapists may decline to use email with clients who intend to email from work.

Finally, different diagnoses can have vast implications for correspondence via email. ISPs can review emails and certain phrases or key words (e.g., political delusions) may be "red flags" that trigger increased monitoring or, possibly, surveillance by law enforcement agencies. Email may not be the best option for clients with psychotic symptoms. The case illustration section below provides an example to help guide reflection on these concerns.

Professionalism and Standard of Care

Among the potential problems cited with using email for psychotherapy is the inability to detect nonverbal cues such as crying or alcohol on a client's breath. While this is admittedly a drawback to the medium, there are also benefits. Clients can describe problems in more detail and can write *when* they are upset instead of waiting until they are calm, so they may be better able to recall details. Similarly, the therapist can respond carefully, editing their reply to contain thoughtful reflection instead of "canned" responses or first impressions. Furthermore, clients can be asked to record their feelings in real time and at different points of time during the day. Email can have positive or negative implications for the standard of care.

Communication via the Internet may affect transference and countertransference in therapy. Inaccurate first impressions and stereotypes are more likely to persist over email than when communication occurs by voice transmission (Epley & Kruger, 2005). People often overestimate their ability to communicate effectively via email (Kruger et al., 2005), believing that others will "hear" the same intent and context that they feel when composing a message. The overall tone of an email is very important in determining how the message will be perceived (Turnage, 2008) so therapist and client alike may need to work on clarifying meaning and affect in emails until they have developed more skill at conveying tone. Subtle humor and sarcasm, for example, may be easily misunderstood by email recipients and may need clarification (for example, a "just kidding" or "jk" after a joke). Granberry (2007) and Matison (2012) provide helpful suggestions for practical considerations involved in the use of email, such as decisions about signature blocks, electronic stationery backgrounds, conveying emotion, and the use of emoticons and common Internet abbreviations.

An oft-cited characteristic of email is its tendency to elicit disinhibited communication (Suler, 2004). Depending on the situation, this may result in candor, honesty, and openness; in other situations, it may lead to lying, dishonesty, and deception. Conversely, the asynchronous, distant nature of email communication may also prompt excessive, self-conscious control of one's behavior or self-image. Researchers refer to this phenomenon as impression management and it is common in cyberspace (Chester & Bretherton, 2007).

Administrative Issues

Many administrative issues have a bearing on ethical aspects of counseling by email. Although they are too numerous to detail here, several issues are important to mention. Licensure and regulatory problems may emerge, particularly if the therapist and the patient reside in different states or countries. Some areas require the therapist to be licensed in the patient's jurisdiction in order to provide any type of therapy, including e-therapy. Furthermore, some jurisdictions have laws regulating telemedicine and

cybermedicine, including therapy via email. Therapists should investigate the relevant laws prior to beginning a course of email therapy and one should develop a system for finding out when laws have changed, possibly through an evolving trusted wiki. Malpractice insurance providers are often helpful with such questions.

Reimbursement is another issue that has provoked much debate. Many providers express concern that using email will require an excessive time commitment without adequate financial reimbursement. Initial reports, however, have not supported this fear. On the contrary, email has been credited with improving practice efficiency (Rosen & Kwoh, 2007), by reducing both telephone workload and unnecessary office visits. The question, then, becomes one of what fees, if any, will be charged for email and how fees will be set. Clients and therapists should agree upon the fee structure prior to beginning a course of therapy.

Communications with third parties and "prospective clients" can be problematic. Therapists must decide how to respond to those clients who send unsolicited email requests for advice or appointments. Baur (2000) suggests that one address these contacts in the same way that one would respond to equivalent contacts via telephone calls. Although this chapter is primarily concerned with email between therapists and clients, additional ethical concerns apply to the use of email with colleagues and other third parties. Standards of "netiquette" are typically higher for professionals such as therapists than for the general population; Cleary and Freeman (2005) offer email suggestions for mental health nurses that are applicable to numerous other professionals in the mental health field.

CASE EXAMPLES

Example 1

Suppose that Sheila, a fictional client, forwards the following email from her therapist to her husband, who then forwards it to his mother:

Sheila,
From what you have told me about your father-in-law, it sounds as if he may suffer from a psychiatric disorder. I know at times it must seem as though he is being unreasonable, but I would urge you to consider that the way he acts sometimes might be beyond his control.
Hang in there,
Dr. Cyberpsych

Such communications may be common in the context of media psychology, advice columnists, or radio personalities who are offering advice for entertainment purposes, but may be unethical in the context of an established therapist-client relationship. While the therapist can decide to whom she forwards or sends email, whether to delete the email and so forth, she cannot control what her client does with email once it has been sent. Being mindful of this, communications should be "sanitized" to some degree in the same way that progress notes and comments during therapy sessions may be censored. While verbal statements similar to those in Dr. Cyberpsych's email, above, may be commonplace in face-to-face therapy sessions, different implications arise when such thoughts are put into writing. Dr. Cyberpsych's response, above, could be tactfully revised as follows:

Sheila,
It must be very difficult for you to face these family struggles so often. While every family goes through its ups and downs, there are some things we could talk about in our next

session at my office that might help you to understand a little better why you are feeling so frustrated and why it seems so hard for you and your father-in-law to communicate.
Hang in there,
Dr. Cyberpsych

Example 2

The following example illustrates some of the difficulties and ethical questions raised by different clinical scenarios and symptom-specific problems:

John A., a young man who operates a forklift at a distribution center, is referred for therapy following an altercation with a coworker at the warehouse. Mr. A. reports that he has previously been disciplined for similar incidents and conflicts with his coworkers. You observe that Mr. A. avoids eye contact, mumbles, and often responds inappropriately to subtle social cues, such as humor and sarcasm. You suspect that Mr. A. may suffer from autism spectrum disorder, level 1, and you recommend psychotherapy directed at developing stronger interpersonal communications skills to reduce the incidence of workplace misunderstandings. Mr. A. says that he will not be able to attend weekly therapy appointments and he inquires about the possibility of conducting the appointments online, via email.

In this example, email communications may not adequately address Mr. A's difficulties with face-to-face, nonverbal communication. As a general rule, if a client's difficulties cannot be addressed in somewhat generalized, cautious language, with the limited capabilities of email communication, then it may be prudent to question whether email is the appropriate medium for the particular discussion. A patient struggling with anxiety and stress related to corporate fraud at work, for example, may not be the best candidate for email therapy, as courts would be interested in the content of the emails if a criminal investigation is involved. Similarly, a manic client may be unable to recognize appropriate boundaries and may not hesitate before including the therapist's email address in a list of recipients for a chain-letter type of mass email. The decision whether, and how, to use email communications in therapy should be made on a case-by-case basis.

CONCLUSION

Rates of adoption of email are still low and many therapists who use email with clients either do so for incidental or adjunctive, symptom-tracking uses, or rely on clients who can afford to pay out of pocket for this option. Recently, there have been some efforts at reimbursement through major insurance companies allowing reimbursement for "web visits," i.e., clinician-patient communication via online, secure messaging. If these options are well received by clinicians and clients, they are likely to spur reimbursement for other forms of electronic communication, including email. Further research is needed to help elucidate the benefits, pitfalls and safeguards to help ensure that clients and therapists alike are able to use email to their benefit. In the meantime, in the absence of many published research studies, providers should develop policies to help guide decisions and procedures related to the clinical use of email. In formulating such policies, therapists may refer to existing published guidelines promulgated by professional organizations.

REFERENCES

Anthony, K. (2004). Therapy Online – The Therapeutic Relationship in Typed Text. In G. Bolton, S. Howlett, C. Lago & J. Wright (Eds.), *Writing cures.* Hove: Brunner-Routledge.

Anthony, K., & Goss, S. (2009). *Guidelines for online counselling and psychotherapy including guidelines for online supervision* (3rd ed.). Lutterworth: BACP.

Armson, S. (1997). Suicide and cyberspace: Befriending by email. *Crisis, 18*(3), 103–105.

Baur, C. (2000). Limiting factors on the transformative powers of email in patient-physician relationships: A critical analysis. *Health Communication, 12*(3), 239–259.

Brooks, R. G., & Menachemi, N. (2006). Physicians' use of email with patients: Factors influencing electronic communication and adherence to best practices. *Journal of Medical Internet Research* [online], 8(1) e2 [Accessed April 21, 2015]. Available from: http://www.jmir.org/2006/1/e2/.

Caffery, L. J., & Smith, A. C. (2010). A transmission security framework for email-based telemedicine. *Studies in Health Technology and Informatics, 161,* 35–48.

Carlbring, P., Furmark, T., Steczkó, J., Ekselius, L., & Andersson, G. (2006). An open study of Internet-based bibliotherapy with minimal therapist contact via email for social phobia. *Clinical Psychologist, 10*(1), 30–38.

Chester, A., & Bretherton, D. (2007). Impression management and identity online. In A. Joinson, A. McKenna, T. Postmes, & U. F. Reips (Eds.), *The Oxford Handbook of Internet Psychology,* (pp. 223–236). New York: Oxford University Press.

Cleary, M., & Freeman, A. (2005). Email etiquette: Guidelines for mental health nurses. *International Journal of Mental Health Nursing, 14*(1), 62–65.

Cohall, A., Hutchinson, C., & Nye, A. (2007). Secure e-mail applications: Strengthening connections between adolescents, parents, and health providers. *Adolescent Medicine, 18*(2), 271–292.

Collins, G. B., McAllister, M. S., & Ford, D.

B. (2007). Patient-provider e-mail communication as an adjunctive tool in addiction medicine. *Journal of Addictive Diseases, 26*(2), 45–52.

Constantino, R., Crane, P. A., Noll, B. S., Doswell, W. M., & Braxter, B. (2007). Exploring the feasibility of email-mediated interaction in survivors of abuse. *Journal of Psychiatric and Mental Health Nursing, 14*(3), 291–301.

Epley, N., & Kruger, J. (2005). When what you type isn't what they read: The perseverance of stereotypes and expectancies over email. *Journal of Experimental Social Psychology, 41*(4), 414–422.

Fitzgerald, T. J. (2005). Deleted but not gone. *The New York Times* [online], 3 November. [Accessed April 21, 2015]. Available from: http://www.nytimes.com/2005/11/03/technology/circuits/03basics.html.

Grabois, E. W. (1997). The liability of psychotherapists for breach of confidentiality. *Journal of Law and Health, 12*(1), 39–84.

Granberry, N. (2007). Email – from "to" to "send." *AAOHN Journal, 55*(3), 127–130.

Hill, A. & Roth, A. (2014). The competencies required to deliver psychological therapies at a distance. Lutterworth, BACP. [online]. [Accessed July 17th, 2015]. Available from: http://www.bacp.co.uk/research/competences /counselling-at-a-distance.php.

Joinson, A. N. (2004). Self-esteem, interpersonal risk, and preference for e-mail to face-to-face communication. *CyberPsychology & Behavior, 7*(4), 472–478.

Kruger, J., Epley, N., Parker, J., & Zhi-Wen, N. (2005). Egocentrism over email: Can we communicate as well as we think? *Journal of Personality and Social Psychology, 89*(6), 925–936.

Lange, A., van de Ven, J. P., Schrieken, B., & Emmelkamp, P. M. G. (2001). Interapy: Treatment of posttraumatic stress through the Internet: A controlled trial. *Journal of Behavior Therapy and Experimental Psychiatry,*
32(2), 73–90.

Lenert L., Mufloz R. F., Perez J. E., & Aditya Banson, B. S. (2004). Automated email messaging as a tool for improving quit rates in an Internet smoking cessation intervention. *Journal of the American Medical Informatics Association, 11*(4), 235–240.

Leong, S. L., Gingrich, D., Lewis, P. R., Mauger, D. T., & George, J. H. (2005). Enhancing doctor-patient communication using email: A pilot study. *Journal of the American Board of Family Medicine, 18*(3), 180–188.

Lim, V. K. G., Teo, T. S. H., & Zhao, X. (2013). Psychological costs of support seeking and choice of communication channel. *Behaviour & Information Technology, 32*(2), 132–146.

Malater, E. (2007). Introduction: Special issue on the Internet. *The Psychoanalytic Review, 94*(1), 3–6.

Mattison, M. (2012). Social work practice in the digital age: therapeutic e-mail as a direct practice methodology. *Social Work, 57*(3), 249–258.

Nagel, D. M., & Anthony, K. (2009). *Ethical framework for the use of technology in mental health* [online]. [Accessed April 21, 2015]. Available from: http://onlinetherapyinstitute .com/ethical-training/.

Pergament, D. (1998) Internet psychology: Current status and future regulation. *Journal of Law Medicine, 8*(2), 233–279.

Peterson, M. R., & Beck, R. L. (2003). E-mail as an adjunctive tool in psychotherapy: Response and responsibility. *American Journal of Psychotherapy, 57*(2), 167–181.

Recupero, P. R. (2005). Email and the psychiatrist-patient relationship. *Journal of the American Academy of Psychiatry and the Law, 33*(4), 465–475.

Recupero, P. R. (2008). Ethics of medical records and professional communications. *Child Adolescent Psychiatric Clinics of North America, 17*(1), 37–51.

Robertson, L, Smith, M., Castle, D., & Tannenbaum, D. (2006). Using the Internet to enhance the treatment of depression. *Australasian Psychiatry, 14*(4), 413–417.

Robinson, P., & Serfaty, M. (2007). Getting better byte-by-byte: A pilot randomised controlled trial of email therapy for bulimia nervosa and binge eating disorder. *European Eating Disorders Review, 16*(2), 84–93.

Rosen, P., & Kwoh, C. K. (2007). Patient-physician email: An opportunity to transform pediatric health care delivery. *Pediatrics, 120*(4), 701–706.

Roy, H., & Gillett, T. (2008). E-mail: A new technique for forming a therapeutic alliance with high-risk young people failing to engage with mental health services? A case study. *Clinical Child Psychology and Psychiatry, 13*(1), 95–103.

Ruwaard, J., Lange, A., Bouwman, M., Broeksteeg, J., & Schrieken, B. (2007). Emailed standardized cognitive behavioural treatment of work-related stress: A randomized controlled trial. *Cognitive Behaviour Therapy, 36*(3), 179–192.

Sánchez-Ortiz, V. C., Munro, C., Startup, H., Treasure, J., & Schmidt, U. (2011). The role of email guidance in internet-based cognitive-behavioural self-care treatment for bulimia nervosa. *European Eating Disorders Review, 19*(4), 342–348.

Sands, D. Z. (2004). Help for physicians contemplating use of email with patients. *Journal of the American Medical Informatics Association, 11*(4), 268–269.

Stanfill, K. E., Kinn, J., & Bush, N. (2014). Soldiers' preferences for follow-up communications with behavioral health providers. *Telemedicine and e-Health, 20*(8), 742–743.

Stine, K., & Scholl, M. (2010). E-mail security: An overview of threats and safeguards. *Journal of the American Health Information Management Association, 81*(4), 28–31.

Suler, J. (2004). The online disinhibition effect. *CyberPsychology and Behavior, 7*(3), 321–326.

Tate, D. F., Jackvony, E. H., & Wing, R. R. (2006). A randomized trial comparing human email counseling, computer-automated tailored counseling and no counseling in an Internet weight loss program. *Archives of Internal Medicine, 166*(15), 1620–1625.

Turkle, S. (1999). Cyberspace and identity. *Contemporary Sociology, 28*(6), 643–648.

Turnage, A. K. (2008). Email flaming behaviors and organizational conflict. *Journal of Computer-Mediated Communication, 13*(1), 43–59.

Vernmark, K., Lenndin, J., Bjärehed, J., Carlsson, M., Karlsson, J., Öberg, J., Carlbring, P., Eriksson, T., Andersson, G. (2010). Internet administered guided self-help versus individualized e-mail therapy: A randomized trial of two versions of CBT for major depression. *Behaviour Research and Therapy, 48*(5), 368–376.

Watkins, D. C., Smith, L. C., Kerber, K., Kuebler, J., & Himle, J. A. (2011). Email reminders as a self-management tool in depression: A needs assessment to determine patients' interests and preferences. *Journal of Telemedicine and Telecare, 17*(7), 378–381.

Yager, J. (2003). Email therapy for anorexia nervosa: Prospects and limitations. *European Eating Disorders Review, 11*(3), 198–209.

Ye, J., Rust, G., Fry-Johnson, Y., & Strothers, H. (2010). E-mail in patient-provider communication: A systematic review. *Patient Education and Counseling, 80*(2), 266–273.

Yellowlees, P., & Nafiz, N. (2010). The psychiatrist-patient relationship of the future: Anytime, anywhere? *Harvard Review of Psychiatry, 18*(2), 96–102.

Chapter 2

USING CHAT AND INSTANT MESSAGING (IM) TO CONDUCT A THERAPEUTIC RELATIONSHIP

Kathleene Derrig-Palumbo

INTRODUCTION

The term *online therapy* is a broad-reaching term that describes any means of delivering mental health services via the Internet. It includes video conferencing, audio conferencing, chat-room or instant messaging, and secure email dialogues between client and therapist among the many other modalities described in the following chapters. This chapter discusses one of the frequent definitions of online therapy: chat – real-time, text-based online communications using the Internet.

There are multiple terms that refer to the same type of communications delivery – chat, chat room, texting, private messaging (PM), and instant messaging. All indicate real-time communications between client and therapist. The distinction between chat and instant messaging, private messaging, and texting is that chat rooms are usually open "rooms" in which any number of individuals may come and go as they please and communicate with any or all of the attendees of the chat room. The others are usually a private dialogue, occurring between two or more people in a secure chat room to which no one other than the invitees is able to enter. Therefore, "chat" therapy utilizes instant messaging technology for the delivery of mental health services.

Chat therapy involves the exchange of dialogue using the written word and emoticons or "emojis." People who utilize chat will often abbreviate words and use "emojis" to express their feelings, such as being happy, sad, or angry. Emojis can be actual facial expressions that the chat room technology renders, icons, characters, designs or they may even be keyboard characters strung together to resemble facial expressions. For example, happy is :), sad is :(. Therapists who work online must be aware of their client's predisposition toward abbreviation and emojis prior to utilizing them. It is important to observe how the client makes use of the medium and to then mirror that usage as appropriate.

Chat therapy has received its share of scrutiny over the years. There have been a series of concerns surrounding the use of chat in therapy that have been discussed and debated rigorously since the medium was first used for the provision of mental health services. The concerns that were voiced are highly important points to consider carefully, as they all speak to the efficacy of the medium and to the best interests of the clients seeking therapy in this fashion. As of this writing, although many therapists have come to realize the benefits to be had from using chat, online therapy is still being used primarily by early adopters. Many of the original arguments against chat therapy still persist. It is important for therapists new to this medium to realize that much study and analysis has gone into examining chat therapy and many of the concerns that have been voiced have been thoroughly deliberated and addressed.

IDENTITY

The discussion surrounding chat therapy begins with identity, with regard to the identity of the therapist as well as concern about the identity of the client. The primary concern regarding the identity of the therapist is centered on how the consumer can be certain that he or she is meeting with an actual licensed mental health provider. Because chat does not utilize physical facial expression, theoretically a person who is not a therapist could pose as one by simply researching and assuming the credentials of a real therapist. Typically the names and license numbers of therapists are listed on the websites of the state regulatory boards that license the therapists in the United States and other countries list membership of professional organizations. This is where it may be sensible for therapists to use a credible clearinghouse to vet their information and present them to consumers. Some websites, such as www.MyTherapyNet.com, research every therapist that applies, require multiple forms of identification, conduct interviews, check for malpractice insurance, and check that their professional licenses are in good standing with no outstanding complaints. These websites then present therapists to the public who can be relied upon as legitimate, qualified mental health providers who have been trained in the techniques and the legal and ethical issues of online therapy.

There is equally a good deal of discussion regarding determining the identity of the client who engages in online therapy. The one perspective from which client identity is not analyzed is in regards to health insurance coverage. As of this writing (February, 2016), online therapy is now beginning to be looked at by insurance companies in the United States and elsewhere. Some insurance companies are conducting pilot studies and/or are actively providing insurance for their members for online therapy. This is still very new to insurance companies. As a result, many forms of identification are needed as well as additional paperwork in order for online sessions to be covered. At this point, there is no concern that an uninsured client may be assuming the identity of a covered member. However, it is likely that the health insurance industry will lean towards covering online therapy regularly in the United States soon, as with other countries (MyTherapy Net, 2009).

There is also concern amongst providers that by not knowing the identity of their client, there could be legal and ethical ramifications. For instance, if a client is presenting as a child abuser, therapists in the United States, the United Kingdom and many other countries have mandatory responsibilities to report child abuse. Be sure to identify if this law exists in your country of practice and, if the therapist has no idea where the client lives and what the client's real name is, the therapist is unable to make their mandatory report. However, the person using online therapy needs to use a credit card to purchase the session, unless it is provided free of charge. The credit card must have a correct name and correct address attached to it or the charge will not go through. As a result, you will have some information to begin a report. Since child abuse laws exist in most countries it is imperative legally and ethically that you follow through with a report. We are mandated to report suspected child abuse. Be sure to report all the information that you have to your local child protection services. It is then up to them to investigate the report or to refer it out to the state/region in which the suspected child abuse exists. There are many permutations of this, all leading to the necessity of having some information on whom the client is and where they live. However, it is interesting to note that in traditional face-to-face private practice, most providers do not ask for identification from their clients and many clients pay in cash. Therefore, it is also possible that a client in face-to-face therapy is using an assumed name and false contact information on their intake form.

As it turns out, by its very nature, online therapy tends to make it more difficult for a client to be seen anonymously, because the cash pay alternative is removed. Online clients pay for services using a credit card or other electronic means, meaning that the credit card billing address as well as the name of the person on the credit card is provided by the client. By utilizing an established online therapy service, these details are addressed in the proper fashion. In addition to billing information, the online therapy service is able to track the I.P. address of the client, which although on its own does not provide a precise geographical location, in the case of an emergency the Internet Service Provider can relay that information.

Another point that is raised frequently regarding client identity is how is it possible to know that it is actually the client who signed up that is using the service? For example, what if someone signs up to the service who is having issues with domestic violence and subsequently, his or her partner finds out. What prevents the partner from signing on as the victim? When there is no face to go along with the dialogue, it can be near impossible to know with certainty that the person is on the other end. This is where, once again, it may be important to consider utilizing established, credible online therapy clinics, because they will utilize the appropriate security authentication protocols that maximize identity security. However, the responsibility does not end with the service; it ultimately rests on the client. The client must take appropriate measures to protect his or her password, changing it often and utilizing letters, numbers and capitalization schemes that become impossible to guess. If the client takes these precautions and a credible online therapy service is utilized, this issue is mitigated (Derrig-Palumbo, 2005).

So in summary, the question of "how do I know I'm speaking to a real therapist?" is answered in one way by accessing therapists only from established online therapy services. The question of "how do I know the identity of my client?" is answered the same way. Additionally, both parties need to protect their login information and change their passwords regularly in order to reduce the potential for identity theft. Therapists in private practice may ask for copies of a driver's license or passport and/or ask for some sessions to be done in person if possible or ask the client to engage in a video-conferencing session. By following this protocol, people utilizing the Internet to provide and access mental health services can be confident that the issue of identity is addressed.

THE THERAPEUTIC RELATIONSHIP

Quickly following on the heels of the question of identity is the issue of efficacy. There is much captivating debate as to the efficacy of chat therapy. This question is typically broached in a general fashion by asking whether the use of the written word can adequately establish the therapeutic relationship. To answer this, we must take a step back and ask if the written word can adequately communicate the depth and breadth of human experience. For the last few thousand years, the written word has been used to convey a rich palette of human experience with great success. More specific to the case of chat therapy, personal relationships are known to commonly flourish through the exclusive use of the written word. Some pen pals, who have never met in person or spoken by telephone, develop the strongest of bonds. This has carried over to the use of email and chat rooms where, again, people who have never met nor spoken form lasting friendships and business partnerships, resulting in love affairs, marriages and successful business ventures. It is illuminating to look at why these bonds are often so strong because these are the same underlying reasons that can make chat therapy effective.

Relationships that make use of the written word for communication eliminate some of the inherent barriers to honest self-disclosure in a face-to-face setting. Many people who feel inhibited in sharing aspects of their lives in a face-to-face situation lose that inhibition when putting those thoughts and feelings to paper. Disclosing intimate details of one's life while face-to-face with someone often carries a fear of the possibility of judgment. Sometimes the judgment is only perceived. For instance, one person may speak of a personal indiscretion, while the listener grimaces because of a momentary flash of pain. The grimace had nothing to do with the disclosure, but to the person speaking, it appears to be a reaction to what has been said. Even when no outward sign of judgment is perceived, being in intimate proximity with the listener creates a greater sense of anxiety. Therefore, especially with regard to disclosing intimate personal details, using the written word can often free the person to disclose thoroughly. This is advantageous when such communication is used to build a personal relationship and perhaps even more so when in a therapeutic relationship. In general, clients report that chat therapy frees them to get to their root issues much more quickly than if they had been face-to-face with their therapist. In fact, some individuals have reported that after having spent months in face-to-face therapy without getting to their real issues, the switch to chat therapy led them to divulging these issues within the first few sentences of discourse with their therapists. Since the client and the therapist are not in the same room, the compassionate, caring, collaborative, nonjudgmental and accepting attitude needs to carry across through written words and can thus be made even more apparent to the client.

The following are samples of questions and statements that can be used to elicit a certain response from the online client. Most are short and are easy to incorporate into the session (Meichenbaum, 2000; Wachtel, 1993).

Expressing Empathy

- "How sad."
- "How tragic."
- "That is terrible."
- "What an incredible ordeal."

Permission-gathering Statements

- "Is it okay if I ask you some questions about . . . ?"
- "Are you up to some questions now?"
- "Only tell me about what you feel comfortable with."

Normalizing Statements

- "Often it is hard to . . ."
- "Often it is hard not to . . ."
- "It is okay if you . . . This is a lot to go through."

Nurture Collaboration

- "Do you think it would be advisable to . . . ?"
- "As we have both seen. . . ."
- "If you can't have what you want, at least you can feel that you are . . . ."

Colombo-like Statements

- "Correct me if I am wrong."
- "I get the impression that . . ."
- "You seem rather . . . and seem to expect . . ."
- "I have the sense that you . . ."
- "I think you are trying to . . . Am I correct?"

Comments that Pull for Patient's "Strengths" and Nurture Hope

- "All this weighs on you so heavily and yet you somehow go on!"
- "What has allowed you to . . . in spite of . . ."
- "So, somehow you were able to get past the obstacle of . . . Is that correct?"
- "How did you do that?"

Initial Behavior Analytic Interview Questions

- "In order to understand your situation, I would like to ask you some questions."
- "Can you take a few moments and describe the situation you are in now?"
- "What are the problems as you see them?"
- "How would you describe the specific (problem) behavior?"
- "How serious a problem is this as far as you are concerned?"
- "How often does this behavior happen?"
- "Where does the problem behavior usually occur?"
- "How long does it go on for?"

Questions that Focus on Expectations

- "What else do you think I should find out about you and your situation to help you with this problem?"
- "What questions have I not asked that I should ask in order to learn more about you and your situation?"

- "What *other* questions *should* I ask in order to better understand your situation and what we can do to help you?"
- "Do you have any questions you want to ask me?"

Questions to Consider in the Goal-setting Process

- "Why is it important to think about goals before beginning an activity?"
- "Does your goal seem realistic?
- Should you establish sub goals?"
- "Of these goals, which one should you begin with? How should you choose?"
- "How can you go about achieving these goals?"
- "Do you have a plan? Do you need help?"

Questions Designed to Enhance Motivation to Change

- "What is different when the problem is absent or manageable?"
- "How would you like for things to be different?"
- "If you were completely successful in accomplishing what you want, what would be changed?"
- "How would things be different if you followed this idea and did X?"

Questions Designed to Assess and Bolster Confidence

- "How confident do you need to feel to be able to do X?"
- "How sure are you, say on a scale of one to 10, that you can keep doing what you are doing?"
- "What things might get in the way of your being able to follow through on this?"
- "What can you do (or do with the help of others) about this problem?"

Questions Designed to Elicit Commitment Statements

- "What are one or two things you should do first?"
- "How would you know if the effort was worth it?"
- "So, are you saying that you are willing to try doing Y?"
- "Are you saying, and I want to make sure that I get this straight, that you would be able to . . ."

Questions Designed to Highlight Situational Variability

- "Are there some times that you can handle it better than at other times?"
- "What is different when things are not as bad or when you are not experiencing X?"
- "For now don't change anything; just keep track (notice) when things are better."

Questions Designed to Elicit Self-motivational Statements

- "I don't know if this would be too difficult for you, but . . ."
- "Maybe this is asking too much of you."
- "Of the things we have discussed, which are the most important reasons to change?"
- "How are you going to do that in spite of . . . ?"
- "Of these different options, which one would you choose? How did you select that one?"

Questions Designed to Help Individuals Notice Changes that They Have Been Able to Bring About

- "How will you/others be able to tell?"
- "What would be different?"

- "How will we know when the goals have been achieved?"
- "How will you feel about such changes?"

Questions Designed to Help the Individual Take Credit for Change or Improvements

- "How did it go?"
- "How were things different this time as compared to the last time?"
- "What do you think accounts for the change?"
- "What, if anything, did you do differently this time?"
- "How did your 'game plan' work? Were you able to follow your game plan?"

It is apparent that once identity and the ability to create the therapeutic relationship are addressed, the idea of chat therapy becomes plausible. However, chat still must pass muster with the legal and ethical mandates of the profession. There are certainly some overlying legal and ethical questions, such as practicing outside your own region and mandated reporting, but for the purpose of this discussion, the focus will be on those mandates that apply directly to chat therapy.

From the legal perspective, first and foremost there is the question of confidentiality. As opposed to being together in an office where, barring someone listening in outside the door, the words spoken between client and therapist leave no record, using chat via the Internet has the potential of being overheard. The issue of confidentiality provides the blueprint for how security must be handled for systems that enable the process of online therapy. In fact, this issue originates with the intake, transfer and storage of client personal information. In the US, HIPAA (Health Insurance Portability and Accountability Act) compliance lays out underlying requirements for the structure of the online therapy service's company, the software systems that are employed and the data management protocols that are employed. Indeed, most countries have legislation governing these matters, such as the Data Protection Act in the UK. These systems and protocols generally mandate a secure chat environment that not only meets industry standard security protocols for the handling of personal data, but also takes the special needs of therapy into consideration. Some large online therapy service providers employ a proprietary chat system that follows very specific mandates regarding encrypting chat stream identifiers, storage of chat session details and emergency procedures for locating a client's local police and hospitals.

The overriding ethical principle regarding confidentiality and the safekeeping of any sensitive information is that the practitioner must be assured of adequate protection for their clients. In some cases, this will mean that the best option is for the practitioner to be the only keeper of records pertaining to treatment of, for example, transcripts of therapy chat sessions. Back-up to the practitioner's computer can be provided by storing copies of data on a removable storage device (like a pen/flash drive or removable hard drive) and that can then be stored securely. Where a practitioner decides to have data stored by a third party – such as when records of chat sessions are kept by the chat service provider – it is always the responsibility of the therapist to verify that those records are kept in a safe, encrypted manner and will be treated with appropriate regard to confidentiality, almost certainly requiring a written agreement laying out how the information will be treated. In the US, this requires that the service provider is, at least, contracted with the practitioner as a HIPAA compliant business associate, although even this may be insufficient in some areas where additional safeguards may apply. In the UK, it would require the practitioner to be assured of compliance with the Data Protection Act plus the requirements of good practice and the relevant ethical codes. Most

countries, states or regions have their own rules on proper protection of sensitive client information and it is recommended that practitioners seek legal and professional advice on how to proceed in their own practice. In any event, data should always be encrypted and properly stored.

From the ethical perspective, a therapist must be certain that treating a particular client using chat therapy is an appropriate treatment plan for that client. If a client is being considered for chat therapy, the therapist should take care to screen the client and determine the appropriateness of that particular choice of treatment. Is the client a proficient typist? Does typing frustrate the client? Is chat therapy appropriate considering the severity of the client's disorder? Does the client live in a rural area with no other access to a therapist? If the first contact between client and therapist occurs online, the therapist should consider if the client is searching for and interviewing therapists. Has the client ever been in traditional and/or online therapy before? Is this just an experiment of whether the client is committed to the process of therapy? Does the client want a one-time educational and counseling session? Is the client interested in the minimization of symptoms or in long-term therapy? Chat therapy may also serve as a bridge to traditional, in-person therapy, where such interaction is preferred. Consider hypothetically a victim of domestic violence who is virtually held captive in the home. His or her only means of reaching out may be through the computer and working online with a therapist to create a plan may be the only viable first step. Therapists must carefully consider all the presenting factors prior to making a judgment on the appropriateness of on-line therapy for any particular client.

This brings us to the question of who is best served by chat therapy. As always, there are exceptions to every rule, but adolescents and young adults who have grown up on the Internet tend to do very well with chat therapy. They are very used to communicating via the written word, predominantly by using mobile texting, computer instant messaging, chat rooms, blogs and social networks. Many therapists report that when adolescents are "forced" to go to therapy, they tend to sit through the session in silence. However, that same child may type prolifically and discuss every intimate detail of their life when using chat therapy. Online therapy for the younger generation shapes up to be a natural assumption in that they figure that they do nearly every other thing imaginable online, so why not therapy?

Those who live in rural areas also benefit from chat therapy. Often, small rural communities are places where mental health issues carry great stigma. Even if there is a therapist nearby, this is likely to be someone that is well known in the community, which causes great reluctance when considering making an appointment. Although webcam or audio is an option available to someone living in a rural community, a first venture toward getting help is likely to be quite stressful. For many people, eliminating the face-to-face presence reduces their anxiety levels and chat therapy is likely to be the online therapy method of choice for many rural clients.

Chat therapy can also be quite useful in couple therapy. Using chat forces the other party to stop talking, to stop thinking about what to say next, and to just read what their partner is saying. For those couples who function poorly when in the same room, particularly in cases of divorce, chat therapy can be effective. For couples who may not be able to meet in person due to work or any host of reasons, chat therapy can get them into couple's therapy despite geographical challenges.

Chat therapy is also well suited for use by people who lack a private area in their home or office in which they would be comfortable speaking out loud to their therapist, say, by telephone. It is well suited for busy workers who can benefit from short stress interventions or coaching sessions. Businesses are beginning to recognize the financial benefit to providing early interventions for mental health issues, especially in the areas of stress, depression, and relationships. These three areas are the biggest causes of loss of productivity in the workplace and the cost of treatment is far outweighed by the direct and indirect savings.

Some therapeutic approaches are better suited to chat therapy than others. Client-directed Outcome-Informed Clinical Work, Cognitive Behavioral Therapy, Family Brief Therapy, Imago Relationship Therapy, Narrative Therapy, Rational Emotive Behavior Therapy, and Solution-Focused Brief Therapy all work very well when utilized online (Derrig-Palumbo, 2005).

Client-directed, Outcome-informed Clinical Work was founded by Dr. Scott Miller. This theory is based on score generated outcomes at the beginning, during, and at the end of each session. Since this form of therapy has been largely studied through a telephonic EAP setting, it can easily be transferred online. All the forms that are used for this type of treatment can be turned into a web-based program. This form of treatment can be used with adults as well as children (Miller et al., 2004).

Cognitive Behavioral Therapy is a theory that focuses on the connection between thoughts and feeling and how our perceptions influence our feelings (Beck, 1979). It has a large number of interventions that can easily be done online through chat, audio, or video-conferencing. Those interventions that require written feedback from the client can easily be transformed into a web-based document that can be shared online between client and therapist. Your chat room interface must have document share capabilities to share the document.

Family Brief Therapy is best conducted online when all family members log into a group chat room setting (or group video-conferencing session). Each family member can reflect on what is being said by other members as well as the responses from the therapist. Most adolescents chat online and/or through text messaging. This is a natural part of their everyday life. Adolescents may even initially relate better online than face-to-face with their parents due to outward power struggles. Sessions can be conducted online with the intention to bring the sessions face-to-face (Derrig-Palumbo, 2005).

Narrative Therapy is based on the retelling and rewriting of people's stories in their lives. The key is to understanding these stories and assisting the client to re-author their own life story in order to separate their problems from who they are as a person. The writing of one's stories can be a cathartic release. Narrative Therapy relies on the written word of the client's stories; chat is an ideal way to achieve this type of process.

The focus of Rational Emotive Behavioral Therapy (REBT) is to replace irrational beliefs, thoughts, and feelings with rational and more effective ones. Using this theory within the chat room setting is ideal because REBT deals with the present and challenges thoughts with rational short statements to uncover the client's set of beliefs (Ellis, 1994: 1957).

Solution-Focused Behavioral Therapy (SFBT) focuses on promoting solution behavior rather than studying the changing of problematic behavior. SFBT also focuses on the language client's use. This is ideal to use in a chat setting. Chat allows the client to look back and see what exactly was said in order to uncover patterns of language. The success of SFBT is to focus on clear paths towards solution. The most common intervention is "The Miracle Question," keeping the client focused on what they want and the steps necessary to achieve it (deShazer, 1985).

Client Scenario – Joshua

This is a session with a 16-year-old boy who had a difficult time communicating face-to-face. Half of his sessions were conducted online and the rest were carried out face-to-face. Joshua was fearful of relating to other people. His father was always working and his mother suffered from addiction to pain medication and was diagnosed with depression. He felt as though his thoughts and opinions were not important and had severe problems meeting others due to his lack of communication skills and self-confidence. However, he was able to communicate online with others through chat and games. Chatting online with him gave him the opportunity to open up in an environment that was comfortable and which ultimately lead him to feel comfortable face-to-face. Using both types of session allowed him to communicate better with others as well as his parents.

Kathleene: Hello.
Joshua: Hi.
Kathleene: How are you?
Joshua: Good and you?
Kathleene: Pretty good, thanks.
Kathleene: How are things going?
Joshua: Things are going well.
Kathleene: Tell me details about school.
Joshua: School is going well.
Joshua: I am doing good in all my classes.
Joshua I am happy with my homework and quiz scores.
Kathleene: What type of grades are you getting?
Joshua: A's, B+.
Joshua: B's.
Kathleene: GREAT!!!!
Joshua: Yes.
Kathleene: What is your favorite class?
Joshua: Hmm.
Joshua: I really don't have a favorite class.
Joshua: History is a joke this year.
Kathleene: Why is that?

Joshua: Our teacher gets her notes from Google, but then she copies and pastes them to Microsoft word and then states that they are her lecture notes.

Kathleene: That sucks.

Kathleene: How do you know?

Joshua: There are little links in blue on most sites that lead to other sites.

Joshua: They are in brackets most of the time.

Kathleene: I see . . . great detective work.

Joshua: Then we typed in the specific topic on Google and we found her exact notes on it.

Kathleene: Well are they good notes?

Joshua: Of course, they aren't hers, someone else wrote them.

Kathleene: But are they good?

Joshua: Yes, they are good and then she goes on to read almost the whole things, at a fast pcae, which we have to write down on paper for notes.

Joshua: Pace*

Kathleene: Then maybe that is the best that she uses them . . . but that is not good that she just reads them.

Joshua: So, myself and other people said, "screw this" and we find the notes on Google and read them over.

Kathleene: Good idea.

Kathleene: How things going with your parents and you?

Joshua: They are going well.

Joshua: Daniel went away to Washington for 10 days.

Kathleene: Are you spending time with your dad?

Joshua: So we are all savouring each minute.

Kathleene: Really.

Kathleene: I bet you are.

Joshua: Yes.

Kathleene: It must be so quiet there.

Joshua: Yes, it is.

Kathleene: Does everyone seem more relaxed?

Joshua: Yes, I believe so.

Kathleene: SO . . . I hear that you will be moving into your new house in January or so.

Joshua: My mom gets to sleep in now and she doesn't have to worry about picking Daniel up from school.

Joshua: Yes.

Joshua: I am very excited.

Joshua: I am looking foward to my big room.

Kathleene: What color are you going to paint it?

Joshua: I am not quite sure what they are painting the house, maybe just white for now and something else later.

Joshua: Really not sure, going to have to ask them.

Kathleene: Do you want it a specific color?

Joshua: Nah, I really don't care what color they paint it, it's all up to them . . . whatever they get is fine.

Kathleene: Okay.

Kathleene: So how much bigger is the new room than the room you are in now?

Joshua: One hundred times bigger.

Joshua: Even the closet is big.

Kathleene: That is great.

Kathleene: Do you still have someone living with you guys?

Joshua: Well . . . Dave moved out, but now Ucnle Wayne is here with us.

Joshua: Uncle*

Kathleene: How do you feel about that?

Kathleene: Tell me how you really feel.

Joshua: I'm fine, at least he's better than Dave.

Joshua: Uncle Wayne leaves early for work, cleans up nicely and doesn't ever use the computer here at home.

Joshua: Never comes home at 1:00 or 2:00 in the morning.

Kathleene: That is good.

Kathleene: But I know you had problems with him before.

Kathleene: Are you concerned?

Joshua: Not as much.

Kathleene: Good.

Kathleene: Do you have any concerns?

Joshua: No, not really, just as long as he doesn't stay for a prolonged amount of time.

Kathleene: What is a prolong amount of time?

Kathleene: Prolonged.*

Kathleene: Two months?

Joshua: More like 3–4 months.

Kathleene: I got ya.

Joshua: That's just way too long, I mean, he really needs to get his life on track.

Kathleene: So, did you ask how long he is staying?

Kathleene: You are so right.

Joshua: I don't want to ask how long he is staying for because, that is just implying "when will you leave and find your own place?"

Kathleene: No, I meant . . . ask your parents.

Kathleene: What they had in mind.

Kathleene: Do you want him moving with you guys to the new house?

Joshua: I am pretty sure they don't have an answer either, they would probably say, "as long as he needs to."

Joshua: I would really rather not anyone live with us in the new house.

Kathleene: Then it might be a good idea to share your feelings with them.

Kathleene: Maybe talk to your Mom first.

Kathleene: What do you think?

Joshua: Maybe, not quite sure yet.

Kathleene: Okay.

Kathleene: Let me know if you need some help with this.

Kathleene: So how are things going socially?

Joshua: Okay, I wil.

Joshua: Will*

Joshua: Good.

Joshua: My friends and I go to our weekly lunch and movies.

Joshua: On Fridays.

Kathleene: That is great.

Kathleene: Do you feel good about this?

Joshua: Yes, it was a wise idea from the start.

Kathleene: Really . . .

Joshua: Now we have set a precedent for the rest of the year.

Kathleene: Very good.

Kathleene: Do you like having social plans?

Joshua: Yes.

Joshua: I feel it is good to have plans like these.

Kathleene: Why is it good?

Joshua: It is good because we meet each other out of school, away from the working environment, then we just have a fun relaxing time together.

Joshua: The weight of the week has been lifted because it's Friday.

Kathleene: Yes exactly.

Kathleene: Great . . . I am glad that you see the importance of being social on a regular basis.

Kathleene: It is vital for us.

Kathleene: So who goes out with you on Fridays?

Joshua: Alex, Linden, Micah.

Joshua: That's mainly it.

Joshua: We eat, then go see a movie.

Kathleene: Woh is Micah?

Kathleene: Who?

Joshua: Micah is an 11th grader . . . we have known him for a while now.

Kathleene: Is he a good friend?

Joshua: Yes.

Kathleene: You have never mentioned him before.

Joshua: Hmm, I thought I have.

Kathleene: No . . . when did you become friends with him?

Joshua: Last year.

Kathleene: Oh.

Kathleene: Joshua . . . you seem to appear more confident.

Kathleene: Do you feel more confident?

Joshua: Possible.

Joshua: Possibly.

Kathleene: And even more comfortable in this conversation.

Kathleene: Why do you think?

Joshua: Yes.

Joshua: I am really not sure.

Kathleene: Do you feel different?

Kathleene: Have other poeple noticed?

Kathleene: People.

Joshua: I think so, not sure though.

Kathleene: What about others?

Joshua: Not sure, they won't just come up to me and say, "You seem different."

Kathleene: No but I thought maybe in comments to you.

Joshua: Oh, well, no comments.

Kathleene: Anyway, it seems like you are really starting to take some responsibility and you are evolving

Joshua: Thank you.

Kathleene: Stay focused on this track.

Kathleene: I was really concerned after our last session.

Joshua: Ok, I will.

Kathleene: Good.

Kathleene: Two weeks?

Joshua: Okay.

Joshua: 30th?

Kathleene: Monday or Wednesday at 7:30.

Kathleene: What is better?

Joshua: Monday.

Kathleene: Okay . . . go ahead and book it. If there is a problem, please call Paul tomorrow. Thanks.

Joshua: Okay thanks, bye.

Kathleene: Keep up the good work.

Kathleene: Bye.

CONCLUSION

It is obvious that with the twenty-first century, communicating with anyone, anywhere in the world is a mere mouse-click or voice-command away. It is inevitable that in growing numbers, therapists will practice online as the profession comes to accept its efficacy and more and more consumers demand online services. Someday in the not-so-distant future, online therapy may very well be regarded no differently than in-person therapy. In many cases, the distinction for some clients and patients has already faded. It is the responsibility of the current generation of providers to navigate these new waters intelligently and always having the best interest of the clients they serve as their primary consideration.

REFERENCES

Beck, A. T. (1979). *Cognitive therapy and the emotional disorders.* New York: Meridian Books.

Derrig-Palumbo, K. (2005). *Online therapy: A therapist's guide to expanding your practice.* New York: W. W. Norton.

DeShazer, S. (1985). *Miracle question* [online]. [Accessed June 14, 2009]. Available from: http://www.brief-therapy.org.

Ellis, A. (1994: originally published 1957). *How to live with a neurotic.* North Hollywood, CA: Wilshire Book Company.

Meichenbaum, D. (2000). *A clinical handbook for Donald Meichenbaum's presentation at The Evolution of Psychotherapy Conference.* Miami, FL: Melissa Institute Press.

Miller, S. D., Duncan, B. L., & Hubble, M. (2004). Beyond integration: The triumph of outcome over process in clinical practice. *Psychotherapy in Australia, 10*(2), 2–3.

MyTherapyNet (2009). *Homepage* [online]. [Accessed December 2, 2009]. Available from: www.MyTherapyNet.com.

National Board for Certified Counselors. (2004). *Standards for the ethical practice of web counseling* [online]. [Accessed December 2, 2009]. Available from: www.nbcc.org/ethics/wcstandards.htm.

Therapy Hosting (2009). *Homepage* [online]. [Accessed December 2, 2009]. Available from: www.TherapyHosting.com.

Wachtel, P. L. (1993). *Therapeutic communication.* New York: Guilford Press.

Chapter 3

USING MOBILE PHONE COMMUNICATION FOR THERAPEUTIC INTERVENTION

Roy Huggins

INTRODUCTION

Over recent years, the word "phone" has lost meaning as Alexander Graham Bell's world-changing invention was slowly converted into a minor component of complex, powerful, handheld computers that we cheekily call "smartphones." In fact, it's just in a few countries that mobile phones are actually called "phones." Much of the world simply calls them "mobiles," and rightly so.

Socially, we might refer to these gizmos as "phones" for reasons of expediency. Much like "Internet electronic messaging" is called "email," the communications devices we carry around are called "mobile phones" or "smartphones," despite the fact that they are actually personal computers that make deep use of the cellular phone network.

As we explore the use of mobile communication in therapy, it's important to conceptualize these lovely gadgets as what they are: powerful computing devices that have found their way into nearly every aspect of our lives. We will continue to refer to them as mobile phones, but we know what they really are!

How Do Modern Humans Connect?

Imagine with me a fantastical scenario wherein all the space in the space-time continuum suddenly collapses. There is no such thing as "where" anymore, because every location in the universe is now in the same point in space. Not only would it be very confusing at first, but it would also be clamorous. Everyone you wish to connect with (and many you don't) are all there with you all the time under all circumstances.

This is not so difficult to imagine, because we have something akin to that already. For the purposes of communication – and certain kinds of connection – the Internet collapses all the connected places in the world into one spot. The mobile computers we carry each day make us part of that collapsed point in space and we can reach out to the network of people, information and services at any time and from nearly any place.

As such, it's no surprise that people have come to rely on this "non-space" as part of daily life. Those who grew up with it see it as a given and may have difficulty understanding their elders who find it off-putting or simply don't see it the way they do: as a primary medium both for connecting with important others and creating new relationships.

This social order of always-on communication creates some interesting changes for the basic context of therapy:

- Not all clients or practitioners view the boundaries of the therapeutic relationship as being contained in the walls of an office. Clients and practitioners may view therapeutic boundaries as "spaceless."
- Many people expect an instant response to their messages. Social expectations are that mobile phones will deliver our incoming messages instantly, and in some social milieux there is little concept of the idea of "checking messages" – it's supposed to happen automatically. As such, depending on the interpersonal expectations that a particular client or practitioner has developed, therapeutic boundaries may also be "timeless." Even young practitioners, socialized in the networked world, often find this to be intrusive. If not tempered by setting and maintaining proper boundaries with clients, this intrusiveness can become detrimental to the practitioner's self-care needs and possibly to the health of therapeutic boundaries, as well.
- Concepts of privacy and transparency have shifted in recent years. While personal desires for privacy still very much exist, social expectations around what is kept private and how it is kept private have shifted (Boyd, 2010). Classic practitioner training and ethics may be behind the times in this realm.

"MOBILE COMMUNICATIONS," AKA "TEXTING"

"SMS:" the Endangered Species of Texting

The original technology that we called "texting" was a simple innovation called "Short Message Service," or "SMS." SMS messages can communicate short bursts of text. Variations on SMS ("Multimedia Messaging Service," or "MMS") can even send media such as pictures and videos.

SMS is an open system, meaning that anyone with any device can send and receive SMS messages. This means SMS allows everyone to write and read texts to and from each other, so long as their equipment uses the same SMS standards.

SMS is still used because it is the main way for phones to send text messages across brands and across software setups: an iPhone can send an SMS to an Android phone, and different kinds of Android phones can send an SMS to each other. In other words, SMS ensures that we can all text with each other.

That said, SMS is not as popular as it used to be. SMS has limited capabilities, and specialized messaging "apps" are becoming ever more popular.

"Messaging"

At the time of writing, the most popular messaging app was likely to be Facebook Messenger. The number of apps available for texting-like "messaging" is staggering. Snapchat, WhatsApp, Viber, Wickr, and many others make up a growing market of apps whose primary purpose is communication in the style of SMS texting, but with more pizzazz, features and, in some cases, more feeling of community.

The direct messaging features of social media apps are also an important conduit for texting via mobile phones. These include the aforementioned Facebook Messenger, Twitter direct messaging, leaving messages through Venmo (a funds transfer/social media service), "mail" on the LinkedIn app… and the list goes on.

All of the above-mentioned services are what this author calls, "closed systems." Unlike the highly open SMS, these apps are produced, serviced and controlled by the companies that create them. As such, all participants in a conversation using these apps generally need to be using the same app. Also, all communications will generally go through the same company's Internet servers.

The point of this discussion is to highlight the social transition from SMS "texting" to app-bound "messaging." SMS may never disappear completely, but it is already in lesser use than it was in the early twenty-first century. There are some interesting practical consequences to this transition:

- Messaging is more scattered. Digital natives expect that messages can come from a variety of sources and they make choices about which sources to pay attention to.
- A lot of messaging is handled by monolithic private parties. Instead of messages being ferried around by cooperating phones companies, they are handled in-house by a single entity, such as Facebook, Snapchat or whatever private company produces the app currently being used to trade messages.

There are also consequences of interest to practitioners. For example:

- Clients may or may not understand how certain messaging apps might not support the kinds of therapeutic boundaries that their practitioner is working to create and maintain. For example, using Facebook Messenger with a practitioner means being Facebook friends with the practitioner, which is a sticky boundary situation. Similarly, apps like Snapchat and other social messaging apps are likely not an appropriate medium for therapeutic exchanges for a wide variety of reasons, one of which is the record-keeping problems introduced by apps that destroy messages after they are read. Since most people choose only a few apps to attend to, it may be difficult for a practitioner to introduce a new app if the practitioner is the only person the client is meant to use it to communicate with.

- Security may be either improved or worsened. The flexibility of apps means that practitioner and client could specifically choose to use security and privacy-supporting apps for communication. On the other hand, the private ownership of the Internet servers used by "closed system" apps could be more likely to result in privacy breaches should practitioner and client not be sufficiently thoughtful about which app(s) they use together – the companies that produce these apps have control over the messages sent with them, and each company will have its own goals for all that information. Security is discussed in more detail below.

It is worth highlighting that the dominance of messaging apps means that the line between "texting" and social media can be easily blurred if one is not careful. Practitioners should consider social media-related ethical issues when using messaging apps and/or avoid messaging apps that have social media components or are associated with social media services.

Email Through Mobile Apps

Email and texting are viewed as separate things for a number of reasons:

- Email is viewed as potentially more formal, or at least as more appropriate for formal correspondence than texting.
- Email is more heavy-duty than texting. Text messages are mostly text and perhaps some images, while email can be used to send arbitrary file attachments of any kind.
- Email is used through full-blown applications, while texting is done with simple apps or classic cellular phones.

Once again, smartphones are blurring these lines. Reading and writing emails on modern mobile phones could potentially have little practical difference from exchanging SMS messages or using a mobile messaging app. Just like messaging apps, mobile email apps provide notification of new messages and enable participants to compose and read messages on their mobiles as quickly as they can type and tap "send."

The primary advantage of this fact is that it expands the possibilities of available software for practitioners. Specifically, it has the potential to make the use of encrypted email services and secure client portals more accessible to both practitioners and clients by bringing them to our mobile devices.

MOBILE COMMUNICATIONS IN THERAPY

Asynchronous Yet Semi-Interruptive

Mobile communication is "asynchronous," meaning that all participants in a communication need not be actively attending to the conversation at the same time for it to occur. A mobile message can arrive and be ignored for a few minutes or longer, then read and responded to later. A phone call, conversely, is "synchronous." All participants must actively attend to the call simultaneously, lest they lose track of the conversation.

Asynchronous communication is highly popular. It allows for a person to manage many tasks at one time and facilitates constant contact without sustained attention to those contacts.

In addition to being asynchronous, most mobile communication is also semi-interruptive. To explain: a phone call is highly interruptive. When the phone rings, one either attends to it immediately or misses it altogether. Classic email is usually noninterruptive, in that one has to specifically go to "check your email" in order to become aware of the waiting messages.

Most mobile communications (and most modern email apps) are what this author calls

"semi-interruptive." They momentarily interrupt one's attention with a notification signal that means, "You have a new message!" Usually the notification then sticks around in a passive form, as a little icon reminding one to check messages or an "unread messages" count with an ever-increasing number.

This interruptiveness, without synchronousness, means that unread messages take on a cognitive-emotional valence of "must be attended to soon." However, they can still be put off until the recipient is ready for them.

The result is that mobile communications not only reach people wherever they have reception, but they can also reach people's attention at any reasonable moment and in a way that the reader may be likely to tolerate. As discussed below, this feature of mobile communication has clinical applications.

Research on Texting-Based Interventions

As noted in the previous edition of this text by Merz, much of the research on the use of mobile messaging in health care has it used for the following purposes (Merz, 2010):

- *Remote monitoring of clients/patients.* Checking in with clients/patients to determine symptoms and states as they occur outside the office. Remote monitoring tasks can also be accomplished using apps made specifically for this purpose, such as mood monitoring apps.
- *Health education and compliance with treatment plans.* A number of studies have successfully used texting to educate clients/patients about their health conditions and the behaviors that assist in treating those conditions. For many people, compliance with treatment plans is easier when they are reminded to do so, and when they know more about how to do so.
- *Reminders of events, including appointments.* In a number of studies, mobile text

reminders reduced no-show rates for health care appointments.

These interventions benefit from the semi-interruptive, asynchronous nature of mobile communication. Reminders and check-ins can reach clients/patients in their daily lives without requiring appointments or intolerable interruptions.

Merz also discussed evidence of the value of mobile communication in maintaining connection between client and practitioner. While that level of connection may or may not be desirable (more below), consider its applications in the following scenarios:

- An actively suicidal client.
- A client struggling with intrusive trauma flashbacks.

The Always-On Paradigm and Therapy

What do you feel when you think of the idea of being in constant, 24-hour contact with your clients?

For some practitioners, this is nothing new. For others, it may feel positive. For the majority of practitioners, however – including many of those native to the digital world – it does not feel good. It also may not support therapy goals well.

Classically, therapeutic boundaries were matched by physical boundaries – short-term contacts could only occur when in the walls of the office or when near the right landline phones. Currently, those boundaries are defined by social norms and interpersonal agreements – one would not expect a response to a text message received in a movie theater mostly because that is an inappropriate place for it, and not because one wouldn't expect the recipient to be able to receive a message at the theater – it's the rightness of the context, and not the physical logistics of communication, that prevent the message from getting through to the recipient immediately. This is

a significant change in the nature of social availability as compared to the era before ubiquitous cellular phones.

This change in the physical logistics of everyday communication raises a number of clinical questions regarding the use of mobile communications in therapy:

- Is it healthy for clients to have their practitioner be so available? Which clients might benefit from the ability to make contact at nearly any time and which might be harmed by it? Has the practitioner made a conscious, clinically-based decision regarding availability for contact or is s/he unmindfully engaging in mobile communication with clients? Importantly, has the client been enrolled in this communication plan through clear contracting with the practitioner?
- How much availability is healthy for practitioners? How can mobile communications contribute to, or prevent, practitioner burnout? Is the practitioner considering ethical and personal needs around self-care when responding to clients' communication habits? Is the use of mobile communication in therapy deliberate and used to healthfully facilitate the process for both practitioner and client or is it unmindful? Once again, is the client explicitly enrolled in the practitioner's policies around mobile communication?
- How would the practitioner's chosen modality be helped or hindered by allowing (or leveraging) always-on availability? For example, Dialectical Behavior Therapy has strict guidelines around out-of-office contact with clients and calls for written contracts which define what is allowed and how it is limited; psychodynamic approaches generally see time-limited contact as an essential part of forming appropriate boundaries that support the process. Is the practitioner's

approach to mobile communication with clients mindfully designed to support the practitioner's modality and, once again, is the client explicitly enrolled in that communication plan?

When discussing the use of mobile communications with clients, it is important to establish expectations up-front as part of informed consent. Strongly consider including at least the following in your informed consent:

- An official turnaround time for responding to messages. Set a time that is reasonable both for self-care and for setting clinically appropriate therapeutic boundaries.
- Times and circumstances where the practitioner will not respond to messages.
- The appropriate channels to use when messaging the practitioner, including the contact information that should be used.
- The best way to reach out to the practitioner in an emergency.

Discussing these things up-front will help reduce confusion and facilitate a smoother communication flow with clients as well as safeguard boundaries that bolster therapeutic relationships and practitioner self-care. Contracting with clients around how out-of-office communications will be handled is, in many cases, an essential part of healthy therapeutic work in the modern age of ubiquitous mobile communication devices.

ETHICAL AND REGULATORY ISSUES

Professional Boundaries and Standards of Behavior

Texting "Voice"

How do you "talk" when you write text messages?

Written English typically follows a different format and grammar from spoken English. Even in composing this chapter, I tend to avoid personal pronouns. (See what I did there?) In person-to-person speech, an English-speaker would likely sound odd if they avoided saying "I" or "me," or if they overused the passive voice. And if that's not enough, one can imagine the difficulty of trying to simulate the written word by maintaining a mostly flat effect in all verbal communications.

In face-to-face therapy, what would it be like to speak to clients in the same voice used to write papers in school? How would that impact therapeutic effectiveness?

Linguists have described the patterns typically found in text messaging as similar to, or the same as, English speech transcribed into textual formats (Chiad, 2008). Formal writing is not expected in text messages. Formal written English, on the other hand, seeks to convey expression through crafted textual statements. Speed of writing is not a priority, and shortcuts like emoticons are seen as taboo.

In text messaging, however, speed and brevity are priorities. The medium is used to convey speech-like communications through text and low-resolution images such as emoticons and emoji. If one wishes to make a sarcastic statement, an emoticon such as the sideways smile (":)") or a small picture of a smiling face (generally an "emoji") is likely to be necessary to convey the intended meaning.

Another example: consider how one's facial and vocal expressions change the meaning of the question, "what do you mean by that?" One might wish to use such a question in a text message. How would you convey your intended meaning without somehow simulating the effects that are normally produced through facial expression and body language? Consider how the phrase's meaning is conveyed with and without emoticons:

- What do you mean by that?
- What do you mean by that? :)

Before engaging in text messaging in professional contexts, it is wise to investigate standards and guidelines that apply to one's practice for any statements regarding text messages. Sometimes professional standards are different from expected social norms, and specifically restrict the use of certain texting conventions such as emoticons and emoji. In such cases, one should find ways to convey meaning without those tools.

On the other hand, it is worth examining how one's relationships with clients are affected by texting with them. Interpersonal interaction through texting is certainly different from face-to-face interaction and practitioners may need to spend time and energy examining how their behavior in the texting medium impacts professional relationships, just as we do with our face-to-face interaction style. This is especially true of practitioners who are relatively new to texting.

What and When to Text?

Mobile messaging allows for the communication of a wide variety of things. A person on a business trip can take a video of the local sights and immediately send it home to the spouse with a message of, "Wish you were here!"

It is just as easy for practitioners and clients alike to send media of nearly any kind to and from each other and to do so on a whim. So what and when should practitioners and their clients text each other to support therapy and maintain professionally useful boundaries?

There is a danger in this discussion of creating a personal ban on whole categories of content. For example, a practitioner may make it policy that they don't send or receive images and videos at all. One should consider the possible losses that result from categorically denying a whole medium before banning it. On the other hand, sending such media without consideration for its content and meaning could bring unintended consequences.

A related point that has been addressed by several professional organizations is that of personal vs. professional relationships online. While practitioners are in no way banned from using social media, there is a recognized need to keep separate the practitioner's professional interactions from his/her personal interactions.

The Association of Social Work Boards' Model Regulatory Standards for Technology and Social Work Practice, as authored by their international task force, as well as the American Counseling Association's code of ethics, explicitly discourage clinicians from forming personal relationships with clients in social media or through the use of text messaging (ASWB International Technology Task Force, 2015; American Counseling Association, 2014). The Online Therapy Institute's ethical framework for social media also recognizes the need to keep personal and professional social media presences separate (Kolmes, Merz Nagel, & Anthony, 2010).

It seems redundant to remind clinicians that we should not form inappropriate dual relationships with clients. It would appear, however, that several organizations see it as necessary to note that the low-barrier, high-interactivity environment created by the easy availability of always-on connection can make it easy to forget these professional responsibilities around maintaining therapy-affirming boundaries. This is another of many reasons for practitioners to be mindful and proactive about the way we set those boundaries.

It is wise to note that when one feels the desire to share a thought with a client or send them an image or movie, it is indicated to consider one's internal motivation around sending that message:

- Is it an intentional act of therapeutic intervention that is appropriate for the client's needs?
- Does it support or interfere with the therapeutic modality one is employing with that particular client?

- Is there any personal gain – emotional, material, or what-have-you – in sending the message?
- Is there beneficence in sending the message immediately by mobile phone as opposed to waiting for the next scheduled interaction (assuming one has those)?

Additionally, one should also weigh the possible benefits and harms of sending the message:

- What good will be done by creating this connection with the client?
- Is there overall benefit to making the connection immediately?
- How does the medium of mobile messaging create therapeutic benefit that another medium could not create?

The issue of immediacy is an important one in texting. In some social milieux, there is a social expectation that when a text or email is sent, response will be immediate. Even practitioners who resonate with this social norm are unlikely to adhere to it in therapeutic correspondence, however. Communications with clients are generally thought through more deeply and intentionally than personal communications.

The issue of client expectations around practitioner availability is not limited to use of mobile communications, of course. As the British Association for Counselling and Therapy's ethical framework points out, its members ". . . take responsibility for our own wellbeing as essential to sustaining good practice" (British Association for Counselling & Psychotherapy, 2016). This and other reminders of the ethical need for self-care easily apply to making sure we work with clients to find a healthy way of being available via mobile communications.

Practitioner needs are not the only ethical issue in texting immediacy, however. Our interactions with clients set up the norms that they expect. If a client learns that his practitioner will immediately respond to his texts, certain clients can develop a short-term soothing strategy that relies on texting the practitioner. Or others may come to see the practitioner's immediate responses as a necessary sign of a strong therapeutic relationship. Most practitioners cannot or will not maintain this consistently immediate availability and sudden changes in response time could be damaging to clients who build those expectations.

Client expectations around availability should be set and normed early in therapeutic relationships. Like so many ethical issues, informed consent is a key piece for managing client expectations around mobile messaging. The 2014 American Counseling Association code of ethics explicitly requires its members to include in their informed consent an official turnaround time for texts and emails (American Counseling Association, 2014). The Online Therapy Institute's ethical framework for use of technology in therapy asks practitioners in many ways to provide useful information about proper ways to contact the practitioner in various circumstances, including posting proper contact information on websites and ensuring that clients know who to contact and how to contact them in emergencies (Anthony & Merz Nagel, 2009).

In addition to informed consent, it is wise to note and track clients' patterns of interaction via mobile messaging as part of overall clinical assessment of the client. Maintaining clinical awareness can both heighten one's awareness of productive professional boundaries and allow one to take advantage of the medium to discover clinically relevant behaviors and material.

Security

Security is a real concern in mobile messaging, as texting does not generally include a lot of technical security, such as significant use of encryption. It is vital to explore the security of texting from a risk management lens. Behaviors and software settings based on a set of professional "standards" are unlikely to stand up to rapid technological change and will not work consistently across different circumstances. The risk management approach to assessing security in our practices is better suited to creating positive outcomes. When using that lens, all considerations of security start with a "security risk analysis."

Risk analysis is analogous to a community needs assessment: it is a process of objectively and holistically gathering up information about the entirety of one's practice and discovering the security "needs" one has. Here we will explore the kinds of risks that consistently crop up in the use of mobile phones in clinical practice and that should be considered in one's risk analysis.

"Data In Motion" – or, Texts on the Internet

The first security consideration comes in the *transmission* of mobile messages. Techies call this, "data in motion." Mobile messaging data generally does said motion over the Internet. Even though these messages may also spend some time in the telephone network, the bulk (and sometimes the entirety) of their travel is through the global, open network we call the Internet.

In the Internet space, messages may be vulnerable to the following risks:

- Interception. The Internet is a data "bucket brigade" wherein a chain of different telecommunications companies pass our information along from computer-to-computer. While our data passes through each computer, anyone with access to that computer can see what we're transmitting. People with access normally include engineers and administrators. It's also possible that a given computer may have been invaded

by hackers, however, and the data passing through it could be under observation by bad guys.

- Damage or loss. There is a possibility that you could send something that never reaches its destination. Perhaps it gets mangled in transit or somewhere along the bucket brigade it gets dropped. This used to be a significant concern with SMS text messages. Telecommunications companies have increased the reliability of SMS significantly, but lost messages still happen. The problem is that the sender doesn't receive notification when a message is lost – there's no bounce message or other notification that the message never reached its destination.

When in motion, the major risks facing mobile messages are all about interception by bad guys. Based on objective historical information, what are these bad guys generally looking to intercept?

- Financial information such as credit card numbers and bank account numbers.
- Information that can be used for identity theft.
- Passwords.
- Medical information that can be used for identity theft.
- Insurance or other third-party payer information that can be used to submit false claims.
- Any information that they know can be reasonably leveraged for monetary gain.

While other kinds of information could also be of use to bad guys, depending on the nature of the client and the nature of the information, the above items are most vulnerable to interception and their inclusion in mobile messages should absolutely be avoided. Practitioners should enroll clients in understanding this fact, as well.

Many experts advise that administrative issues like appointment times are of low security risk when in motion over the Internet. Therapeutic exchanges may also be of low risk when in motion, depending on the client and the nature of the exchanges (e.g., Internet interlopers may actively watch for information about high-profile clients but ignore others). However, always remember that these risk decisions are to be made by clients after the practitioner provides information about the risks (Huggins, 2013). These risk analysis decisions are not to be made without client collaboration and informed consent. As such, one's policies around mobile messaging security should always include a documented decision-making process that includes the client and emphasizes a full exploration of risks as communicated from practitioner to client.

It is also important, in the case of therapeutic exchanges, to consider that security of information is not the only clinical factor in deciding what medium to use for those communications. Even if interception by Internet interlopers is found to be unlikely, practitioners should consider the emotional value of client confidence in the privacy and confidentiality of their communications with practitioners. For this reason among others, practitioners should strongly consider using technologically secured (e.g., encrypted and digitally authenticated) communication methods for therapeutic exchanges.

Another point about data in motion that should be mentioned is the security of cellular voice calls. This chapter has had little discussion of voice calls, but historically there has been great concern over third parties intercepting and listening in to cellular calls. In the past, one needed only a simple radio to listen to cellular calls that were happening within range of the radio. This is no longer the case.

In the modern era, all or nearly all cellular devices do something to protect the cellular signal. Anyone listening with a radio would hear only digital noise. Eavesdropping on cellular calls now requires somewhat sophisticated equipment that is illegal for civilians to use in nearly all parts of the world. It may be used by law enforcement and intelligence agencies, however, depending on jurisdictional laws and law enforcement policies.

As an aside: a simple Internet search will turn up numerous websites claiming to sell products that allow the user to eavesdrop on any cellular phone they wish. These products are either completely bogus or require that one be able to physically access the targeted phone and install software on it. As such, the claim that they allow you to "eavesdrop on any phone" is somewhat hyperbolic.

"Data at Rest" – or, Texts on One's Gear

The second security consideration comes in what happens with mobile messages while they sit on our phones and computers. Techie folks call this "data at rest."

Any messages exchanged with clients will reside on the equipment of both practitioner and client, including mobile devices and computers, where applicable. They may also reside on the Internet servers that provide services for both practitioner and client.

A tricky part of this risk analysis is getting a solid picture of all the places where messages end up. Mobile messaging services are sometimes more complex than classic SMS text messaging and those messages could pop up on phones, computers and tablets –depending on what app you're using to send and receive messages. What's more, it's even possible for the behavior of text messages to change from client to client. For example, practitioners who use iPhones will discover that messages exchanged with other iPhone users will be sent using Apple's iMessage service. iMessage messages can be read with any device including computers and tablets. If the same practitioner texts with a client who has an Android phone, classic cellular phone, or anything that isn't an iPhone, the message will be sent using classic SMS service instead. iMessage will not be involved at all. (Hint: iMessage messages are colored blue on the screen, and SMS messages are colored green. There is no other visible difference between the two when accessed on an iPhone, however.)

Regardless of how the messages are sent and received, at least the following risks should be considered when discussing mobile messaging with clients:

- Who has access to the client's equipment during the course of a given day?
  - Would the client want any of these people to view messages to/from the practitioner? What harms might occur if any of them did?
  - The practitioner should also consider this question in regards to his or her own equipment.
- Who has the necessary credential (e.g. passwords) to get into the client's gear and/or to log in to the client's online accounts?
  - Can any of these people send messages to the practitioner that appear to come from the client? Would any of them do so? What harms might occur if any of them did?
  - The practitioner should also consider this question in regards to his or her own equipment and online accounts.
- What account(s) does the client use for mobile messaging? Is that account owned by an employer or educational institution? If so, the employer or school administration can access the messages.
  - The practitioner should also consider this question in regards to his or her own equipment and online accounts.

"Authentication" – or, Figuring Out Who You're Texting With

As hinted at in the previous section, a significant security concern with mobile messaging is ensuring that the person on the other end of the conversation is who they claim to be. One may receive a mobile message that comes from a client's phone number or other account, but that isn't a guarantee that the client is the one who wrote and sent the message.

The strength of mobile devices – their mobility – is also a security vulnerability. If a client has bad guys in his or her life, those bad guys may find occasion to pick up the client's mobile and try sending a fake message to the practitioner. If a practitioner has reason to suspect this has occurred, some kind of "authentication" action is indicated.

"Authentication" is the act of ensuring that someone is who they claim to be. After receiving a suspicious mobile message, there are a number of ways to authenticate the sender. The best option depends on one's circumstances.

- If it's a text message coming from a phone number, call the sender and inquire about the message. It's advisable not to reveal any therapeutic relationships in the process of doing this – a simple "I got a message from this phone number" may work. However, depending on the bad guys in the client's life, this method may or may not introduce new dangers to the client's confidentiality.
- Find a different way to contact the client – one that is unlikely to be accessible by others in the client's life – and check if the message came from them.
- Use a code word or code phrase. This is a method that must be set up beforehand. If client and practitioner see that bad guys might try to butt in on the therapeutic relationship, they can set up special phrases or words to use in their messages that signal that the message is authentic.
- Wait until the next scheduled interaction to ask the client if they sent the message.

Other Security Measures

Here we'll talk about two kinds of approaches to managing the risks discussed above. One is technical approaches, or risk reduction methods that involve techie things like encryption, passwords and the like. The other is behavioral approaches, or methods that rely on agreeing to engage in certain behaviors and activities that keep risks to an acceptable minimum.

These technical approaches can help with the risks discussed above:

- **Encrypting messages**. Encryption is where one's computer uses secret codes to make messages unreadable by bad guys who intercept them. This is a perfect method for managing the "data in motion" risks. It may or may not be useful for "data at rest" issues. If bad guys have the necessary passwords to access clients' messages (or your messages), then those passwords could also unlock encryption. One way to manage this could be to use a special app for encrypted messaging that only client and practitioner know about.

    Encryption is not something that a practitioner can put in place without client collaboration. Practitioner and client must both engage in the encryption process. This generally means that both parties must use the same secure messaging app.
- **Mobile device security**. A major part of protecting "data at rest" is putting measures in place on mobile devices that prevent third parties from accessing them. A full discussion of mobile device security is outside the scope of this chapter, but such measures generally include at least the following:
    - Remote tracking: software that allows the device owner to track its location if it is lost.
    - Remote lock and remote wipe: software that allows the device owner to lock down the device when it goes missing or, if necessary, cause the device to wipe out its own data banks so that the information becomes unavailable to third parties who may get their hands on the phone.
    - Passwords: All smartphones, and many classic phones, can be set to require a password or password-like action for access.
    - Device encryption: Modern smartphones can be set up to encrypt their data storage. This encryption is only as effective as the device's passcode/password, however. Dependence on device encryption indicates the enactment of passcodes, passwords, or pass patterns with much more than the typical four characters/points.

In addition to the technical approaches, practitioners and clients are advised to enact at least these behavioral measures:

- **Limit or expand communications based on evaluated risks**. When practitioner and client discuss the risks in the client's life that may be triggered by mobile messaging, it becomes easier to collaborate and decide on rules that balance clinical benefits of those communications with needed management of security risks. Many practitioners ask that clients limit any nonencrypted communications to schedule changes and other administrivia. For some clients, however, even these communications could be risky. Bear in mind that any mobile communications with clients that do not use strong technical security (e.g., encryption and digital authentication) should only be done at the client's request after the client has been clearly informed of the risks of those communications and has decided that the risks are acceptable and that the mobile communications are desired.

In some cases, the benefit of therapeutic mobile messaging might outweigh the risks and thus practitioner and client may decide that it is appropriate for them. One needs to consider the client's security risks and clinical needs as well as the practitioner's ethical and legal requirements. Depending on the professional-political environment, however, some practitioners may not be allowed the option to communicate anything beyond administrivia without using encryption, regardless of clients' desires or informed consent.

• **Create and agree on communications policies**. Informed consent should include discussion of the practitioner's policies around communication, including the best methods to use when communicating with the practitioner, the kinds of communication methods available to the client and the official turnaround time the client can expect for responses from the clinician. This not only helps clients know what to expect, but can also generate important discussions that reveal security risks in the client's life (what's more, these security issues are frequently also clinical issues).

Conflicting Interests: Confidentiality vs. Record-Keeping

One method of ensuring the confidentiality of information is to simply destroy it. Classic spy shows used this method liberally: "This message will self-destruct in five seconds!"

In practitioner life, however, confidentiality is not the only security concern. We must also keep records. So when considering methods of engaging in mobile communications with clients, practitioners also need to consider how to maintain records of those communications.

Practitioners have room to be creative here. Perhaps if one is using a secure texting app that also destroys messages after a set time (e.g., Wickr), one could retain a record of the messages by taking screen shots of them.

Two caveats:

1. If clients have reason to expect that messages with their practitioner are going to be destroyed after a time (such as when they're using an app, like Wickr, that normally destroys messages), then they should be informed if the practitioner intends to do something to foil the destruction mechanism and retain the messages. It's probably also wise to tell the clients how this will be done.

   For example, a practitioner who uses Wickr to do secure texting with a client should tell the client something like, "Wickr allows us to 'text' each other using a high level of security and provides strong privacy protections. To protect privacy, Wickr can destroy the messages we exchange with each other after they're read. I have to maintain a record of our communications, however, so I will use a 'screen capture' or other method (such as by-hand transcription) to retain all the messages we exchange."

2. Whatever method is contrived to maintain records of communications it should be reliable. For example, taking screen shots of text messaging apps might work, but it also requires that the practitioner be vigilant about doing it.

   One should also consider that if the chosen method of retaining messages requires using a "workaround," such as taking pictures of the phone's screen, then the workaround may cease to work at some point when the software is updated.

Professional Standards of Confidentiality

Discussions of risk management approaches to security and privacy tends to look at confidentiality as purely an issue of reducing risks of harm. The ethics of confidentiality are not purely about nonmaleficence ("do no harm"), however. They are also there to nurture beneficence ("do good").

While research on whether or not confidentiality is a necessary element of effective therapy is mixed (Remley & Herlihy, 2012), it is generally regarded as essential to therapy outcomes within our own professional standards and of vital importance in most areas of mental health care.

When planning a security strategy for mobile messaging with clients, practitioners should consider the fact that proper use of encryption facilitates creation of a "private space on the Net." It's worthwhile to consider framing the proper use of encrypted and digitally authenticated communications as a tool to create "safe space" for therapeutic work in mobile messaging.

Retaining Text Messages in Records

Speaking technically, any message one exchanges with clients is a part of the client's record. Practitioners need to maintain records, so it can be assumed that practitioners must maintain all text messages.

Because text messages are textual in nature, it is possible to retain the whole message. That is, one could argue that a summary of a message or a summary of a conversation isn't sufficient record-keeping because it should be possible to retain the original messages.

On the other hand, many textual communications are trivial in their content. Some practitioners might not document a one-minute phone conversation in which they negotiate the timing of an appointment. In such a case, why would a text message doing the same need to be documented?

Practitioners should retain any and all textual communications that are clinically relevant. When deciding on a retention policy for other communications, however, consider at least the following:

- The laws, rules, and professional guidelines that apply to one's practice.
- The manner in which one's records are used. Practitioners who anticipate they will have their records subpoenaed, or who are working with clients who are likely to be litigious, might wish to be more rigorous about retaining mobile communications verbatim.
- The ease of retention. All risk management decisions should include a cost-benefit analysis. If the secure retention of mobile communications is relatively easy, then it is advisable to do so. There is a benefit, however small, in retaining all communications verbatim. If the cost is low, then cost-benefit analysis would indicate that it's worth doing.

CONCLUSION

Mobile communication is likely to keep growing in size and importance. It is difficult to predict the directions that mobile technology will grow in. However, we can see at the time of writing that wearable computing devices, such as smart watches and smart glasses, are a rapidly growing market.

As mobile computing expands, so will the seamlessness between the globally shared virtual world and the actual world. We can't predict the precise outcome of this change, but it is likely that practitioners will need to continue developing our understanding of the clinical and ethical implications of technological development. Specifically, we need to remember:

- Therapeutic boundaries are heavily built on agreements. Practitioners should mindfully and proactively contract with clients to engage in boundary behaviors that are health-affirming for both client and practitioner.
- Practitioners should develop a sense of what kinds of mobile communications are therapeutically appropriate and under what circumstances. That is, we should develop a mindful sense of how and what to "text" and when.
- Practitioners need to be prepared to inform clients of risks and benefits in mobile communication, including those that affect the therapeutic relationship, clinical outcomes of the work, and the security of the client's sensitive information.

Keeping up with these tasks may require an increased level of effort. It is likely worth that effort, however, both to keep up with the environment that our clients live in and to be sure we can leverage modern communications technology for clinical benefit.

REFERENCES

American Counseling Association. (2014). *Code of ethics and standards of practice.* Alexandria, VA: Author.

Anthony, K., & Merz Nagel, D. (2009). *Ethical framework for the use of technology in mental health.* Retrieved July 5, 2015, from Online Therapy Institute: http://online therapyinstitute.com/ethical-training/.

ASWB International Technology Task Force. (2015). *Model Regulatory Standards for Technology and Social Work Practice.* Associated Social Work Boards.

Boyd, D. (2010). Making sense of privacy and publicity. Austin, TX: *SXSW.*

British Association for Counselling & Psychotherapy. (2016). *Ethical framework for good practice in counselling & psychotherapy.* Retrieved July 17th, 2015, from http://www.bacp.co.uk/admin/structure/files/pdf/14237_ethical-framework-jun15 final.pdf.

Chiad, M. O. (2008). Structural and linguistic analysis of SMS Text Messages. *Journal of Kerbala University, 6*(4).

Huggins, R. (2013, October). *Clients have the right to receive unencrypted emails under HIPAA.* Retrieved October 17, 2013, from Person-Centered Tech:http://www.personcentered tech.com/2013/10/clients-have-the-right-to-receive-unencrypted-emails-under-hipaa/.

Kolmes, K., Merz Nagel, D., & Anthony, K. (2010). *Ethical framework for the use of social media by mental health professionals.* Retrieved July 5, 2015, from Online Therapy Institute: http://onlinetherapyinstitute.com/ethical-framework-for-the-use-of-social-media-by-mental-health-professionals/.

Merz, T. (2010). Ch. 3: Using cell/mobile phone SMS for therapeutic intervention. In K. Anthony, D. M. Nagel, & S. Goss, *The use of technology in mental health: Applications, ethics and practice.* Springfield, IL: Charles C Thomas.

Remley, T., & Herlihy, B. (2012). *Ethical, legal, and professional issues in counseling* (4th ed.). Upper Saddle River, NJ: Merrill Prentice-Hall.

Chapter 4

THE RISE OF SOCIAL NETWORKS AND THE BENEFITS AND RISKS TO THE MENTAL HEALTH PROFESSION

Allison Thompson

INTRODUCTION

Social media gives the ability for any person to "create, share and comment on information on a variety of platforms" (Kolmes, 2010) and interact with one another through the site. Since the publication of the previous edition, Facebook has emerged and overcome Myspace in popularity where it has over 400 million users at this time (May 2015). "Social networking sites, such as Facebook and Twitter, are now used by 1 in 4 people worldwide" (Whiteman, 2014). On average, "Americans spend 7.6 hours a month using social media" and "63% of American Facebook users log on to the site daily" (Whiteman, 2014).

Not only has Facebook come out as a top market for social networks but numerous new sites have emerged, such as Twitter, Snap Chat, Instagram, Youtube, and so forth. With the advent of online technology through cellular (mobile) devices, many more new programs and sites have emerged with additional opportunities to connect with individuals with quicker speed and far reaching distance parameters. Such technology can offer additional opportunities with the mental health profession reaching new audiences and educating or providing support. However,

with the intensity of the rise, could there be risks that could affect the counseling relationship and overall ethics? And are there ways social networks can safely provide opportunities for growth in sessions while balancing professional ethics and laws? In this chapter there will be an overview of the changes in social network updates in ethics and the risks of social networks, and future research implications.

AMERICAN COUNSELING CODE OF ETHICS

A discussion still exists on the balance between professional and personal and questions still remain as to how to "integrate Facebook and other social media sites to your work while keeping in mind ethics and client boundaries" (Belmont, 2012). Since the previous edition of this book, The American Counseling Code of Ethics (2014) now has a specific social media section. An overall point they make is that counselors need to understand that they may be subject to the laws of not only their location but their client's location. Our personal pages on social

43

network sites are not expected to follow the codes of ethics. However, once your page becomes a professional identity, code of ethics do apply to you, online activities. "Counselors avoid potential interactions outside of the professional setting that could be harmful to the client. This applies to both in-person and electronic interactions or relationships" with current counseling relationships (ACA, 2014, p. 5). "We are told to practice within areas of competence. We need to be competent within the areas in which we practice. And that extends to our use of technology . . . We need to remain alert to the ways in which our online presence complements or conflicts with our professional self" (Chernack, 2013). It is important to stay updated on changes in laws and ethics in both the primary practice site and areas where the practitioner is serving their clients.

Providing knowledge about your presence on social networking sites, how they are used in your practice and how you will communicate with clients on these sites, is a necessary and preventative way of assisting the informed consent of clients. Counselors with a social network presence must take precautions in distinguishing between a personal and professional space and avoid disclosing confidential information (ACA, 2014). The American Counseling Association clearly states that "Counselors are prohibited from engaging in a personal virtual relationship with individuals with whom they have a current counseling relationship (e.g., through social and other media)" (2014, p. 5) due to creating dual relationships or compromising the client's confidentiality. Some counselors are addressing this ethical concern and potential boundary crossing through social media consent forms. This can also provide the opportunity to process and discuss with your client their thoughts on this subject and could be an opportunity to engage the client in further helpful discussions in their treatment.

NATIONAL ASSOCIATION OF SOCIAL WORKERS ETHICS

It is important to remember that our client deserves and desires privacy and confidentiality as much as we clinicians do. Through social media, it is possible that a client may be exhibiting a different side of their self they may not wish to share clinically at their current stage. There are many parts to an individual personality and how one defines them in various venues can often differ (National Association of Social Workers, 1999). Since January 2009, one social worker has been blogging the intimate details of her clients' lives, including an incident in which an ostensibly intoxicated baby was placed in her office after a "drug raid." This social worker showed a lack of integrity and such actions may be considered a violation of a client's privacy and confidentiality in addition to risking the client's dignity and self worth (Robb, 2011).

For mental health workers of any kind, our ethical code is an integral part of who we are and we must adhere to the code to ensure the validity of the profession. When the core values slide into a gray area it can call into question the integrity of not only the clinician but professional workers as a whole. The most important aspect to remember is the client should be respected and treated with dignity and worth because they are trusting us to help them in their time of need. "The code is unambiguous. We must respect the inherent dignity and worth of the individual as sacrosanct. Sharing personal information is anything but respecting the client's dignity. Why would anyone even want to give the appearance of compromising social work's core values?" (Robb, 2011, p. 8).

Practitioners should not engage in dual or multiple relationships with clients or former clients in which there are risks of exploitation or potential harm to the client. Maintaining healthy boundaries with clients is imperative in helping them feel safe and confident in the therapeutic relationship. Without assuring the client an exclusively, professional relationship this cannot be achieved and is not beneficial to the client or the practitioner.

> Social workers [and other practitioners] sometimes receive electronic requests from clients who want to be "friends" or contacts on social networking sites such as Facebook and LinkedIn. I have consulted on several cases where social workers learned painful lessons after the fact about boundary, dual relationship, confidentiality, privacy, informed consent and documentation problems that can arise if they interact with clients on such networking sites. (Reamer, 2011)

Practitioners must engage in self-care and other actions to ensure their private lives do not impact on their professional responsibility to their clients. There is an inherent need in humans for connection and as typically curious creatures we have a need to explore. It is important to remember the possible ramification that relationships on social media can trigger, such as possible liability, violations of the code of ethics, and failure to respect client's rights.

> Professional social workers must be mindful of social media use because information shared on social media platforms can be used by clients, other professionals and the general public to shape opinions about you and social workers as a whole. Maintaining primary social work values like client privacy and confidentiality are of utmost importance, and upholding one's reputation is critical to competent, successful practice. (University of Wisconsin – Madison School of Social Work, 2013)

Social media has given individuals a way to connect with friends and family in a way that was not possible many years ago.

However, it has also caused concerns when dealing with professional conduct. It is important to recognize that what we post on the Internet is not private without the correct settings and even *then* it is not 100% private. It is important to remember that anyone motivated to do so can access a large amount of information about someone with very little effort. A practitioner's conduct on social media can not only have an effect on their personal life, but can also affect their professional life. Private Facebook pages have been used during job interviews and police investigations. If you yourself wonder if something is appropriate for you to post the answer is mostly "No." This is a new age and a time which brings new ideas and resources to the field. Competence needs to extend to social media where individuals can find news, alerts to social justice and professional networking. Another key aspect of social media that pertains to the field is the prevalence and impact of cyber bullying (see below). Technology can be a tool to help within the field; however, there is always a thin line. Only one thing is clear; the importance of being true to the profession and ensure the best care will always remain of the utmost importance.

MENTAL HEALTH ETHICAL ISSUES AND SOCIAL NETWORKS

Use of social networking sites such as Facebook as a social networking tool, has presented mental health professionals with ethical issues with regards to protecting their private identity. One tool Facebook provides to protect privacy for its users is through the "blocking" option where you can "prevent them (users) from starting conversations with you or seeing things you post on your profile" (Facebook.com, 2014). Being able to hide our identities from clients would initially appear to be a safe way of protecting ethical issues like boundary crossing; however, there are different ethical issues that arise from the action of directly blocking clients from personal pages. "Blocking particular addresses assumes that you know which email address a person is using to access their Facebook profile . . . blocking the mail address does not completely ensure that someone doesn't have access to you" (Kolmes, 2009, p. 1). Kolmes (2009) additionally points out that "forcing users to choose the Block feature as the only way to restrict others' access to their profile is simply another means in collecting data." In order to "block" a client, you must literally type the full name of the person into the search engine. By doing so, we are giving a name and identifying a connection that could be perceived to violate the client's privacy. The ACA Code of Ethics states, "Counselors respect the privacy of their clients' presence on social media unless given consent to view such information" (2014, p. 18). Social media brings up even further issues related to confidentiality and potential feelings of rejection and trust with your clients (ACA, 2014). In protecting private identity while maintaining confidentiality and the welfare of our clients, a way to cope with this is to incorporate the use of technology and social networks in a professional disclosure in order to fully inform clients about what would occur if they initiate contact in a social networking site.

Another way to reduce confidentiality and boundary issues is by creating a specific page rather than a profile on Facebook that is a separate function used to promote organizations or businesses. It is possible to hide who has "liked" or become a fan of the page and it is not as easy to see who posts messages onto the main page of the organization's page. However, the potential mixing of professional pages and clients can bring new ethical issues in the mental health field. For example, if a client "likes" your professional page, it could be perceived as raising up the potential ethical dilemma of it being considered a "testimonial" and most current codes of ethics

prohibit testimonials from clients due to "their being vulnerable to our influence" (Kolmes, 2009, p. 1). There can be a discrepancy to what knowledge and understanding practitioners have in regards to understanding social media and privacy settings, which can affect decision-making and how to maneuver with clients in this issue (Zur & Zur, 2011). Be cautious when using social network sites and what information you post. It is also important that "Clients should be informed about the concerns and issues surrounding privacy and confidentiality" (Zur & Zur, 2011, p. 15). Without communication and helping clients to understand potential risks involved with communication and use of social networks, this can potentially lead to a disruption in the therapeutic relationship and process. "The possible impact on trust and potential harm to the therapeutic relationship are great if there is no specification of the parameters of such involvement and if therapists do not make clear distinctions between their professional and personal lives" (Giota & Kleftaras, 2014, p. 2249). Know and understand the privacy setting and what information can be seen by the public and communicate this to clients to help reduce negative impact and potential ethical dilemmas faced with using social networks personally and professionally.

USES FOR SOCIAL NETWORKS IN MENTAL HEALTH

Groups on Facebook, having a YouTube account to make videos, creating boards on Pinterest and so forth have created a platform for our clients to have an outlet to speak and seek support for mental health. Even organizations like the National Alliance on Mental Health support utilizing web pages to promote mental health issues, advocate, and educate the public. In a recent study, "47% of people aged 21 and under said they find it easiest to talk about their mental health problems online" (Cresci, 2015). Social network sites provide opportunities for support groups, immediate feedback from posting about one's feelings and obtaining articles relevant to mental health issues. They also bring opportunities to engage in dialogue with clients where that does not pose a risk for boundary crossings or dual relationships. Social networking sites can help teach social skills to introverts where they do not initially have to deal with face-to-face communication and can take their time in creating responses without hitting send or posting a comment on a link (American Psychological Association, 2011). Knowing the variety of social media and the use of them can help us with our clients to "develop appropriate effective methods of intervention to counteract possible negative repercussions" (Williams, 2012).

A concern regarding social media use is cyber bullying where "95% of teenagers who use social media have witnessed forms of cyber bullying on social networking sites and 33% have been victims" (Whiteman, 2014). Therapists can help build coping and problem-solving strategies with clients in regards to cyber bullying, identifying social supports and exploring ways to increase the teen client's self-efficacy by using tools on the site, such as blocking and reporting, which can assist with increasing self-efficacy and helping to create a positive outcome. Clients don't always realize the consequences of making a post on a social networking site and how quickly their post can be spread or that what they post can't always be deleted.

Once something is posted, it is a lot harder to delete the information and the potential outcome could result in something the client did not anticipate. Facebook and Internet Keep Safe Coalition joined to create a resource called "Facebook for School Counselors" that teaches "social counselors how to use Facebook and teach students best practices on the social network" (Lytle, 2012).

Providing additional psychoeducation and skill building to clients, parents and school staff can help open a dialogue and create action steps to help address cyber bullying before additional mental health issues arise (e.g., anxiety and depression).

Facebook is also looking at more direct ways of providing interventions and support within the site and not just with psychoeducation. In February 2015, Facebook introduced a new feature that aids in suicide prevention where users can report any concerns for a user's safety and provides options for the reporter "to contact the friend, contact another friend for support or contact a suicide hotline" (Lien, 2015). A handwritten note or phone call from someone in distress can be put on delay until the person has access to these items. However, if someone posts a threat of self-harm, there is a potential reduction in the response time to the person in need. "As platforms for self-expression, social networking sites . . . are sources of real-time information that could aid in suicide prevention" (Kattalai Kailasam & Samuels, 2015, p. 37).

Further studies are being made in exploring how technology can assess language and body language through digital self-portraits, commonly known as a selfie (Sierra, 2015). Algorithms, or a computer program written to tell the computer what and how to do something, can be programmed to identify and alert on alarming posts made by Facebook users and initiate action steps to provide crisis management to the post. With using social networks as a form of data collection, the "activity logs leave behind a digital train of quantifiable and objective data and can be an analogous or complementary to observing individuals in their natural environment" (Toseeb & Inkster, 2015, p. 1). With each "like" or post on pages, a user creates an electronic identity. Facebook already will utilize the history of a user to determine which advertisements will appear on the user's profile page.

Another group, the Samaritans, launched a similar program to alert Facebook or Twitter users to other users they follow that publish posts with alarming phrases, such as indicating self-harm or distress. After one week, 4,000 people had activated the program (Singer, 2014). Unfortunately, a little over a week after the app was introduced, the company disabled it (Singer, 2014). One complaint of the app was geared towards privacy where users did not want their posts uploaded onto the Samaritans website for other users to view. Another concern was of untrained users confronting users voicing distress with outcomes of this interaction potentially more harmful to the person in need of help. Even though the introduction of this program did not go as initially planned, additional research and information is being gathered to help in the diagnosis and treatment of depression, suicide and substance abuse that could impact the future use of social networks in mental health treatment (Peek, 2015).

Researchers are curious about exploring whether this digital information can be utilized in helping to assess moods and/or prevent suicides from occurring. However, there is currently not enough research in this area to make concrete conclusions at this time. Posts on social networking sites and emotions are subjective and it is quite difficult to program a computer to understand emotions or the intent of a specific post. In addition, not all posts are "public," meaning users can set up privacy settings where only people they have identified as "friends" can see information they post on their profile. Even though the outcomes of studies have not initiated long-term use of apps or programs, research continues to be presented that provides hope in being able to incorporate social networking as a tool in addressing mental health issues.

FUTURE RESEARCH IMPLICATIONS

Since the publication of the first edition of this book, a great deal of research and many articles have been written to explore ethical issues in relation to social networking. Recent studies and articles have emerged exploring ways to incorporate technology into data collection as well as creating online programs to assist with mental health matters within social networks themselves. However, there is still a lack of research regarding directly utilizing social networks within the therapeutic relationship or using social networks indirectly in a practice. Possible questions to continue to examine are:

- What percentages of counselors belong to social networking sites and what have been the benefits and pitfalls?
- What is the current research with social networking sites?
- Ongoing monitoring of the role of professional organizations in limiting the personal lives of counselors in or outside of the membership;
- More exact percentages of how many counselors and/or agencies are using social networks as a tool to build clientele or reach those in need of counseling?
- Studies of the effectiveness of counselors who are using social networks as tools in counseling and determining if the tool is helpful or harmful in developing therapeutic relationships and achieving treatment goals.
- What specific agencies or professionals are using social networks as a form of communicating or counseling clients? What are the ethical issues that have occurred? Has this been successful?

CONCLUSION

Research addressing the above questions

could benefit the counseling profession in future ethical decision-making as well as having an influence on how organizations around the world may monitor the private lives of counselors who belong to online-communities. It could also influence potential online resources or programs to alert and provide crisis management support. Again, without credible research on online communities and counselors who participate on these sites, it is hard to predict the current and ongoing effects of these sites. Future research to target more direct use of social networking sites could help reduce the potential for anxiety some service providers have about using social networking while maintaining ethical codes by identifying benefits and exploring how the use of social networks could benefit the therapeutic alliance.

REFERENCES

American Counseling Association. (2014). ACA code of ethics. [online]. [Retrieved on April 23, 2015]. Available from http://www.counseling.org/resources/aca-code-of-ethics.pdf.

American Psychological Association. (2011). Social networking's good and bad impacts on kids. *ScienceDaily*. Retrieved April 26, 2015 from www.sciencedaily.com/releases/2011/08/110806203538.htm.

Belmont, J. (2012). Quick social media tips for counselors using facebook, pintrest, twitter, and blogs. ACA Blog. [online]. [Retrieved February 15, 2015]. Available from http://www.counseling.org/news/blog/aca-blog/2012/08/13/quick-social-media-tips-for-counselors-using-facebook-pinterest-twitter-and-blogs.

Cresci, E. (2015). #timetotalk: is social media helping people talk about mental health? *Theguardian*. [online]. [Retrieved March 31, 2015]. Available from http://www.the guardian.com/technology/2015/feb/05/timetotalk-is-social-media-helping-people-talk-about-mental-health.

Episode 110 – Dr. Kathryn Chernack: Social Media Use and Social Work Practice: Boundary and Ethical Considerations. (2013, January 7). *inSocialWork® Podcast Series*. [Audio Podcast] Retrieved from http://www.insocialwork.org/episode.asp?ep=110.

Facebook.com. (2014). What is blocking? what happens when I block someone? [online]. [Retrieved on April 28, 2015]. Available from https://www.facebook.com/help/131930530214371.

Giota, K. G. & Kleftaras, G. (2014). Social media and counseling: Opportunities, risks, and ethical considerations. *International Journal of Social, Management, Economics, and Business Engineering*, *8*(8): 2248–2250. [online]. [Retrieved on February 15, 2015]. Available from http://www.academia.edu/8440967/Social_Media_and_Counseling_Opportunities_Risks_and_Ethical_Considerations.

Kattalai Kailasam, V., & Samuels, E. (2015). Can social media help mental health practitioners prevent suicides? *Current Psychiatry*, *14*(2): 37–51. [online]. [Retrieved March 30, 2015]. Available from http://www.currentpsychiatry.com/home/article/can-social-media-help-mental-health-practitioners-prevent-suicides/5ffdeb8492dac956c36d9e954d4a7027.html.

Kolmes, K. (2010). A psychotherapist's guide to facebook and twitter: Why clinicians should give a tweet! *Psychotherapy.Net*. [online]. [Accessed on February 15, 2015]. Available on https://www.psychotherapy.net/article/psychotherapists-guide-social-media.

Kolmes, K. (2009). Should mental health professionals block clients on facebook? [online]. [Retrieved on February 15, 2015]. Available from http://drkkolmes.com/2009/12/11/should-mental-health-professionals-block-clients-on-facebook/.

Lien, T. (2015). Facebook updates feature for suicide prevention. *Los Angeles Times*. [online]. [Retrieved on February 27, 2015]. Available from http://www.latimes.com/business/technology/la-fi-tn-facebook-suicide-prevention-20150225-storyhtml.

Lytle, R. (2012). New facebook efforts targets educating school counselors: A new guide strives to help counselors better understand facebook. *US News.Com*. [online]. [Retrieved on April 29, 2015]. Available from http://www.usnews.com/education/high-schools/articles/2012/04/16/new-facebook-effort-targets-educating-school-counselors.

National Alliance on Mental Health Illness. Tools for leaders. [online]. [Retrieved on April 26, 2015]. Available from http://www2.nami.org//Content/Navigation-Menu/State_Advocacy/Tools_for_Leaders/Media_Tool_Kit_Using_Social_Networking_Tools.htm.

National Association of Social Workers. (1999). NASW Code of Ethics. [online]. Retrieved on April 25, 2015. Available from http://www.socialworkers.org/pubs/code/code.asp.

Peek, H. (2015). Harnessing social media and mobile apps for mental health. *Psychiatry Times*. [online]. [Retrieved July 20, 2015]. Available from http://www.psychiatrictimes.com/cultural-psychiatry/harnessing-social-media-and-mobile-apps-mental-health/page/0/2.

Reamer, F. (2011). Eye on ethics: Developing a social media ethics policy. *Social Work Today*. [online]. [Retrieved on April 25, 2015]. Available from http://www.socialworktoday.com/news/eoe_070111.shtml.

Robb, M. (2011). Pause before posting: Using social media responsibly. *Social Work Today*, *6*(36): 1–4. [online]. [Retrieved on April 25, 2015]. Available from http://www.socialworktoday.com/archive/020911p8.shtml.

Sierra, L. (2015). New app would monitor mental health through "selfie" videos, social media: Newscenter. *University of Rochester*. [online]. [Retrieved on March 30, 2015]. Available from http://www.rochester.edu/newscenter/mental-health-monitoring-through-selfie-videos-and-social-media-tracking-87632/.

Singer, N. (2014). Risks in using social media to spot signs of mental illness. *The New York Times*, p. B1. [online]. [Retrieved July 20, 2015]. Available from http://www.nytimes.com/2014/12/27/technology/risks-in-using-social-posts-to-spot-signs-of-distress.html?_r=0.

Thompson, A. (2008). Counselor's right to privacy: Potential boundary crossings through membership in online communities. *Counseling Today*, *51*(2): 44–45.

Thompson, A. (2010). Using social networks and implications for the mental health profession. *The Use of Technology in Mental Health [applications, ethics, and practice]*, 39–46.

Toseeb, U. & Inkster, B. (2015). Online social networking sites and mental health research. *Frontiers in PSYCHIATRY*, *6*(36): 1–4. [online]. [Retrieved on April 1, 2015]. Available from http://journal.frontiersin.org/article/10.3389/fpsyt.2015.00036/full.

University of Wisconsin-Madison School of Social Work. (2013). Social media considerations for social-work students. *University of Wisconsin – Madison*. [online]. [Retrieved on April 25, 2015]. Available from http://socwork.wisc.edu/using-social-media-social-work-student.

Whiteman, H. (2014). Social media: How does it really affect our mental health and well-being? *Medical News Today*. [online]. [Retrieved on March 30, 2015]. Available from http://www.medicalnewstoday.com/articles/275361.php.

Williams, R. (2012). Facing the facebook

ethics. *ASCA schoolcounselor.* [online]. [Retrieved on March 30, 2015]. Available from https://www.schoolcounselor.org/magazine/blogs/november-december-2009/facing-the-facebook-ethics.

Zur, O., & Zur, A (2011). The facebook dilemma: To accept or not to accept? Responding to a clients' "friend requests" on psychotherapists' social networking sites. *Independent Practitioner, 31*(1): 12–17. [online]. [Retrieved on July 20, 2015]. Available from http://www.zurinstitute.com/face booktherapy.pdf.

Chapter 5

USING FORUMS TO ENHANCE CLIENT PEER SUPPORT

Meyran Boniel-Nissim

INTRODUCTION

Support groups operated through the Internet have existed since the middle of the 1990s, exploiting modern technology in continuation of traditional, face-to-face support groups (aka self-help or mutual-aid groups), which have been employed since the 1930s. The Internet has provided a special platform for operating these groups.

Initially online support groups were constructed through e-mail lists and relatively primitive server-based software that created newsgroup sites. Technological developments, as well as users' experiences and desires, contributed to more advanced web-based platforms that created highly dynamic support communities characterized by advanced and rich design. The result is that today hundreds of thousands of online support groups are active worldwide, trying to meet users' expectations and provide some relief to human difficulties.

DEFINITION AND DESCRIPTION OF ONLINE SUPPORT GROUPS

An online support group connects people who share a common problem, difficulty or area of distress. Online support groups known for their convenience; anonymity and privacy; textuality; richness enhanced by the option of use external links, pictures, movies, and sound; availability almost anywhere, anytime; relative inexpensiveness or even free; and broad social acceptability. Moreover, the Internet more readily enables the matching of group participants who possess similar needs. For many, this is apparently a unique opportunity to communicate and associate with people who share their concerns.

There are various types of online infrastructure that enable group communication. *Synchronized communication* allows all online participants to take part in the communication at the same time through chat rooms. Those groups offer the advantages of immediacy and spontaneity of interactions. Many Internet-based chat support groups are time limited and managed by a professional facilitator (Binford-Hopf et al., 2013).

In many ways, synchronized communication is similar to face-to-face communication in terms of instantaneous response, because the responses of other participants are immediately presented in the chat window and associated with the name of the participant who posted them. This form of online communication, which enhances spontaneity and authenticity, brings the obstacle that participants are dependent on the presence of other group members in the chat room at a given time. Group sessions need, of course, to be scheduled in advance. In addition, the size of a synchronous group must be taken into consideration: it is difficult to hold a chat discussion with more than a few participants because of the lack of visibility and nonverbal communication cues. In contrast, a forum structured around a-synchronous postings from members who contribute at any time may – in principle – successfully serve a very large group of participants (Hsiung, 2000, 2007). The immediacy of synchronized communication makes it necessary for participants to be more aware of their wording, the length of their writing, their response time and the need to refer and direct comments to a relevant participant.

Many of the difficulties presented by synchronized communication are easily resolved through *asynchronous communication*. Asynchronous communication provides a vehicle for participants to communicate without the necessity of simultaneous participation. Usually, online support groups are asynchronous, operated through an Internet forum ("bulletin board") platform, which provides an anonymous, text-based and generally free virtual social environment. In this environment – typically run by means of server-based software (meaning that participants access a website by using a regular Internet browser) – people share information and personal experiences, communicate with one another and form interpersonal interactions with the purpose of obtaining emotional relief, on the one hand, and supporting others in need, on the other.

Some forums are chronologically reversed, so that the most recent main message is presented first. A main message heads a thread of messages in which participants interact with one another. A participant may post a message at any time and of any length. The delay in asynchronous communication allows messages to be edited with care before they are submitted, if the person so chooses. Use of attachments and links is often possible too. Forums are often open to anyone and their history can usually be browsed freely.

In addition to the active members of the group, passive, reading-only participants (called lurkers) may read and stay informed about developments within the group. While lurkers do not actively take part, they frequently experience a commitment to the group and obtain support from it (Nonnecke & Preece, 2002). A study comparing participants who post messages (posters) to participants who only read messages (lurkers) showed that posters scored significantly higher in the degree of interactional empowerment than lurkers. Thus, posters strengthened interpersonal relationships and awareness of mutual support and community as a basis for empowerment, and therefore showed greater impact on their external social structures. However, no difference was found in terms of interpersonal empowerment (meaning the cognitive state that can be grasped with competences, control, and self-efficacy) (Petrovčič & Petric, 2014).

A smaller number of asynchronous support groups take place through an e-mail list – which is another way of creating asynchronous group communication online. Although forum-based groups are more advantageous from the perspective of both technology and usability, some people prefer joining an e-mail-based group because it saves the necessity of accessing a website in order to read messages. While a forum is operated through a website and is usually open to anyone, an email list offers more private communication, since only members of the list can receive or send messages.

In any of these versions of online support groups, online participants can often have the option of using nicknames in order to retain full privacy and secrecy unless they choose to identify themselves or disclose personal information. The degree and type of participation in a group is usually a matter of choice, the participants themselves deciding how often to participate, how deep their writing is to be and to what degree to support others. However, intimate disclosures are quite normative as is both asking for and providing help and advice to others in the group.

ONLINE SUPPORT GROUPS VS. FACE-TO-FACE SUPPORT GROUP

Two of the special features that distinguish online from offline support groups are the textual nature of online communication and the variety of technical aids for the use of participants. Early theorizing predicted that computer-mediated communication would be impersonal because of its invisibility and anonymous nature and the fact that it is not possible to directly observe nonverbal bodily cues or facial expressions (unless deliberately indicated). However, the huge number of individuals who choose to take part in this type of communication seems to contradict that notion (Tanis, 2007). People adapt their linguistic and textual behaviors in an attempt to overcome limitations created by written-only communication; in this way, communication becomes more personal and tends to resemble face-to-face communication. Some of the tools available to online writers constitute attempts to substitute nonverbal communication, such as highlighting text by color, size, or boldness; use of emoticons; creative use of punctuation marks to create faces and symbols; links to other online materials, integrating pictures and sounds with text; and the use of personal signatures. These tools help get the message across in a richer way and with greater accuracy. Additionally, written communication facilitates the creative use of written language through the employment and integration of lingual creative applications, such

as rhymes, metaphors, poems and original (invented) terms (e.g., Provine et al., 2007).

DISTINCTION BETWEEN GROUP THERAPY AND SUPPORT GROUPS

There is much confusion between group therapy and support groups, whether online or offline. This misunderstanding has developed apparently because these two forms of providing psychological help to people in need have certain common denominators. However, it is important to emphasize that despite several similarities, they are two different entities, have different goals and expose clients to different procedures and protocols.

Four of their major distinctions are as follows: first, an online support group is fundamentally based on mutual-help among its participants, not on facilitated or professionally led intervention (by one or another psychotherapeutic approach). Second, an online support group is neither necessarily managed nor supervised by a trained professional. Third, the procedures and policies of many online support groups do not follow necessarily the standards of professionalism and ethics or the legal obligations. Fourth, unlike therapy groups, most online support groups are open to anyone and no prescreening is conducted; similarly, members may be able to leave and return at will.

MOTIVATIONS TO PARTICIPATE IN ONLINE SUPPORT GROUPS

Online support groups allow people in need to receive help in numerous areas of distress: physical medical conditions, such as a certain disease or syndromes (e.g., diabetes, breast cancer, tinnitus, epilepsy); emotional difficulties (related to various issues, such as bereavement, divorce, being fired, school failure, sexual assault); coping difficulties (e.g., smoking cessation, diet and weight loss, immigration); living with disabilities (e.g., hearing impairment, dwarfism, limb amputation); and relatives of people with certain difficulties (e.g., parents of children with autism, children of Alzheimer patients).

Still we know that not all in need engage in a support group. For example, most women using online support groups for pregnancy loss are white, while African-American women seem to be underrepresented despite being at higher risk for stillbirth. Moreover, most of the participants are well educated, even though pregnancy loss in well-educated women is relatively low (Gold et al., 2012). Many women with breast cancer do not participate in online cancer support groups. A comparison between women with breast cancer who use support groups and nonusers revealed that users were more likely to be Caucasian than African Americans (Hen et al., 2012).

It seems that online support group users make selective use of varied features depending on their needs. People with strong motivation for social interaction make more one-to-one connections with other participants. However, people with strong motivation for information seeking may tend to limit their use to informational discussions in forums (Chung, 2014). Age is also an important factor that influences motivation to participate in the group. Baams et al. (2011) investigated same sex attraction support groups, in order to reveal whether younger and older participants differ in their motivation to enter the group and remain in it. Results showed that younger compared to older participants were more motivated to receive online social support, whereas older participants were more likely to use the group for sexual purposes. Another research study on a forum for patients with systemic lupus erythematosus also showed varying purposes for engaging in the group, such as

starting a new relationship, seeking information, receiving emotional support and giving a contribution (Mazzoni & Cicognani, 2014).

Chung (2013) tried to identify potential factors leading to preferences for online support groups rather than face-to-face groups. An online survey on a sample of online support group users revealed that for those who lack satisfactory support from offline social contacts and those who develop close relationships online, online support can become an alternative source of support.

FACILITATION OF ONLINE SUPPORT GROUPS

There is no consensus or standard that directs the management and supervision of online support groups. Some groups are conducted with no officially designated administrator; in others, the administrator is one of the members, chosen either by the group or by its owner (e.g., the portal's administration, a professional association, etc.) to oversee and supervise proceedings so that group procedures are successfully maintained. A research study on online cancer support groups by Lieberman (2008) clearly pointed to the advantages of professional facilitation as superior to peer facilitation when judged by several criteria.

Coulson and Shaw (2013) investigated the benefits and challenges for facilitators. In a qualitative study design with open-ended questions, 33 facilitators shared their experiences. Thematic analysis identified three themes: emergence, empowerment and nurturing. Emergence revealed the reasons for setting up an online support group (e.g., no existing forum catered for people with a particular condition, to help educate people living with rare conditions, sharing experiences etc); A sense of empowerment resulted from their gratitude for being able to give something back and offer others the benefit of their experience as well as from becoming an expert in their own condition and offering support to others: an opportunity for moderators to share their received wisdom. Nurturing was evident in the abilities required of the facilitators to set up the forum initially and mange it (e.g., technical abilities, personal boundaries, safe space for their members).

Indeed, facilitators' responsibilities have multiple aspects. First and foremost, they should promote cohesiveness, as this is one of the most important and influential factors at work in a group (Yalom & Leszcz, 2005). It is a mission, however, that is particularly complex to achieve in an online group, which is characterized by physical distance and sometimes also by anonymity and a sense of personal invisibility. A second important role played by facilitators is to maintain the rules and practices of the group procedure in regard to ethics, such as preventing unwanted exposure or 'outing,' use of harsh language and 'flaming,' deleting problematic or misleading messages, negotiating with and solving the problems of frustrated or embittered members, making attempts to prevent impersonation and 'phishing,' and so on. Facilitators may take such actions openly or, sometimes, secretly in back communication channels. A third function is to make sure that published information is well-founded and based on credible sources and to prevent it from misleading and misguiding people in need and distress. Obviously, in a busy forum with lots of messages posted every day, group facilitators cannot check every piece of information and advice provided, but they should take steps to guide participants and so minimize the effect of any problematic and harmful information that is published and should take action immediately if misleading or false information is brought to their attention. An additional role of the group facilitator entails stimulating discussions related to the group's common topics, raising intriguing questions and posting materials of interest. Another function is to ensure that the group atmosphere is as positive, supportive, and constructive as possible. This may be done by both modeling appropriate messages and responses and by providing feedback to members (usually through private communication) (Till, 2003).

As the multiple and responsible role of a group facilitator can easily become highly time and energy consuming, the different tasks involved could be divided among several people who share the mission and have suitable skills and experience – preferably backed up with training whenever applicable. Moreover, one of the strengths of online groups is the continuous communication between the members of the group and leadership characteristics can come from participants other than the facilitator. Kodatt et al. (2014) investigated the leadership qualities in an online support group by analyzing posts from a support group for men with HIV. Results showed that only 10% of the posts reflected leadership types. However, the most common leadership style was mentoring and providing feedback, followed by providing encouragement, offering inspirational motivation, intellectual stimulation and through idealized influence.

PSYCHOLOGICAL PROCESSES IN ONLINE SUPPORT GROUPS

Being part of a group enables participants to go through a process in which they can learn about themselves and about how others see them and receive an opportunity to express themselves authentically. Yalom and Leszcz's (2005) conception regarding therapeutic forces that operate in groups and facilitate change is highly relevant here. These forces include instilling hope, inducing a sense of universality, imparting information and knowledge, offering advice and guidance, developing altruistic attitudes, encouraging interpersonal learning and providing a convenient space for catharsis.

Qualitative and quantitative research on online support groups shows that these forces operate in virtual groups just as they do in face-to-face groups. However, additional processes characterize online support groups. Because communication takes place in a virtual arena, as noted above, some forums allow one to participate while preserving anonymity and invisibility. This unique situation operates as an accelerator of disinhibition and consequent self-exposure. These processes go some way to explain why new members feel comfortable soon after joining the group in sharing personal experiences and relatively quickly develop feelings of intimacy in relationships with other group members. Disinhibition, furthermore, induces dynamic progress in the group by encouraging sharing, self-expression and introspection. It should be noted, at the same time, though, that disinhibition can also be a source of damage by promoting flaming, acting out and judgmental attitudes (Suler, 2004; Barak, Boniel-Nissim, & Suler, 2008; Tanis, 2007).

Communicating through writing, in contrast to speech, leads to significant cognitive and emotional self-processes. For example, writing has been found to contribute to the process of thought arrangement and subsequent emotional relief (Pennebaker & Seagal, 1999). Writing is a way for a person to express and share thoughts, emotions and experiences that may not be otherwise expressed. In addition to mere ventilation, the writer is focused on herself or himself while writing, allowing for an examination and re-examination of thoughts for clarification, explanation and eventually – unlike in face-to-face interactions – the choice of whether to transmit the text to the group. This reflective process contributes to self-awareness, awareness of others and a developing sense of control, all in a safer place than the participants' offline environment (Barak, Boniel-Nissim, & Suler,

2008; Barak, Boneh, & Dolev-Cohen, 2010; Hoybye et al., 2005).

As noted above, evidence that has accumulated shows that involvement in an online support group empowers participants, in addition to providing emotional relief (as opposed to healing users). Several specific processes have been identified as responsible for creating a sense of personal empowerment: the exchange of relevant information and knowledge, undergoing the psychological impact of writing, providing and receiving emotional support, accepting social recognition, sharing personal experiences, developing interpersonal relationships, helping others in need, being assisted in making decisions and taking consequent action and experiencing amusement and fun. These processes produce specific outcomes: clients become better informed, more confident, better accepting of their condition, more optimistic, more active, and have generally improved well-being (Barak et al., 2008; van UdenKraan et al., 2008).

POSITIVE AND NEGATIVE ASPECTS ON ONLINE SUPPORT GROUPS

Research shows consistent advantages of participating in an online support group. Mostly the fact that specific groups with special conditions can meet together virtually in order to share and support each other (e.g., Attard, & Coulson, 2012; Aho, Paavilainen, & Kaunonen, 2012; Mo & Coulson, 2012; Becker, 2013; Sherman & Greenfield, 2013).

Positive aspects of online support groups includes emotional support (e.g., sharing oppressive feelings, supporting well-being, sympathy), sharing experiences, informational support (e.g. referring to sources of help, information sharing), empathy and understanding, friendship formation, encouragement, validation, resilience and positive thinking (Attard & Coulson, 2012; Aho, Paavilainen,

& Kaunonen, 2012; Becker, 2013).

As a result of these positive aspects of online support groups, empowering processes can take place (Barak, Boniel-Nissim, & Suler, 2008). Aardoom et al. (2014) found when studying an online support community for eating disorders that exchanging information, finding recognition and sharing experiences were the empowering processes most often reported by participants. The most pronounced and empowering outcome of these things was feeling better informed, a finding confirmed by Bartlett and Coulson (2011) in their study of chronic illness online support groups. Mo and Coulson (2012) examined an online support group for people living with HIV/AIDS, finding that greater use of online support groups was associated with more frequent occurrence of empowering processes including receiving useful information but also from social support, finding positive meaning and helping others.

Limitations and negative aspects of online support groups relate mostly to their virtual nature. For example, messages may sometimes be answered only after a significant time lag – and in all asynchronous forms of communication at least some lag will be present. Some members of online support groups find that the public nature of online support groups leads them to share limited personal information, despite others demonstrating the marked disinhibition noted above. Lack of nonverbal information can sometimes cause members to misunderstand the meaning of messages and make flaming or hostile comments. Moreover, because of the dynamic nature of forums, members may leave the group without any warning. The potential diversity of group membership can be seen as a benefit, but may also act as a disadvantage when it leads to disagreements and rejection. For some members, online support might not be enough as they still feel alone in their offline environment. Moreover, very frequent visits to the group can

sometimes be seen as a form of social avoidance (Aiken & Waller, 2000; Attard & Coulson, 2012; Bartlett & Coulson, 2011; Lawlor & Kirakowski, 2014; Sherman & Greenfield, 2013).

RESEARCH ON ONLINE SUPPORT GROUPS

Much research has been conducted on processes, behaviors, communication characteristics, personal expressions, emotional experiences and other process-related variables that occur in the dynamics of online support groups. Some research has focused on psychological factors that take place in online group processes (e.g., universality) and found that, indeed, the act of identifying and comparing oneself with similarly distressed people contributes to emotional relief (e.g., Attard & Coulson, 2012; Aho, Paavilainen, & Kaunonen, 2012; Mo & Coulson, 2012) and empowerment (van Uden-Kraan et al., 2008; Aardoom et al., 2014; Bartlett & Coulson, 2011; Mo & Coulson, 2012). Generally, this research shows that online support groups are as dynamic, lively and engaging as offline support (and therapy) groups.

Outcome research attempts to examine the impact of interventions; that is, the effects and changes that intervention procedures have caused in participants. However, whereas the goal of therapy in therapeutic interventions is generally known and clear, the objective of support groups is much less clear, as their purpose often seems to be more general than to foster specific therapeutic change. Moreover, as indicated by Barak et al. (2008), in contrast to psychotherapy, which is usually aimed at well-defined, pre-planned changes relating to an area of distress, support groups strive to improve general feelings relating to well-being and empowerment.

As a result, studies and literature reviews that refer to therapeutic changes caused by participation in online support groups have usually shown little evidence of actual, distress-specific improvement (e.g., Horgan, McCarthy, & Sweeney, 2013). However, publications report much empirical evidence from interviews and questionnaires, and also from observations of actual support group writings, and support the notion that participants can gain generally positive feelings directly related to their experiences in the group. These elevated feelings pertain to increased self-confidence and a sense of independence and decreased anxiety, loneliness, and depression – all of which indeed relate to the concept of well-being (e.g., Barak & DolevCohen, 2006; Beaudoin & Tao, 2007; Buchanan & Coulson, 2007; Stewart et al., 2013; Aardoom et al., 2014). The result can be a better ability to make decisions related to one's distress condition, a better knowledge of, or at least acquaintance with, relevant information resources and the promotion of self-assurance in regard to difficulties – in other words, experiences related to the concept of empowerment (Barak, Boniel-Nissim, & Suler, 2008) – even when the goals of therapy, as opposed to the less-precisely defined but still beneficial goals of support groups may not be met.

It seems that these results imply that, for many people, the combination of specific professional therapeutic intervention, on the one hand, and participation in a relevant online support group, on the other, could provide optimal help for their problems (Bartlett & Coulson, 2011; Bender et al., 2013).

These days, support groups have expanded to social networks such as Twitter and Facebook (De la Torre-Diez, Diaz-Pernas, & Anton-Rodriguez, 2012) and through applications developed for smartphones. More research is needed to investigate the potential of support in those communities as they have different characteristics than the traditional online support forum.

CONCLUSION

The advent of online support groups in the 1980s and 1990s has positively changed the mental condition of many people suffering from various types of personal distress. People who experience emotional hardship – caused by, for example, disease, failure, social circumstances and other stressful and painful situations – can now easily find others with whom to share their miseries and to consult, to be helped by and to offer help to. By participating in such virtual groups, not only have many people improved their condition, but they have also gained a sense of personal empowerment that directly contributes to their general well-being.

Thus, online support groups may serve as an important social agent in enhancing quality of life for disadvantaged, marginal, weak and unhealthy populations. Moreover, online support groups may serve as a significant aid to therapists by complementing therapeutic services. Obviously, not all support groups are equally valuable and successful; it takes the leadership of a good moderator, advanced and suitable online technology and design, involved group partners and appropriate participants to yield a constructive online support group (McKenna, 2008). With a thoughtful and well-planned approach, however, these groups may make a great contribution to the well-being of many members of society (Barak et al., 2008; Tanis, 2007).

REFERENCES

Aardoom, J. J., Dingemans, A. E., Boogaard, L. H., & Van Furth, E. F. (2014). Internet and patient empowerment in individuals with symptoms of an eating disorder: A cross-sectional investigation of a pro-recovery focused e-community. *Eating Behaviors, 15,* 350–356.

Aho, A. L., Paavilainen, E., & Kaunonen, M.

(2012). Mothers' experiences of peer support via an Internet discussion forum after the death of a child. *Scandinavian Journal of Caring Sciences, 26,* 417–426.

Aiken, M., & Waller, B. (2000). Flaming among first-time group support system users. *Information and Management, 37*(2), 95–100.

Attard, A., & Coulson, N. S. (2012). A thematic analysis of patient communication in Parkinson's disease online support group discussion forums. *Computers in Human Behavior, 28,* 500–506.

Baams, L., Jonas, K. J., Utz, S., Bos, H. M. W., & van der Vuurst, L. (2011). Internet use and online social support among same sex attracted individuals of different ages. *Computers in Human Behavior, 27,* 1820–1827.

Barak, A., Boniel-Nissim, M., & Suler, J. (2008). Fostering empowerment in online support groups. *Computers in Human Behavior, 24*(5), 1867–1883.

Barak, A., Boneh, O., & Dolev-Cohen, M. (2010). Factors underlying participants' gains in online support groups. In A. Blachnio, A. Przepiorka, & T. Rowiński (Eds.), *Internet in psychological research* (pp. 17–38). Warsaw, Poland: Cardinal Stefan Wyszyński University Press.

Barak, A., & Dolev-Cohen, M. (2006). Does activity level in online support groups for distressed adolescents determine emotional relief? *Counselling and Psychotherapy Research, 6*(3), 186–190.

Bartlett, Y. K., & Coulson, N. S. (2011). An investigation into the empowerment effects of using online support groups and how this affects health professional/patient communication. *Patient Education and Counseling, 83,* 113–119.

Beaudoin, C. E., & Tao, C. (2007). Benefiting from social capital in online support groups: An empirical study of cancer patients. *CyberPsychology and Behavior, 10*(4), 587–590.

Becker, K. L. (2013). Cyberhugs: Creating a voice for chronic pain sufferers through

technology. *CyberPsychology, Behavior, and Social Networking, 16,* 123–126.

Bender, J. L., Katz, J., Ferris, L. E., & Jadad, A. R. (2013). What is the role of online support from the perspective of facilitators of face-to-face support groups? A multi-method study of the use of breast cancer online communities. *Patient Education and Counseling, 93,* 472–479.

Binford-Hopf, R. B., Grange, D. L., Moessner, M., & Bauer, S. (2013). Internet based chat support groups for parents in family-based treatment for adolescent eating disorders: A pilot study. *European Eating Disorders Review, 21,* 215–223.

Buchanan, H., & Coulson, N. S. (2007). Accessing dental anxiety online support groups: An exploratory qualitative study of motives and experiences. *Patient Education and Counseling, 66*(3), 263–369.

Bunde, M., Suls, J., Martin, R., & Barnett, K. (2007). Online hysterectomy support: Characteristics of website experiences. *CyberPsychology and Behavior, 10*(1), 80–85.

Chung, J. E. (2013). Social interaction in online support groups: Preference for online social interaction over offline social interaction. *Computers in Human Behavior, 29,* 1408–1414.

Chung, J. E. (2014). Social networking in online support groups for health: How online social networking benefits patients. *Journal of Health Communication, 19,* 639–659.

Coulson, N. S., & Knibb, R. C. (2007). Coping with food allergy: Exploring the role of the online support group. *CyberPsychology and Behavior, 10*(1), 145–148.

Coulson, N. S., & Shaw, R. L. (2013). Nurturing health-related online support groups: Exploring the experiences of patient moderators. *Computers in Human Behavior, 29,* 1695–1701.

De la Torre-Diez, I., Diaz-Pernas, F. J., & Anton-Rodriguez, M. (2012). A content analysis of chronic diseases social groups on Facebook and Twitter. *Telemedicine and e-*

Health, 18, 404–408.

Han, J. Y., Kim, J.-H., Yoon, H. J., Shim, M., McTavish, F. M., & Gustafson, D. H. (2012). Social and psychological determinants of levels of engagement with an online breast cancer support group: Posters, lurkers, and nonusers. *Journal of Health Communication: International Perspectives, 17,* 356–371.

Horgan, A., McCarthy, G., & Sweeney, J. (2013). An evaluation of an online peer support forum for university students with depressive symptoms. *Archives of Psychiatric Nursing, 27,* 84–89.

Hoybye, M. T., Johansen, C., & Tjornhoj Thomsen, T. (2005). Online interaction: Effects of storytelling in an Internet breast cancer support group. *Psycho-Oncology, 14*(3), 211–220.

Hsiung, R. C. (2000). The best of both worlds: An online self-help group hosted by a mental health professional. *Cyber Psychology and Behavior, 3*(6), 935–950.

Hsiung, R. C. (2007). A suicide in an online mental health support group: Reactions of the group members, administrative responses and recommendations. *Cyber-Psychology and Behavior, 10*(4), 495–500.

Gold, K. J., Boggs, M. E., Mugisha, E., & Palladino, C. L. (2012). Internet message boards for pregnancy loss: Who's on-line and why? *Women's Health Issues, 22,* 67–72.

Kodatt, S. A., Shenk, J. E., Williams, M. L., & Horvath, K. J. (2014). Leadership qualities emerging in an online social support group intervention. *Sexual and Relationship Therapy, 29,* 467–475.

Lawlor, A., & Kirakowski, J. (2014). Online support groups for mental health: A space for challenging self-stigma or a means of social avoidance? *Computers in Human Behavior, 32,* 152–161.

Lieberman, M. A. (2008). Effects of disease and leader type on moderators in online support groups. *Computers in Human Behavior, 24*(5), 2446–2455.

Lieberman, M. A., & Goldstein, B. A. (2006). Not all negative emotions are equal: The role of emotional expression in online support groups for women with breast cancer. *Psycho-Oncology, 15*(2), 160–168.

Mazzoni, D., & Cicognani, E. (2014). Sharing experiences and social support requests in an Internet forum for patients with systemic lupus erythematosus. *Journal of Health Psychology, 19,* 689–696.

McKenna, K. Y. M. (2008). Influences on the nature and functioning of online groups. In A. Barak (Ed.), *Psychological aspects of cyberspace: Theory, research, applications.* Cambridge, UK: Cambridge University Press.

Mo, P. K. H., & Coulson, N. S. (2012). Developing a model for online support group use, empowering processes and psychosocial outcomes for individuals living with HIV/AIDS. *Psychology & Health, 27,* 445–459.

Nonnecke, B., & Preece, J. (2002). Silent participants: Getting to know lurkers better. In C. Lueg & D. Fisher (Eds.), *From Usenet to Co Webs: Interacting with social information spaces.* London: Springer.

Pennebaker, J. W., & Seagal, J. D. (1999). Forming a story: The health benefits of narrative. *Journal of Clinical Psychology, 55*(10), 1243–154.

Petrovčič, A., & Petric, G. (2014). Differences in intrapersonal and interactional empowerment between lurkers and posters in health-related online support communities. *Computers in Human Behavior, 34,* 39–48.

Provine, R. R., Spencer, R. J., & Mandell, D. L. (2007). Emotional expression online: Emoticons punctuate website text messages. *Journal of Language and Social Psychology, 26*(3), 299–307.

Sherman, L. E., & Greenfield, P. M. (2013). Forging friendship, soliciting support: A mixed-method examination of message boards for pregnant teens and teen mothers. *Computers in Human Behavior, 29,* 75–85.

Suler, J. R. (2004). The online disinhibition effect. *CyberPsychology and Behavior, 7*(3), 321–326.

Stewart, M., Letourneau, N., Masuda, J. R., Anderson, S., & McGhan, S. (2013). Impacts of online peer support for children with asthma and allergies: "It just helps you every time you can't breathe well". *Journal of Pediatric Nursing, 28,* 439–452.

Tanis, M. (2007). Online social support groups. In A. Joinson, K. McKenna, T. Postmes, & U. Reips (Eds.), *The Oxford handbook of internet psychology.* Oxford, UK: Oxford University Press.

Till, J. E. (2003). Evaluation of support groups for women with breast cancer: Importance of the navigator role [online]. *Health and Quality of Life Outcomes.* 1(16). [Accessed May 6, 2009]. Available from: http: //www.hqlo.com/content/1/1/16.

van Uden-Kraan, C. F., Drossaert, C. H. C., Taal, E., Shaw, B. R., Seydel, E. R., & van de Laar, M. A. F. J. (2008). Empowering processes and outcomes of participation in online support groups for patients with breast cancer, arthritis, or fibromyalgia. *Qualitative Health Research, 18*(3), 405–417.

Weis, R., Stamm, K., Smith, C., Nilan, M., Clark, F., Weis, J., & Kennedy, K. (2003). Communities of care and caring: The case of MSWatch.com®. *Journal of Health Psychology, 8*(1), 135–148.

Yalom, I., & Leszcz, M. (2005). *The theory and practice of group psychotherapy* (5th ed.). New York: Basic Books.

Chapter 6

USING CELL/MOBILE PHONE SMS TO ENHANCE CLIENT CRISIS AND PEER SUPPORT

Stephen Goss and Joe Ferns

INTRODUCTION

This chapter explores the development and use of SMS (short message service) text messaging systems in counselling and support services with particular attention to the way in which this technology has been applied by Samaritans in the UK. In particular, it will look at the way in which the service was developed, give a brief outline of how the service operates, explore the experience to date and give examples of case material. Samaritans offers 24-hour emotional support services aimed at those in distress including people at risk of suicide. It is perhaps best known for its telephone service, one of the oldest in the world having been founded in 1953. More recently, Samaritans developed email (in 1994) and SMS (in 2007) as additional channels through which their services can be accessed. The number and variety of SMS text message-based services for a variety of mental health concerns, and in a variety of settings, has slowly increased over the years, including as a means of providing follow-up to care to reduce rates of relapse, self-harm, and suicide (e.g., Chen et al., 2010; Berrouiguet et al., 2014) as well as for a variety of other applications (e.g., Spohr et al., 2015) and reviews of the evidence base to date suggest that their use can be effective, at least when well directed and provided by properly trained and prepared personnel (e.g., Buhi et al., 2013; Hall et al., 2015).

Messages restricted to just 160 characters, as is commonly the case with SMS, would appear at first sight to place a major block in the way of creating a freely flowing, in-depth, supportive relationship. Certainly, both participants need to be highly focused, making the most efficient possible use of the space available. However, as with a number of the other technologies described in this book, the very restriction of communication breadth has been found not only to have less effect on the help that can be offered than might be thought, but also to have some distinct advantages. Not least is the perception of anonymity, privacy and ease of contact in both practical and emotional terms for the user but there are also advantages in the level of focus and precision required. Furthermore, it should be noted that there is evidence that even very limited forms of contact through short messages – even postcards, let alone text messaging – can provide a sense of contact which is in itself supportive as well as encouraging clients to continue to (or return to) working with services in other ways (e.g., Carter et al., 2005). While the evidence regarding the impact of post-discharge contact is somewhat mixed (Evans et al., 2005), overall trends indicate positive benefits (Luxton, 2013) and, furthermore, there is evidence to suggest that SMS support can, in some circumstances, provide an alternative to face-to-face interviews with practitioners (Bopp et al., 2010). Supportive text messages can be perceived to have positive effects by service users (Agyapong et al., 2013) but such simple contacts can, however, readily be continued and expanded to make use of SMS text messaging to provide more detailed, extended care and an on-going relationship with practitioners, repeated messaging becoming a form of continuing care in itself.

SMS systems to provide emotional or psychological help, whether for those in crisis or for longer-term difficulties began to be introduced some years ago. Increasing numbers of services now use them, such as What Now?, a youth-oriented service in the North of England and numerous others are planned, such as that for the Campaign Against Living Miserably (CALM), who focus on suicide prevention and facilitating ease of access to mental health support for young men, a population who are generally underrepresented in mental health support services while disproportionately vulnerable to suicide.

SMS text messaging is also particularly relevant to the needs of services in countries with emerging economies (Chipchase, 2007) where the infrastructure of mental health support may be less well developed. Mobile phones are rapidly becoming ubiquitous, or nearly so, in many such countries (e.g., ITU, 2009; Textually.org, 2009) the fastest growing mobile phone market in the world being Africa (Arnquist, 2009). A number of projects have demonstrated the feasibility of reaching populations hitherto very poorly served by mental health professionals (e.g., Gadebe, 2006) and while further evaluative research is still required, the possibilities opened up – particularly for harder to reach and rural populations or those in developing countries – are highly encouraging (Déglise, 2012).

In the case of Samaritans, 201 branches are staffed by around 15,500 volunteers in the UK. Samaritans has a federal structure, with each branch operating with a fair degree of independence and autonomy. Between them, they handle over 2.8 million contacts each year that involve meaningful dialogue. Many more contacts are very brief (e.g., a caller hanging up as soon as the call is answered) or comprise testing or "prank" calls as people "dip their toe into the water" and use such initial contacts as a way of finding out what the service is like. This is of particular relevance to contact methods like SMS or email, as Samaritans service users have indicated that they have used them as a means of discovering the kind of response they will get, before building up courage to speak to a practitioner directly, live and on a one-to-one basis. Thus, it could be argued that at least some text-based services can operate as a gateway to accessing other forms of helping and may be particularly important for those who would not otherwise turn to helping services at all.

It is interesting to note that many of the same comments that the organization has received regarding its SMS and email services were similar to those received when Samaritans was first established well over half a century ago, when the concept of offering support services by telephone was reacted to with skepticism and, in some quarters, outright resistance.

ADVANTAGES OF SMS

"Distraction"

Sometimes, especially when people are in crisis, it is helpful to have something to do not least as a way of calming immediate emotional turmoil but also to allow increased opportunity for reflection and considered expression. In comparison with making a telephone call, text messaging is a more physically and mentally involving activity that has greater capacity to take the person out of their current state, temporarily, by providing a task that must itself be concentrated upon through the need carefully to key in the correct characters and so on. Manipulating the technology thus becomes a kind of distraction technique in itself, often helpful for those at risk.

Confidentiality

It is arguable that text messaging is a more confidential means of contacting support services than most other means. Consider the example of children or young people who may not be able to use a phone with privacy and may also be unable to access their own computer for email use without parental supervision. It is very difficult to see what text message someone else is sending, unless looking directly over their shoulder and, if deleted after sending, communications can remain completely undetectable unless a third party directly intercepts the message or is paying the bill and obtains access to the

numbers contacted. Even then, the content of messages is usually unavailable.

HOW SAMARITANS' SMS SERVICE WAS DEVELOPED

The Samaritans SMS service was developed in a detailed, carefully planned way on the principle that any emotional support, especially for those who may be in crisis, should be done well or not undertaken at all. The care with which this process was undertaken stands as an exemplar of the approach to introducing technologically mediated mental health support services and is one that could be readily and helpfully emulated by practitioners seeking to introduce any of the technologies discussed in this volume. Its thoroughness serves users far better in the long run than rushing to introduce technologies. A service once offered that then has to be withdrawn may have potentially disastrous results for those who could then find themselves suddenly cut off.

Table 6.1 outlines the process undertaken by Samaritans to introduce their SMS service in a safe, carefully planned way.

Table 6.1
DEVELOPMENT PROCESS OF SAMARITANS' SMS SERVICE IN THE UK

Phase 1	Desk research: Consultation with focus groups (aged 13–25 years). Consultation with other service providers.
Phase 2	Internal role plays and consultation with volunteers. Development of basic training systems. Basic software development.
Phase 3	Live trials at music festivals to provide contained, time limited community to test take up rates, utility, systems and training needs.
Phase 4	Limited live 3 month trial by 10 branches.
Phase 5	6 month pilot to test ability to offer 24/7 emotional support by SMS and to test systems and demand levels.
Phase 6	Final troubleshooting phase to address problems of providing an integrated 24/7 SMS service.
Phase 7	Development of an accreditation system whereby branches are accredited to run the SMS service. Gradual roll out of service across Samaritans branches.

Phase One: Desk Research

It is important not to duplicate the work of others in mental health service provision, so that services do not overlap and to ensure that the learning afforded through their development and implementation is not lost. A great deal of effort was put into an initial "desk research" phase, ensuring that the systems and service design were based on a full understanding and awareness of the potential of this method of working, its pitfalls, the current state of the best technological solutions available and the experiences, both published and unpublished, of those who already used SMS communication as part of any kind of support mechanisms. This phase also involved detailed consultation with service users themselves through a series of focus groups, especially with 13–25-year-olds, the primary anticipated target audience.

Phase Two: "It's a Lot Easier Than We Thought It Was"

The second phase involved development of response protocols, methods, and training in collaboration with a sample of the practitioners who would be providing the service. Initial concern regarding the ability to provide adequate support within 160 characters was steadily replaced by recognition that it was indeed possible to create meaningful, empathic, and helpful responses through text messaging. Examples of training activities included deliberate circumvention of the technology itself to enable clearer focus on the detail of the process of responding in such short communications by using role-play simulations of contacts in which volunteers playing both client and practitioner roles used paper with 160 boxes in which to write each character by hand. By removing the technology itself, replacing it with the most familiar means of written communication, it was possible to obtain very direct feedback

on the ability to express the necessary content in the space available. Participants reported that it was much more possible to do so and to do it well than they had expected prior to such exercises, a typical response being "it's a lot easier than we thought it was going to be."

Another example of the learning gathered through Samaritans' experience of introducing their SMS service has been that while practitioners were keen to be given guidance on how to use "text speak" (abbreviations, emoticons, and so on), service users themselves indicated that they strongly preferred a "plain English" approach as it appeared to show more respect and, perhaps, represented the genuine voice of the practitioner more accurately. While some contractions or simple abbreviations (e.g., "2" for "too" or "4" for "for") were fine, it was found to be important to avoid these when expressing feelings and especially strong feelings.

Phase Three: Limited Initial Trials in Contained, Temporary Community Setting

The next phase of development was to offer the SMS service at a small number of events with the service being carefully promoted to ensure that it was understood to be only for that time and place. Music festivals were deemed to be ideal for this purpose not only because they attracted a relatively young section of society, anticipated to be the main users of SMS support services, but also because they created a community of sufficient size to create a significant level of demand while being small enough to prevent the new service being overwhelmed. The service would also not be expected to continue after the end of the event providing containment of the public trial, so potential service users would not be left without a means of support on which they might have expected to rely.

Phase Four: Limited Three-month Trial at Selection Locations

Ten branches of Samaritans were then selected to offer the SMS service on a trial basis for a period of three months. This meant that the service could be tested in a more typical public setting than that of music festivals but on a scale at which take-up rates would not be overwhelming and whereby any difficulties or harm caused, should there be any, would be limited. It also provided a further opportunity for analysis of the experience and for another iterative stage of development for the service. A number of community groups who provided support to young people in crisis, including those who self-harm, were asked to disseminate publicity material about the SMS service. Data was collected and the experience reviewed before progressing to the next phase.

Phase Five: Full Six-month Pilot Phase

At this stage, Samaritans was approaching the "point of no return" with the service and made the decision to commit to adding SMS to its suite of services. Phase five involved a further trial on a national basis for an initial period of six months. Usage levels were monitored and data was collected regarding the nature of the service with special attention being paid to difficulties that were encountered. Formal systems of training, supervision, and caller care were developed in order to facilitate the eventual roll-out.

Phase Six: Final Troubleshooting

Some systems were changed and then tested to ensure that any issues were identified before bringing additional branches into the service.

Phase Seven: Roll Out of the New SMS Service

The SMS service formally moved out of development and into implementation. An accreditation system was put in place to ensure that branches who wished to begin delivering the SMS service were sufficiently robust and received the support they needed.

OUTLINE OF THE SMS SYSTEM USED

The Samaritans' SMS system can be outlined very simply (see Figure 6.1). A caller sends a text. This goes to a SIM Host – a

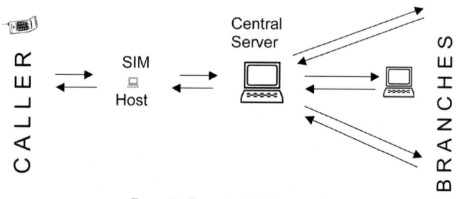

Figure 6.1. Samaritans' SMS system.

computer that acts as a "hub" to pass on the message. This is then translated into an email that is sent to the organization's central server in encrypted form. At that point the telephone number is stripped out as a further protection of privacy.

When volunteers at Samaritans' branches are ready to answer the next contact, they "pull" the next SMS message from the server. This reliance on "pull," rather than "push," technology is based on the same system Samaritans uses to deal with emails. It has the advantage of managing the rate at which volunteers deal with contacts; ensuring that they are not overwhelmed and that each message receives proper consideration. However, one operational disadvantage is that it results in "pull" services feeling less urgent than the telephone (a "push" service). During the early stages of the SMS development project, when SMS accredited branches were scarce, there were some issues in persuading volunteers in these branches to prioritize SMS contacts above phone contacts (since phone contacts would ultimately trip on to another branch and be answered).

Individual service users can be "assigned" to a branch, ensuring that they receive consistent responses from within the same group. Each branch of the organization thus has a list of existing service users to whom on-going support is provided and new contacts to add to that list. A very similar system is used for dealing with emails received by the organization. First developed in 1994, it has required very few changes since its inception.

Initial incoming SMS messages are responded to within 60 minutes with subsequent messages being responded to much faster. This is facilitated in part by the system automatically identifying where an on-going conversation is taking place and putting responses from service users to volunteers' texts at the front of the queue. Thus, a service user demonstrating a desire to have continuing contact is able to receive it. For comparison, emails received by the organization are responded to within 24 hours as a maximum, with a typical response time usually being around 12 to 13 hours. Smaller scale services with lower-level demand often manage to respond even faster than this.

Since the initial trialing of the SMS service began in April 2006 (going fully operational around a year later), 51 branches now offer the SMS service and they have responded to over 413,000 messages from around 7,600 unique mobile numbers in the 36-month period to April, 2009. Volume of demand is also reported to be continuing to rise with a further 25 percent increase in volume predicted in the rest of 2009.

This level of demand is all the more telling given that it has been achieved without the SMS service ever having been advertised nationally since the initial pilot, other than being noted on Samaritan's website. The influence of Web 2.0 style viral transmission of the number to use and knowledge of the existence of the service itself, is clearly evident in the information sharing among peer groups, forums, discussion lists and so on. As branches are accredited, some limited local publicity is undertaken with schools and colleges, but this is carefully controlled so as not to overwhelm capacity.

The greatest levels of demand have been consistently found to be highest at around lunchtime, when schools finish, and then peaking dramatically at around 9 pm to 10 pm, an important factor when planning service responsiveness. This is in contrast to usage of the telephone service which peaks between 10 pm and 2 am.

It has been a noticeable trend in this service that the average number of text messages per user has been steadily increasing over time. This suggests that the service is developing enduring contacts with the number of exchanges between caller and practitioner averaging around 60 messages. These figures underline that despite the restricted number of characters per message, seen as a whole series they can and do develop into something much deeper than a simple request for information. This is evidence contrary to the impression that text messaging is an inadequate environment in which to support relational helping.

CASE EXAMPLES

The following are examples of the opening sequence of incoming and outgoing SMS messages from Samaritans' service. All have been thoroughly anonymised and are reproduced here with permission. Note that incoming messages can exceed the 160 character limit because some mobile phones allow this functionality; however, outgoing messages remain within the standard limit.

Case 1: A Young Woman Sends a Text, Early One Thursday Evening

Caller: My friend is suicidal.

Jo: I'm sorry to hear that. How are you feeling about it? Has she or he spoken to Samaritans?

Caller: No, she doesn't really want to talk to anyone it's only me and another friend that no she has been cutting herself and thinking about pills.

Jo: How are you feeling about that?

Caller: Pretty shitty, I don't know what to do. She was meant to be going to uni but dropped out 'cause she missed home. She didn't say anything about why she is like this.

Jo: That's a lot for you to cope with – has she tried to kill herself?

Caller: She cuts herself and has thought about overdosing but didn't . . . does my number get stored?

Jo: No, don't worry – I can't see your number and this is completely confidential to Samaritans. This is a safe space for you to talk about it if you want to.

Caller: What's your name? Sorry I like to know who I am talking to. Do you know if she can go on medication?

Jo: You can call me Jo. I don't know whether she can go on medication – that's not something we can help with – has she spoken to you about medical help?

Caller: Okay . . . can you see my texts from the past?

Jo: Yes, we can read your previous messages. How are you feeling tonight?

Caller: I suppose I'm okay . . . I don't mean to sound selfish but all of this has made my relationship with my boyfriend complicated.

Jo: Would you like to tell us more about how things are with your boyfriend?

Caller: Well, my mate is suicidal and I have been trying to help which means spending most my time with her and not him.

This case continued the exchange and included the service user obtaining help with her relationship with her boyfriend as well as with her suicidal friend.

Case 2: A School Age Caller Sends a Text at 4:20 PM on Monday Afternoon

Caller: I cannot find enough time for homework.

Jo: Hi . . . not enough time for homework . . . Is this a problem for you? How are you feeling today?

Caller: I'm not too good. Friends ignoring me. Teacher sendin' way too much homework. I don't have a lot of time to do it.

Jo: That can't be easy for you – I wonder how long has it been like that–do you feel able to tell me a little more about how you are feeling right now?

Caller: It has been goin' on since I started high school. It makes me feel rejected.

Jo: You seem to have had a tough time since you started at this school. Do you know the reason why?

Caller: I went to a different school, then the rest of my close friends. They can't even help with homework.

Jo: I understand you miss your friends and this makes you feel bad. Have you ever felt suicidal?

Caller: Yes I have felt suicidal.

Jo: Are you feeling suicidal now?

Caller: Not really. It only happens when I'm alone in the house.

Jo: Are you alone in the house often? If so, is there a reason you are alone often?

Caller: My mum and dad work a lot so I go home alone 'cause I am an only child.

Jo: Do your mum and dad know how you feel? Is it easy to talk to them about the things that matter to you?

Caller: It is not easy to talk to them 'cause they'll ignore me when somethin' better comes up.

Jo: Who can you talk to when you feel lonely?

Caller: No one.

Jo: No? Then I hope you will find this a safe and confidential space where you can share your most difficult feeling. Does it help to text?

This case continued into a much longer conversation. Note the more intense use of "texting language" with this younger person.

SERVICE USER PROFILE

It is a generality that most mental health services find that their clientele is disproportionately composed of women. Atypically, however, just over half of the callers to Samaritans' telephone service are male. While men are more likely than women to own a mobile or smart phone, particularly in poorer countries, not only is this set to change in the coming years (GSM Association, 2014), it is already quite wrong to think that SMS text messaging is particularly suitable for men. This is a common – but sexist – assumption given that women actually make greater use of SMS messaging (e.g., Balakrishnan, 2009; Geser, 2006; Proitz, 2004). Men and women do seem to make *different* use of text messaging (e.g., Potts, 2004; Rafi, 2009; Tossel, 2012), which should be born in mind by service providers. Furthermore, SMS text messaging also brings the clear benefit of being able to present a means of access to young people which is attractive and accessible (e.g., Ling, 1999; Kaseniemi & Rautiainen, 2002, Chandra, 2014).

In practice, Samaritans' SMS service has found that, as expected, the largest group have indeed been aged under 24 (67%). Eight percent were aged 25–34 with the same proportion aged 35–44 and only 9 percent over 45 (the remaining 8% representing missing data). This is a much younger age group than use the telephone support service.

In general, the main reasons for contacting the SMS service are similar to those across other Samaritans services. Among the SMS service users the main variation has been a greater proportion of issues that would be expected to arise among this younger audience with more emphasis on peer group pressures, bullying, and so on.

However, Samaritans has noted that contacts via any text-based means appear to come from a higher risk group than those who access the service by telephone, with a higher proportion being actively suicidal rather than simply distressed. This may be because it is easier to be open by email (the disinhibition effect, cf Suler, 2004) or that the population is actually different or, to some extent, that those who make "testing" or abusive calls to the helpline have not yet begun to do so by email or text message. In the SMS service, the severity of contacts and proportion of service users in crisis (e.g., the likelihood of the service user being actively suicidal) is *even* greater than with email. This is possibly due to the SMS number having been passed on through crisis services rather than being to do with the nature of SMS use in itself, but neither possibility can be ruled out at the time of writing (December, 2015). Certainly, this evidence is also contrary to the opinion that SMS is not appropriate for those with severe or acute needs.

IMPACT

Of those who contacted the service, 75 percent felt that doing so helped make a decision not to self-harm. 66 percent felt that Samaritans had helped them make a decision not to end their life, at least on that occasion. Feedback from service users has also included comments such as:

- "The text service is great, it helped me build up the confidence inside of me to phone up and speak to someone."
- "It's made me delay self-harming as I know a response is on its way."
- "The text service has been my savior. Sometimes a feel that if I hadn't contacted the Samaritans I may have seriously harmed/killed myself."
- "I think the text service is really good because I have phoned Samaritans before and ended up hanging up because I didn't have the courage to speak aloud."
- "I think it is a great idea to be able to text and not necessarily having to speak to someone."

While this is not the "hard," randomized controlled trial evidence that would accurately demonstrate the full impact of this kind of service, comments that demonstrate that it

has saved or extended a person's life by averting or delaying serious harm testify to its value in ways that are rarely achieved by composite statistics or changes in psychometric scores. Clearly, SMS support services will need to undertake further research to establish outcomes among their own user group. However, even these fairly straightforward findings establish a helpful indicator of how service users reply when asked how helpful an intervention has been, in this case providing a ringing endorsement of the service.

CONCLUSIONS

High quality services are essential for all mental health interventions and the same is true of SMS and other technologically mediated means of access. In short, it is better not to run a service at all than to run it badly.

An inherent risk in developing such services is that the technology becomes the primary focus. Over and above the technical system needs, there is also a need to make sure that people are adequately trained and prepared. Furthermore, resources must be sufficient to ensure that response times are adequate and systems are sufficiently robust. The experience of Samaritans has underlined that while there are many "off-the-shelf" packages which can help handle incoming SMS messages in volume, most, if not all, are unlikely to be sufficient for the needs of mental health and crisis care where any difficulties or limitations in functionality can have a serious impact for service users. Specific services will have specific requirements and it is vital for people seeking help that their needs are fully taken into account in system design and implementation. Delivery times of messages, for example, can extend to more than an hour at peak times. High volumes of messages can also create problems (Samaritans' service received over 800 messages in its first hour) unless the resources are made available to ensure that the system is sufficiently robust to handle demand.

It is also important that where a variety of means of contact are possible; they must be integrated with clear policies for how the different channels of communication may be combined. For example, if a person makes contact by SMS clearly indicating that they are in crisis but then ceases to respond to the messages they are sent, is it appropriate for the service to make contact by telephone? How is that handled if a user indicates a preference *not* to use the telephone? Services should also consider whether the introduction SMS services in particular are to be seen as gateways to other kinds of provision or as a service delivery method in themselves. Despite initial expectations to the contrary, the latter proved to be the case for Samaritans. Different services will have different answers to these questions but careful consideration and policy development leading to effective combination of technologies is likely to be a key factor for all.

That meaningful emotional support and mental health interventions are possible through SMS has undoubtedly been demonstrated by Samaritans' service. It appears that, as in the case of many other technologies, the initial doubts of many are being steadily dispelled. Demand from service users is vast and likely to continue to grow.

Developing new means of contact is a challenging and time-consuming process. It must be done because there is a clear need rather than simply because the technology is "there" and it must be done in a way that is "safe" and thoughtful. We must be guided in this by the people who use our services, their needs and their preferences in how to make contact.

To use any form of emotional support service requires a huge amount of courage from an individual. It is an act of trust which places on the service provider a duty to continue to improve and to strive to develop more and better ways to enable contact. Therefore, while it may be a time-consuming and difficult process, it is not one which we can afford to neglect.

ACKNLOWLEDGMENT

NB This chapter is based in part on a presentation by Joe Ferns, *The Work of The Samaritans Online*, at the OCTIA 2009 Conference, Leicester, 25th April 2009.

REFERENCES

Agyapong, V. I., Milnes, J., McLoughlin, D. M., & Farren, C. K. (2013). Perception of patients with alcohol use disorder and comorbid depression about the usefulness of supportive text messages. *Technology in Health Care, 21*, 31–39. DOI: http://dx.doi.org/10.3233/THC-120707.

Arnquist, S. (2009). In rural Africa, a fertile market for mobile phones. *New York Times* [online]. [Accessed December 21, 2009]. Available from: http://www.nytimes.com/2009/10/06/science/06uganda.html?_r=3 &ref=science.

Balakrishnan, V. (2009). A look into SMS usage patterns among Malaysian youths. *Human IT*, 10(2), 55–80.

Berrouiguet, S., Alavi, Z., Vaiva, G., Courtet, P., Baca-García, E., Vidailhet, P., Gravey, M., Guillodo, E., Brandt, S., & Walter, M. (2014). SIAM (Suicide intervention assisted by messages): The development of a post-acute crisis text messaging outreach for suicide prevention. *BMC Psychiatry 14*, 294. doi: 10.1186/s12888-014-0294-8.

Buhi, E. R., Trudnak, T. E., Martinasek, M. P., Oberne, A. B., Fuhrmann, H. J., & McDermott, R. J. (2013). Mobile phone-based behavioural interventions for health: A systematic review. *Health Education Journal, 72*, 564-583. doi: 10.1177/00178969 12452071.

Bopp, J. M., Miklowitz, D. J., Goodwin, G. M., Stevens, W., Rendell, J. M., & Geddes, J. R. (2010). The longitudinal course of bipolar disorder as revealed through weekly text messaging: A feasibility study. *Bipolar Disorders, 12*(3), 327–334.

Carter, G. L., Clover, K., Whyte, I. M., Dawson, A. H., & D'Este, C. (2005). Postcards from the EDge project: Randomised controlled trial of an intervention using postcards to reduce repetition of hospital treated deliberate self poisoning. *British Medical Journal, 331*(7520), 805.

Chandra, P. S., Sowmya, H. R., Mehrotra, S., & Duggal, M. (2014). 'SMS' for mental health – feasibility and acceptability of using text messages for mental health promotion among young women from urban low income settings in India. *Asian Journal of Psychiatry, 11*, 59–64. doi: 10.1016/j.ajp.2014.06.008.

Chen, H., Mishara, B. L., & Liu, X. X. (2010). A pilot study of mobile telephone message interventions with suicide attempters in China. *Crisis: The Journal of Crisis Intervention and Suicide Prevention, 31*(2), 109–112.

Chipchase, T. (2007). Jan Chipchase on mobile phones. *Ted.com* [online]. [Accessed December 21, 2009]. Available from: http://www.ted.com/talks/jan_chipchase_on_our_mobile_phones.html.

Déglise, C., Suggs, L. S., & Odermatt, P. (2012). Short message service (SMS) applications for disease prevention in developing countries. *Journal of Medical Internet Research, 14*(1), e3. doi:10.2196/jmir.1823.

Evans, J. l., Evans, M., Morgan, H. G., Hayward, A., & Gunnell, D. (2005) Crisis card following self-harm: 12-month follow-up of a randomised controlled trial. *British Journal of Psychiatry, 187*, 186–187.

Gadebe, T. (2006). SMS help for teens in distress. *SouthAfrica.info* [online]. [Accessed December 21, 2009]. Available from: http://www.southafrica.info/services/health/teensindistress.htm.

Geser, H. (2006). Are girls (even) more addicted? Some gender patterns of cell phone usage. *Sociology in Switzerland: Sociology of the Mobile Phone* [online]. [Accessed December 21, 2009]. Available from: http://socio.ch/mobile/t_geser3.htm.

GSM Association. (2014). Women & mobile: A Global Opportunity – A study on the mobile phone gender gap in low and middle-income countries. London: GSM Association. [online]. [Accessed August 8th, 2015]. Available from: http://www.gsma.com/mobilefordevelopment/wp-content/uploads/2013/01/GSMA_Women_and_Mobile-A_Global_Opportunity.pdf.

Hall, A. K., Cole-Lewis, H., & Bernhardt, J. M. (2015) Mobile text messaging for health: A systematic review of reviews. *Annual Review of Public Health, 36*, 393–415.

ITU. (2009). *The world in 2009: ICT facts and figures* [online]. [Accessed December 21, 2009]. Available from: http://www.itu.int/ ITU-D/ict/material/Telecom09_flyer.pdf.

Kaseniemi, E., & Rautiainen, P. (2002). Mobile culture of children and teenagers in Finland. In J. E. Katz & M. Aakhus (Eds.), *Perpetual contact.* Cambridge, UK: Cambridge University Press.

Ling, R. (1999). 'We release them little by little': Maturation and gender identity as seen in the use of mobile telephone. In *International Symposium on Technology and Society (ISTAS 99) Women and Technology: Historical, Societal and Professional Perspectives.* July 29–31, Rutgers University, New Brunswick [online]. [Accessed December 21, 2009]. Available from: http://www.telenor.no/fou/program/nomadiske/articles/11.pdf.

Luxton, D. D., June, J. D., & Comtois, K. A. (2013). Can postdischarge follow-up contacts prevent suicide and suicidal behavior? A review of the evidence. *Crisis: The Journal of Crisis Intervention and Suicide*

Prevention, 34(1), 32–41. http://dx.doi.org/10.1027/0227-5910/a000158.

Potts, G. (2004). *College students and cell phone use: Gender variation* [online]. [Accessed December 21, 2009]. Available from: http://personalwebs.oakland.edu/$gapotts/rht160.pdf.

Proitz, L. (2009). The mobile gender: A study of young Norwegian people's gender performances in text messages. In *Mobile communication and social change.* International Conference, Seoul, Korea.

Rafi, M. (2009). SMS text analysis: Language, gender and current practices. *Tesol France Online Journal* [online]. [Accessed December 21, 2009]. Available from: http://www. tesol-france.org/Online Journal.php.

Spohr, S. A., Taxman, F. S., & Walters, S. T. (2015). The relationship between electronic goal reminders and subsequent drug use and treatment initiation in a criminal justice setting. *Addictive Behaviors, 51*, 51–56.

Suler, J. R. (2004). The online disinhibition effect. *Cyberpsychology and Behavior, 7*(3), 321–326.

Textually.org. (2009). Mobile phone use soars in Africa, unevenly. In *Textually.org* [online]. [Accessed December 21, 2009]. Available from: http://www.textually.org/textually/archives/2009/10/024783.htm.

Tossel, C. C., Kortum, P., Shepard, C., Barg-Walkow, L. H., Rahmati, A., & Zhong, L. (2012). A longitudinal study of emoticon use in text messaging from smartphones. *Computers in Human Behavior, 28*, 659–663.

Chapter 7

USING WEBSITES, BLOGS, AND WIKIS IN MENTAL HEALTH

John M. Grohol

INTRODUCTION

One of the leading transformational technologies in the past few decades has been the Internet. It is where people regularly turn to get answers to their questions, collaborate with others, get advice and support and to be entertained. It should not be surprising then to learn that most people at one time or another have investigated a health topic online (Fox & Duggan, 2013; Fox, 2006; iCrossing, 2008). More people turn to the Internet first than to their own doctor or a friend to get information related to a health concern (Fox & Duggan, 2013; iCrossing, 2008).

While many things have changed in the online landscape in the past five years, much remains the same. Websites still provide the bulk of health information online, although the way people access them has changed substantially (via a mobile device instead of a desktop or laptop computer). A website is simply an ordered collection of information that can sport many features, including a blog, links to other resources or social networks and static pages of information arranged by topic. Websites may also be community-enabled, meaning that they allow for social networking to take place. Websites may just be a single page of information (for

instance, advertising one's practice), or can be a huge information store containing tens of thousands of articles and features (such as WebMD.com or PsychCentral.com). A website's mainstay – the static article – is usually authored by a single individual, edited and published without comment or further editing by visitors.

Mental health websites today generally contain information about a condition's symptoms, commonly accepted treatments, news and research information on conditions (including clinical trials), links to other online resources of interest to that condition, related book reviews and symptom checkers (sometimes in the form of online screening quizzes). There are many to choose from and most generally offer similar types of resources to users. Two examples of mental health websites are HelpGuide.org and PsychCentral.com.

A blog (from the term, "web log") is a topical online website or journal consisting of individual entries that are arranged in reverse-chronological order. Blogs may be characterized by their links to other information or opinions online, usually with commentary and perspective by one of the blog's owners. Blogs also usually allow for reader commentary and discussion, which makes the blog a two-way conversation between the author and his or her readers. Most bloggers appear to be hobbyists who blog for fun, but "health" is a focus of 14 percent of bloggers (Sobal, 2010). A specific and popular type of blog is an online journal, which many people use to diary their daily life. Two examples of mental health blogs are World of Psychology (www.psychcentral.com/blog) and Practice of the Practice (www.practiceofthepractice.com).

Blogs can be public or private; private blogs require a password to access and are not indexed by search engines, such as Google. Whether out of ignorance or a desire for attention and popularity, most blogs are kept public, even when people are discussing the most intimate details of their lives. This can lead to some unintended consequences if the blog's author doesn't take into account that what they may write on the blog could someday be linked back to their real name (even if they use a pseudonym to create the blog).

A wiki is a type of web page that allows any authorized user to contribute or edit content on the page. The most famous example of a wiki is the free online encyclopedia, Wikipedia. Wikis can be stand-alone websites on their own, or a part of a larger website. Because any authorized user can edit a wiki page, wikis keep copies of every edit ever made. If a malicious edit is made to a wiki page, it can quickly and easily be reverted to a previous untainted version of the page by an editor overseeing the wiki. Each wiki page also has an attached discussion page, allowing users to collaborate on the content on the page.

Wikis are primarily used as a collaboration or education tool when a person wants a community of users to help edit or add content on a specific topic. For instance, in companies, wikis are often used as an online space to manage all of the details that go into a project, encouraging employees and co-workers to collaborate. They can be used anywhere online collaboration is needed amongst a set of people (who don't even need

to be on the same continent). In addition to the workplace, they are most often used in educational settings, as a classroom collaborative writing tool (Hadjerrouit, 2014). They have experienced mixed success in this environment, with some research finding that students prefer not to be required to use a wiki (Witney & Smallbone, 2011). Except for Wikipedia, wikis' popularity as a general, public website publishing platform has largely peaked; few people or websites use them any longer to publish information online. This decline in popularity is likely due to problems in maintaining wikis against spammers and a lack of participation interest in editing them. Wikis and blogs are considered prime examples of empowering Web 2.0 tools. Web 2.0 tools allow for the easy editing or adding of content to the Internet with little or no technical knowledge or skill. For instance, free services like Wordpress.com allow any individual to set up a blog in less than five minutes and start blogging immediately. The world's largest free encyclopedia, Wikipedia (en.wikipedia. org), allows anyone to edit virtually any article on the site (such edits, however, may quickly be undone by a volunteer Wikipedia editor who disagrees with the edits). Web 2.0 tools such as these also encourage a two-way dialogue between content creator (whether it be a blog or wiki) and visitors who read the content. Blogs and wikis allow for discussion amongst the readers of an entry – a feature that remains largely absent on traditional websites (such as government websites like nimh.nih.gov).

APPLICATION

Websites, blogs and wikis are all primarily used in mental health to help educate people about relevant mental health issues in their lives. They can help a reader learn about a relaxation or mindfulness technique, or share another person's story of their daily battles living with a mental illness. Psychoeducation can form a cornerstone of psychotherapy and in helping an individual understand their own or a loved one's mental health concern and the types of treatments commonly used. By learning about their mental health concern, the individual becomes an informed and educated patient (referred to as an "e-patient"), one that can play a more active and engaged role in the transformative process (Khin-Kyemon, 2013). Valuable therapy time can be used to focus on the client's individual needs and issues, rather than in explaining basic components of mental illness or its treatment.

Using such educational tools in therapy is best done as a collaborative process. Clients may be encouraged to research their mental health issues online and also print out pages that speak to them or seemed to offer them valuable insights into their own change process. These pages could then be brought into a future session with the therapist and discussed. Alternatively, clients can e-mail links to websites or individual pages they found interesting.

Not all websites are created equal. Since anyone can publish anything online, it can be challenging to determine whether the information found online is relevant, accurate and reliable. Keys to the validity and usefulness of a given website or information found online can be had from:

- helping the client identify the publisher,
- the author of the article,
- whether the article cites any scientific research or not,
- generally whether the site is a mainstream publisher, or a personal site and just somebody's opinion.

While all different types of sites and information found online may hold potential, clients may need help understanding the difference between well-accepted treatment strategies found online versus scientifically suspect strategies (such as magnet therapy or vitamin therapy). The only difference between a website and a wiki is that usually anyone can edit a wiki. But since creating and publishing a website is only slightly harder, there is very little actual difference between these two forms of online publishing when it comes to psychoeducation.

Multiple studies have demonstrated the validity and value of online health information, provided both by mainstream for-profit websites, as well as nonprofit websites (Grohol et al., 2014; Guara & Venable, 2011). Most of the websites listed on the first two pages of popular search engines also appear to provide reliable and valid information about most mental health concerns (Grohol et al., 2014). Clients should be made aware that as long as they stick to mainstream websites that appear on one of the first two pages of search results, they generally will find reliable information.

People can vet information found on a website, blog, or wiki by looking for confirmation of that information on other websites. For instance, if one site says that depression is often treated by antidepressants and psychotherapy, other sites should be in general agreement. Clients can also be counseled to look for some telltale signs of legitimate website publishers – a privacy policy, terms of use, information about who runs the site (including contact information and an address), authorship and dates on all articles, and ideally, a seal such as the Health on the Net badge (HONcode) that denotes the site is aware of the unique issues regarding publishing health and mental health information. These are minimal requirements for a mental health site and they don't guarantee any type of quality. But they do immediately help a person distinguish a potentially beneficial site from a potentially unbeneficial or even dangerous site. Personal sites and blogs can also hold a lot of value. They can help a person feel less alone by reading about others' experiences in coping with a mental illness or psychological problem. But they may not be the best place for a person to conduct their primary, personal research on a disorder or condition and its treatments.

Beyond simple psychoeducation, blogs offer an additional therapeutic benefit – they provide people with an online "space" in which to diary or chronicle their grappling with a specific mental health concern. A survey conducted by America Online in 2005 reported that nearly 50 percent of those people who blogged used blogging as a form of self-therapy (Tan, 2008). Online journaling has been conducted for well over a 15 years at the time of writing and while there have been no studies specifically chronicling the benefits, they would likely be similar to those detailed for writing in general (e.g., significant physical and mental health improvements, see Pennebaker, 1997) and journal writing in particular (Thompson, 2004). People intending to blog may view blogging as a potential way to alleviate distress, especially when they lack typical social support in their environment (Baker & Moore, 2008). Blogs allow their authors to convey a significant range and depth of emotional experiences and can increase feelings of connection to family and friends (McDaniel et al., 2012). Because blogs also allow an author to receive feedback from others on what they write, it can set up a self-reinforcing mechanism to continue blogging, especially if the feedback is positive (Miura & Yamashita, 2007).

Beyond simply keeping a journal online, blogging may have additional therapeutic benefits. Increased disinhibition online (Joinson, 2007) suggests that blogging can possibly provide an author with a platform on which to write where their writing is even more honest and open than if writing to only oneself in a traditional paper journal. Additionally, since most blogs allow others to comment on each entry, readers can provide beneficial (or harmful) feedback to the author

about what they've written (Nagel & Anthony, 2009). This continuous feedback loop provides another level of potentially therapeutic work outside of the therapy session.

Even if a person has no interest in writing on their own blog, simply reading about other people's experiences can also be beneficial to a client (Richards, 2008). While this sort of psychological benefit is usually gained in reading done in online support group communities, it can also be gained by reading people's blogs who are writing about coping with depression, anxiety, or some other concern.

ETHICAL CONSIDERATIONS

Because the Internet is the world's largest information resource today, it is also potentially the world's largest *mis*information resource as well. Well-meaning people can stumble upon inaccurate or even potentially harmful information online (although there yet remains to be a documented case in the research literature of someone doing so that resulted in serious harm). There are, however, groups on the Internet that help provide a great deal of information and support for committing suicide, anorexic food intake control, self-harm methods, and similar disturbing topics. So while the potential for good is far greater than harm, the implications of consuming online health information remains a legitimate concern that should be addressed.

Any website, blog, or wiki can be a potential instrument of misinformation and harm. Websites that appear to be legitimate can simply be advertising portals trying to get the reader to purchase a bottle of placebos, purchase a feel-good audio CD, or become a patient at an expensive inpatient facility. Blogs can provide people with all sorts of potentially harmful (or, at the very least, useless) personal opinions that may carry some apparent legitimacy if the blog is popular (regardless of whether the information is good or not). For instance, popular websites such as the Huffington Post and Forbes allow virtually anyone to blog on any topic imaginable, regardless of their expertise or background in the topic. Because the article appears on such well-known websites, readers may mistakenly believe the authors have somehow been vetted. Additionally, there is a burgeoning industry of companies created to purportedly help people "enhance" their minds (through online tools, blogs and apps), but with little scientific data supporting their techniques.

Wikis are likely seen as potentially the most harmful form of information online, because anyone can edit one. Yet because they remain fairly rare (a person is far more likely to come across an ordinary website or blog), their potential for harm is probably the least. The most popular wiki, Wikipedia, seems to have enough interested people working as article editors to keep most articles relatively accurate and relatively unbiased at any given moment. So while an article may contain misinformation for small amounts of time, most articles on Wikipedia appear to offer mostly valid information on most mental health conditions. People are often encouraged to use a wiki such as Wikipedia as a jumping off point to understand the basics of a condition, but to research the condition further on specific mental health websites.

Health bloggers regularly use anonymity strategically to protect their identity because of embarrassment about their illness or stigma associated with it (Rains, 2014). Nonetheless, potential bloggers should be made aware of privacy issues related to their sharing of information on a blog or a website. Even while writing under a pseudonym or alias, such information has the possibility of being traced back to one's real identity. Such identity leakage may occur if a person uses a similar username, pseudonym or alias on other, unrelated nonmental health sites, or as a part of one's email address or general online identity. Professionals should discuss such concerns

with their clients and make them aware of the limits of such privacy protections, so that if they do choose to share, they do so in a way that limits potential future harm.

CLIENT SCENARIO

Jane is a 42-year-old housewife, married with two children. Lately she's been feeling more run down than usual and sometimes looks at her life and wonders, "What if?" She complains of having little to no energy or motivation to do the daily chores to keep the household running in the manner in which she usually likes it. When asked by her husband "what's wrong?" or what can he do to help, she has no real answer and instead just brushes off his suggestions and offers of help. While she used to enjoy meeting with her friends every week for coffee and sometimes to go to a movie or shopping, she hasn't seen most of her friends now for over two months. When they call, she avoids picking up the phone to talk, because she doesn't feel like it and has no answers to why she's avoiding them. She spends a lot of time checking her Facebook feed to see what her friends and other family members are up to, but rarely posts anything of her own. This only makes her feel worse. She feels sad, lonely and distracted. Jane has trouble concentrating and feels her memory is slipping.

After feeling this way for more than two months, Jane decided to see if there was anything online that could help her understand what her problem was. Like most people, she began her search at Google, a popular Internet search engine, and just typed in many of her symptoms: sad, lonely, problems with memory and concentrating. Within the search results, she found many articles about these symptoms, some indicating that perhaps her concern was something called "depression." She clicked on a few of the articles to learn more and came across a website called PsychCentral.com. While there, she read an in-depth guide to depression that explained the common symptoms, possible causes and treatments available to help her. She was still unsure, however, and a little scared about talking to her husband or doctor about her feelings.

So Jane went back to the search results and looked for a blog on depression (now that she knew what term she was looking for). She found a blog called Sunny Spells and Scattered Showers (sunnyspellsandscattered-showers.blogspot.com/), which detailed one person's experiences with depression. She enjoyed reading it and found she could relate a lot to what the author wrote. It also gave her some perspective and confidence that this was a condition that could be helped through getting the right treatment.

Jane picked up the phone and called her family physician to schedule a checkup. While at the doctor's office, she talked about her feelings and inability to just "snap out of it." She also mentioned that she had done some research online and thought that maybe she was depressed. Did he know of any professional he could refer her to? The doctor listened, asked a few follow-up questions related to Jane's symptoms and gave her a standard physical to rule-out any physical issues that might be the cause of her symptoms. After being satisfied that Jane was suffering from a mental health concern, he gave her the names and numbers of some mental health professionals to call.

When Jane met with her therapist for the first time, she explained that she found the information online helped her not only figure out what might be the problem, but also gave her the strength and courage to ask for help. The therapist encouraged her to continue researching and learning from her online experiences. The therapist also encouraged Jane that if she ever had any questions about something she read online, she could print out a copy and bring it to the next session to review.

Jane returned home later that night and accessed the Internet again, looking for more resources and information about depression. She found a self-help book online entitled *Psychological Self-Help* (www.psychologicalself-help.org), written by a psychologist. In the book, she read the chapter about depression and happiness and then a few pages about things she could do to help change her behavior. She thought that while her therapy and medication would help her depression, it wouldn't hurt to continue working on her problems outside of therapy, too. She found the exercises challenging and resolved to talk to her therapist in the next session about the point of the cognitive-behavioral techniques she was practicing.

Jane's experience is typical of most Internet health users – they first search for a health or mental health concern online, starting with a regular search engine such as Google. They often don't know the exact name of the condition they are searching for, instead typing in symptoms they know they (or a loved one) have. While such a strategy often provides hit-or-miss results, it is usually sufficient to lead a person to a reputable resource that has scored highly within the search results (Grohol et al., 2014). It is then the user's journey of learning and discovery begins.

CONCLUSION

The Internet continues to grow at a rapid pace, with tens of thousands of new blogs and websites created each day. People will continue to use these resources primarily as they were intended – as an educational tool meant to inform and reduce the stigma traditionally attached to mental health concerns. Websites, wikis, and blogs help inform people who otherwise may not recognize a mental health problem or concern and provide them with specific steps and resources to find help. It also gives a person the opportunity to engage in conversations on blogs and wikis with other people who can help answer a question they may have about a symptom, life event, or other concern.

In rare circumstances, websites, wikis and blogs can also be platforms for misinformation. Most people know to be skeptical about information they find online if they can't verify it through other websites, or through some other means (such as reviewing it with a professional). It helps to review signs of legitimate websites and information versus those that may be suspect with a client. It also helps to encourage clients to review primary information on well-known and respected mental health websites first before exploring the entire Internet for additional resources.

As video and data sharing become more commonplace, it is likely we will see even more people sharing their mental health experiences through video and their personal health data. Privacy concerns notwithstanding, people seem more inclined to share even the most sensitive information about themselves first and ask questions later. A therapist can help their client understand the potential problems with such sharing and ensure they understand that pseudonyms are not a foolproof anonymity mechanism.

Websites are increasingly becoming not only an information tool, but also an important part of one's social connectedness. People are turning to the Internet not just for information, but also for community and support from others with similar concerns. The Internet is making people feel less isolated and stigmatized because of their mental health issues and the reach and connectivity the Internet fosters will only expand in the years to come.

REFERENCES

Baker, J. R., & Moore, S. M. (2008). Distress, coping and blogging: Comparing new Myspace users by their intention to blog. *CyberPsychology, Behavior and Social Networking, 11,* 81–85.

Fox, S. (2006). Online health search 2006. *Pew internet and American life project* [online]. Retrieved 11 Apr, 2015 from: http://www.pewinternet.org/2006/10/29/online-health-search-2006/.

Fox, S., & Duggan, M. (2013). Health online 2013. *Pew internet and American life project* [online]. Retrieved 11 Apr 2015 from: http://www.pewinternet.org/files/old-media//Files/Reports/PIP_HealthOnline.pdf.

Grohol, J., Slimowicz, J., & Granda, R. (2014). The quality of mental health information commonly searched for on the Internet. *Cyberpsychology, Behavior, and Social Networking.*

Guada, J., & Venable, V. (2011). A comprehensive analysis of the quality of online health-related information regarding schizophrenia. *Health and Social Work, 36,* 45–53.

Hadjerrouit, S. (2014). Wiki as a collaborative writing tool in teacher education: Evaluation and suggestions for effective use. *Computers in Human Behavior, 32,* 301–312.

iCrossing (2008). *How America Searches: Health and Wellness* [online]. Retrieved 11 April, 2015 from: http://www.icrossing.com/icrossing-has-health-wellness.

Joinson, A. N. (2007). Disinhibition and the Internet. In J. Gackenbach (Ed.), *Psychology and the Internet: Intrapersonal, interpersonal and transpersonal implications* (2nd ed.). San Diego, CA: Academic Press.

Khin-Kyemon A. (2013). A book review and a conversation with e-Patient Dave. *Healthcare, 1,* 149–151.

McDaniel, B. T., Coyne, S. M., & Holmes, E. K. (2012). New mothers and media use: Associations between blogging, social networking, and maternal well-being. *Maternal and Child Health Journal, 16,* 1509–1517.

Miura, A., & Yamashita, K. (2007). Psychological and social influences on blog writing: An online survey of blog authors in Japan. *Journal of Computer-Mediated Communication, 12*(4), 1452–1471.

Nagel, D. M., & Anthony, K. (2009). Writing therapies using new technologies – the art of blogging. *Journal of Poetry Therapy, 22*(1), 41–45.

Pennebaker, J. W. (1997). Writing about emotional experiences as a therapeutic process. *Psychological Science, 8*(3), 162–166.

Rains, S. A. (2014). The implications of stigma and anonymity for self-disclosure in health blogs. *Health Communication, 29,* 23–31.

Richards, D. (2008). Towards an informal online learning community for student mental health. *British Journal of Guidance and Counselling, 36*(1), 81–97.

Sobal, J. (2010). State of the Blogosphere, 2010. Retrieved 11 April, 2015 from http://technorati.com/state-of-the-blogosphere-2010/.

Tan, L. (2008). Psychotherapy 2.0: MySpace® blogging as self-therapy. *American Journal of Psychotherapy, 62*(2), 143–163.

Thompson, K. (2004). Journal writing as a therapeutic tool. In G. Bolton, S. Howlett, C. Lago, & J. Wright (Eds.), *Writing cures.* New York: Brunner-Routledge.

Witney, D., & Smallbone, T. (2011). Wiki work: Can using wikis enhance student collaboration for group assignment tasks? *Innovations in Education and Teaching International, 48,* 101–110.

Chapter 8

THE ROLE OF BLOGGING IN MENTAL HEALTH

DeeAnna Merz Nagel and Gregory Palumbo

INTRODUCTION

Since the introduction of the Internet, there has been an evolution in human communications. One of the corollaries to this reinvention is that there is a resurgence in the use of the written word. The Internet has inspired collaboration on a scale never before imagined and messaging between people has evolved to take advantage of the unique characteristics of this new medium.

The common theme supporting online communications is sharing and interactivity. Prior to the Internet, the written word was static. Books, magazines, and newspapers provided unidirectional communication. Information could be disseminated but interactivity was not supported by these media, other than the occasional letter to the editor. The Internet brought change not only to how people could distribute their writings, but also to how those writings could remain dynamic and alive. Text stored online cannot only be accessed by anyone, anywhere, but there exists the potential for that text to be edited by those who view it. There are various forms of technology that support such interactivity and one of the most popular forms is called the "blog."

Definition

The term "blog" is short for "web log" but can be used as a noun or a verb. As example, noun: "Kate is examining Action Research processes on her blog" or verb: "Kate has just blogged about the woes of getting the Victoria Line to Hanger Lane" (Anthony, 2004). A blog is a form of website that is customarily maintained by an individual who regularly posts commentary, event descriptions, or other materials such as graphics or videos. Blogs can provide commentary or news on a subject or they may function as personal online diaries. Typically, blogs will combine text, images, and links to other blogs, web pages and other related media. Many blogs provide an opportunity for readers to submit their personal comments, inspiring an interactive and evolving dialogue.

Blogging is a standardized form of online communication and as such, its various elements – which include title, description, keywords, author, date, and content – are usually coded with a programming language called "xml" so that the content can be accurately categorized and searched in a standardized format. This standardization gave birth to a new way for the information to be delivered to interested readers – RSS feeds. RSS stands for Really Simple Syndication. RSS is a web "feed" or "channel" to which readers may subscribe. Thus, as blog content is updated, the "feed" is instantly delivered to all subscribers, eliminating the need for the reader to continually check the blog for new updates.

RSS benefits publishers by providing a way for them to syndicate their content automatically. It benefits readers who want to be updated by their favorite websites and aggregates all of their updates into one place – their RSS reader.

By definition, blogs are regularly updated websites that facilitates interactivity. Because they are regularly updated, their content tends to be current. Additionally, the interactivity lends itself to readers providing additional insight and information on the subject, enhancing the relevancy of the content.

BUSINESS APPLICATIONS OF BLOGGING

By Gregory Palumbo

This combination of current information and interactivity naturally gave way to search engines favorably ranking blogs. In fact, blogs may rank on the first page of search results, alongside major websites. So although blogging began with individuals discussing favored topics, businesses took note of their popularity with readers and favorability with search engines and began to implement blogs as part of their marketing strategy.

The popularity of blogging for business purposes revolves not only around search engine popularity but also around the unique way that blogs allow publishers to maintain a close relationship with their subscribers. Businesses depend upon long-term customer retention. Companies dedicate large portions of their advertising budgets to marketing to previous customers. Blogs allow companies to provide their previous customers with useful information. Their customers appreciate the on-going support and develop strong bonds with these companies. The businesses are able to inform their customers of additional products, services and promotions to entice customers to make new purchases. As opposed to traditional mailers or telemarketing campaigns, the company incurs virtually no cost to disseminate their offers. This allows companies to focus more on providing useful content that helps cement the bonds with their customers and less on the "hard sell" that is typical of print and telemarketing campaigns.

Businesses that implement blogs find that their cost of acquiring a new customer is further mitigated by the increase in long-term business that results from the enhanced relationship afforded by the blog. Instead of focusing on new customer acquisition, companies focus on retention and implementing new products and services that complement the customers' original purchase. Since each subscriber is predisposed to having interest in the company's content, products, services and promotions, they are interested in hearing about additional solutions to challenges that they may be having. In television advertising, it is generally accepted that it takes approximately 13 exposures to a commercial before a new customer is inspired to make a purchase. Blogging provides a very similar kind of repeated exposure to a company's marketing message, with the distinct advantage of not costing the company to distribute it.

Marketing by using a blog also provides other advantages to businesses. Although the "hard sell" is still a viable approach, recent trends suggest that people are more willing to purchase products and services from companies that provide helpful information and resources. This is a "soft sell" and is very effective in that companies that create compelling content are able to convert people looking for free information into paying customers. Therefore, potential new customers are able to gain useful data from a company which creates an affinity with the company. They may even recommend the company to others without having purchased products or services themselves. Well thought out blogging campaigns can create excitement amongst subscribers and can result in great PR – even coverage by traditional media outlets (Palumbo, 2008).

Blogs can be used by businesses to help their customers connect with one another. By enabling and encouraging communities around their products and services, companies create a "social network" that allows customers to support one another. This is not meant to replace traditional customer service but is an adjunct to it that provides an additional outlet for customers to find the answers for which they are looking. This "social network" can also be a source for customers to connect with like-minded people. By providing value to the customer beyond that which is derived directly from a company's products and services, the company creates a "home" for the customer which fosters customer loyalty and brand allegiance.

Additionally, blogs as of this writing, are used with a high degree of success to create significant revenue streams.

The primary way that blogs are monetized is through advertising products or services directly on the blog.

This can be done two ways.

The first way involves the typical banner advertisements that are seen in the columns of blogs. The banners are linked to "sales pages" that sell a product or service. The owner of the blog either makes money directly from the sale of the product or service, or from an "affiliate commission" – a commission that the blog owner is paid from the provider of the product or service for sending a customer to their company.

The second way is by promoting the product or service directly in the text of the blog.

Buyer beware! Consumers are not as responsive to the "hard sell", as mentioned earlier. Blog posts that promote a product or service should feel informative, build interest and intrigue and then simply provide a way for the reader to learn more (e.g. by sending them to the sales page) and suggesting that they do so.

This type of "content rich" sales page ("content rich" meaning informative and helpful to the reader), is highly effective at "converting" readers into customers.

In fact, it is so effective at converting readers into eager buyers, that successful, savvy marketers send advertising traffic directly to those pages, instead of to the sales page for the product.

When you send someone who clicks on one of your ads to such a blog post, this is referred to as "Native Advertising." And again, Native Advertising is a highly effective method of generating significant revenue. For many marketers it is their primary method of selling.

MENTAL HEALTH APPLICATIONS OF BLOGGING

Mental health providers are typically latecomers to adopting new technologies. A therapist's work is a unique service predicated upon confidentiality and discretion. At first glance it may seem difficult, even ill advised, for a therapist to create a blog for their business. However, it is imperative to look at the big picture. Within a few short years blogs have gone from novelty to necessity for any business looking to maximize its reach and relationship with their customers. Therapy is not an exception. The prerequisite is that the goal and parameters of the blog are clearly defined before setting out, but that should be the case for any business. Therapists know their business; they are clear on what is appropriate, ethical and legal. Within those bounds, therapists will find that there are a few very effective uses of blogging.

One effective use of blogging is to share knowledge that will benefit readers. Self-help articles and articles related to the therapist's niche area are two viable uses of blogs. The therapist has the opportunity to utilize his or her expertise while educating the lay and/or professional audience. See the following blog post as an example of sharing relevant self-help information:

When Infidelity Happens, It Takes Both to Pick Up the Pieces . . .

April 5th 2012

By DeeAnna

Recent articles in the *New York Times* . . . and the *Wall Street Journal* . . . suggest that couples therapy is not always the answer to fixing a broken relationship, and I tend to agree. Instead, understanding one's own sense of self, becoming grounded and focused – that becomes the recipe for moving forward, whether you were the one involved in an affair, cyberaffair, cybersex, or other activity that was not in the relationship contract, or the one who was blindsided by your partner's behaviors. It takes both people working on healing the hurt to get the relationship on track. It is not uncommon for the person who has been betrayed to take the stance that they did no harm so they do not need therapy . . . and that works fine . . . almost never.

Why? Because when deep betrayal rips at the fabric of a relationship, both parties end up hurt. While the person betrayed may not have any obvious part in their partner's indiscretions, that person unfortunately becomes the collateral damage of those indiscretions. The relationship is essentially involved in a train wreck. Regardless of who caused the train wreck, both people have been hurt and damaged and to get back on track, both people

need to heal. Whether that healing is through individual therapy or coaching, couples counseling, intentional meditation, self-help books or workbooks – those are just the details. The most important thing is to heal from the wounds of the betrayal and feel good about oneself. Both must do this.

In many ways, infidelity and betrayal in a relationship becomes an opportunity for growth. Certainly we hope we embrace opportunities that don't always come to us in the midst of crisis, but often, the crisis becomes the impetus for change. If only one person seeks to grow, the other person is left behind and instead of the couple getting back on the train, one party steps onto the bitter bus.

Regardless of whether a couple stays together after the infidelity, healing and understanding are essential so the patterns are not repeated as the relationship continues, or into future relationships. People change after crisis and surviving the crisis of infidelity is no different. Knowing that the change can be for the better – that each party can decide to embark on a journey of self-growth that will enhance their future is the best chance at saving the relationship (Nagel, 2012).

While blogging is not the proper method of delivery for therapeutic exchanges (Nagel & Anthony, 2009a) a therapist's effective use of blogging potentially increases client caseload, drawing potential clients to a therapist's particular specialty or location. A blog also serves as an altruistic offering of information to people in an easily accessible, easy to use format. Therapists can not only use a blog as a website, a blog can be used to create community. Therapists can create a blog post and ask participants of a workshop to connect with each other via comments on the blog. Counselor educators can post homework assignments or handouts on a blog (Truffo, 2007). Blogging can be a personal notebook, providing the life and times of, say, a psychology graduate student; blogging can be used as a teaching tool, suggesting that psychology and counseling students find a particular blog topic and comment; blogging can be used as a public service reaching many people about a single topic. Finally, blogging can be used to create a virtual community whereby like-minded people come together around a particular interest (Clay, 2009a). In the blog post example below, the Online Therapy Institute rallies like-minded professionals around pertinent issues related to the promotion of online therapy.

How Professionals Can Promote Online Therapy

By DeeAnna

Yesterday I completed facilitation of a two-day Distance Credentialed Counselor training in Springfield, IL. Every time I do a training I meet great people and I learn. In this training there was much concern expressed about therapists being able to cross state lines; how to know what each state's law says, and whether there is a "clearinghouse" for such information.

So in this training I heard of two more states that may have implemented restrictive language into their law regarding online counseling – not allowing a licensed practitioner in that state to offer online therapy services to anyone outside the state (Massachusetts and Nebraska). I am hoping I can get more clarification and actually see a copy of their language.

And so on my drive back to the hotel, it occurred to me that one way we can effect change as professionals in our various states and countries is to become active in our professional organizations. If you are in the states and you are member of APA, ACA, NASW, get involved. Join taskforce committees. To have influence in your state, join a state chapter. Volunteer to be on the board. Be part of a government relations or ethics committee. Become the ethics chair of your state chapter. That is how we can begin to educate our

colleagues about the value of online counseling. I do not think we should be legislating WHERE online counseling can occur. I think we should be legislating competency.

It is obvious to me that state licensing boards are way behind the curve when it comes to understanding the global community – and global e-commerce. Placing practice restrictions on licensed professionals does not allow consumers choice in treatment, and seems to be a rather paternalistic stance. And clearly, state licensing boards have no clue about the online culture. Most states require practitioners to have taken a class on multiculturalism to obtain a license to practice, yes? Yet the boards do not understand that we have an entirely new culture of people who live within a mixed reality, choosing to receive professional services online through their global community. So if we look at the online community as a culture, then we could make the claim that in this instance, our state boards are not being very culturally sensitive, could we not?

While this issue of "crossing state lines" is rather U.S.-centric, my point in this post is to encourage professionals to become involved in their local professional organizations no matter what country, so that we can all make a difference. We want online therapy to be a viable option within the global community!!

Have a great summer day! (Nagel, 2009a).

Blogs may be used by organizations to provide their members with timely, relevant, and thought-provoking commentary while exposing the organization's mission and work to nonmembers as well. In this way, the organization provides education in the form of a public service to nonmembers and information to members. Nonmembers may in turn decide to join the organization after reading information provided on the blog. One such organization that is utilizing a blog in this manner is the American Counseling Association Weblog found at http://www.counseling.org/news/

blog. At the ACA blog's inception, four individuals regularly blogged for it. Two of the individuals represented the membership and two were employees of the organization. Occasionally, a guest blogger would be hosted as well. Now ACA's blog has several regular bloggers who represent ACA's membership and the counseling profession at large.

Therapists may also offer their own or other blogs to existing clients as additional reading regarding various topics. Therapists should educate clients about the boundaries and parameters of the use of blogs. For instance, clients should understand that the therapist would not accept (i.e., publicly post to the website that hosts the blog) a blog comment from an existing or former client. To that end, therapists should monitor blog comments prior to official posting. Therapists can explain that a client's post on a therapist's blog may potentially threaten confidentiality of the therapeutic relationship and explain, conversely, that the therapist will not comment on a client's blog for the same reasons.

Additionally, therapists are in a unique position to educate clients about the use of blogs and as well as other Web 2.0 applications. The following blog post is an example of how a therapist can inform the general public and yet specifically target clients who may or may not be the therapist's own client. For instance, this blog post from 2009 still receives traffic as of this writing in October 2015, receiving 105 unique visitors in the past 30 days.

Are You in Counseling? Would You "Friend" Your Therapist?

Jun 28th, 2009

By DeeAnna

I have spent time lately training therapists and writing about a therapist's boundaries online. And so now I am curious from the other perspective, what people think about connecting with their therapist online via social media sites like Facebook, MySpace, or other similar social networks?

I guess it might help for those of you who are not in the counseling profession to talk first about our code of ethics – what we as therapists, counselors, psychologists, social workers and psychotherapists must carry out to remain ethical. Regardless of the discipline, we all have a code of ethics that we are expected to follow and with a few differences in intent and wording, there are some ethical tenets that remain universal. Two of these tenets are with regard to confidentiality and dual relationships.

While most ethical codes have not yet addressed social media in their codes, some of us in the field have interpreted the existing codes as applied to social networking as follows:

Friending a client on Facebook or MySpace could potentially breach confidentiality. While the client may agree or even initiate the connection, others who are friends of the therapist and/or the client may "connect the dots" and assume or confirm that the person is indeed a client of the therapist.

Friending a client on Facebook or MySpace could be interpreted as a dual relationship. As a therapist I do not socialize with my clients. I don't meet my clients for coffee and I don't go to their home for dinner. Inviting a client to my Facebook page is like inviting a client into my living room.

Feedback anyone? What do you think?

Have a beautiful summer day! (Nagel, 2009b)

Blogging may also be used as a form of journal writing or self-help intervention therefore teaching the client about the effects of posting information into cyberspace can be critical (Nagel & Anthony, 2009b). For instance, clients that post personal information to the Internet may not immediately think through the potential hazards of doing so. Many people who use journal writing as a form of self-help may imagine a perceived audience as they write. This works well, but with blogging as a form of journaling, the perceived audience becomes the World Wide Web audience, bringing a person's personal information into the psyche of the general public. Therapists can help clients understand the permanence of information posted to the Internet and discuss the impact of posting particularly personal information for everyone to access. Some people now use blogs as a way to conduct self-therapy (Tan, 2008) and not merely as a form of self-help. Take for instance, the case example given in a recent news article in which Stacey Kim blogged about her husband's death to cancer. The day after, she blogged about the experience of holding him in her arms as he died. She said she received many supportive responses from people around the world and several people asked her if she was in therapy following such a traumatic loss. Kim replied, "No, but I have a blog" (Grossman, 2008).

It is also advantageous for therapists to discuss record ownership with the client. Informing the client that the therapist owns verbatim transcripts of the actual sessions mitigates the risk that a client may decide to post the contents of a therapy session in a blog post. While this scenario may be far-reaching, practicing due diligence ultimately keeps the client's personal information confidential and away from the public eye. Likewise, blogs are not the proper venue to discuss case information even in the most generic of terms. Current or previous clients might read the therapist's blog and realize the seemingly innocuous post is about them (Clay, 2009b).

MICROBLOGGING

Complementing the normal kinds of blog is what is commonly referred to as a microblog. Microblogging is a networking service that allows mobile users of cell phones and other Internet connected devices to stay abreast of activities within a group by receiving frequent published updates, typically of 140 characters or less. Text messages are uploaded to a microblogging service such as Twitter, Jaiku, and others and then distributed to group members. All persons subscribed within a specific group are instantly notified of the microblog, enabling groups to keep tabs on one another's activities in real time (Kayne, 2008).

Many of the same reasons exist for microblogging as blogging, from personal to professional, and many therapists use microblogging to build a professional network and as a public service. Twitter is the most popular microblog site. PsychCentral, a website known for providing information about mental health and psychology posted "Top Ten Psych Tweeps" (Kiume, 2009) featuring people who offer useful information about mental health and psychology and many on the list are therapists. Some of the therapists on the list are still tweeting while others are not; nonetheless, Twitter is still very popular. Many people who tweet are sending out information in short 140 character messages that may reflect an interesting article, a thought provoking question or a link to the latest blog post of their personal blog or an organizational blog. For instance, the American Counseling Association has a profile on Twitter displayed as Counseling Views and the American Counseling Association Web-log posts are tweeted at Counseling-Views. Anyone viewing the Counseling-Views profile will have access to blog post links and other relevant ACA information.

Other profiles may represent an individual yet have a username that reflects the majority of the profile content.

As example, Kate Anthony's Twitter username is @TherapyOnline because she tweets mostly about issues related to technology and mental health. Since she blogs at various sites all of her posts can be reached through her profile. Her profile content offers a variety; she offers retweets (reposting a someone else's tweet) of interest; she asks questions; offers links to various news items and tweets self-help content as well. In addition, she announces news related to the Online Therapy Institute, the organization she cofounded.

CONCLUSION

Clearly, the meshing and intertwining of blogs and microblogs along with other Web 2.0 applications such as social and professional networks like LinkedIn and Facebook offer the opportunity for a sense of community to grow and learn from one another.

It is also clear that blogging can be monetized to create revenue streams. This allows readers to naturally progress through the process of being introduced to a product or service, to actually purchasing that product or service.

These applications add to our ability to rely on the collective intelligence and wisdom across the globe, as well as to market our products and services successfully. Whether for professional or personal pursuits, when used responsibly, blogging can make a substantial and positive impact on the counseling profession and the world at large.

REFERENCES

Anthony, K. (2004). The art of blogging. *BACP Counselling and Psychotherapy Journal, 15*(9), 38.

Clay, R. (2009a). Meet psychology's bloggers. *Monitor on Psychology, 39*(11), 34.

Clay, R. (2009b). Think before you post. *Monitor on Psychology, 39*(11), 37.

Grossman, A. J. (2008). *Your blog can be group therapy* [online]. [Accessed August 11, 2009]. Available from: http://www.cnn.com/2008/LIVING/personal/05/07/blog .therapy/index.html.

Kayne, R. (2008). *What is microblogging?* [online]. [Accessed August 10, 2009]. Available from: http://www.wisegeek.com/what-is-microblogging.htm.

Kiume, S. (2009). *Top ten psych tweeps* [online]. [Accessed June 29, 2009]. Available from: http://psychcentral.com/blog/archives/2009/06/29/top-ten-psych-tweeps/.

Nagel, D., & Anthony, K. (2009a). *Ethical framework for the use of technology in mental health* [online]. [Accessed August 10, 2009]. Available from: http://onlinetherapyinstitute.com/ethical-training/

Nagel, D., & Anthony, K. (2009b). Writing therapy using new technologies – the art of blogging. *Journal of Poetry Therapy, 22*(1), 41–45.

Nagel, D. (2012). When infidelity happens, it takes both to pick up the pieces . . . *Havana Wellness Studio* [online]. [Accessed October 26, 2015]. Available from: http://www.havanawellnessstudio.com/2012/04/05/when-infidelity-happens-it-takes-both-to-pick-up-the-pieces.

Nagel, D. (2009a). How professionals can promote online therapy. *Online Therapy Institute Blog* [online]. [Accessed November 20, 2009]. Available from: http://onlinetherapyinstitute.com/2009/07/25/how-professionals-can-promote-online-therapy/.

Nagel, D. (2009b). Are you in counseling? Would you 'friend' your therapist? *Mental Health on the Web* [online]. [Accessed November 20, 2009]. Available from: http://www.havanawellnessstudio.com/2009/06/28/are-you-in-counseling-would-you-friend-your-therapist/.

Palumbo, G. (2008). *Webinar – Blogs and newsletters to drive traffic to your site* [online]. [Accessed August 10, 2009]. Available from: http://www.securetherapy.com/regsTest/webinararchives.asp?EUID=.

Tan, L. (2008). Psychotherapy 2.0: MySpace blogging as self-therapy. *American Journal of Psychotherapy, 62*(2), 143–163.

Truffo, C. (2007). *Be a wealthy therapist: Finally you can make living while making a difference.* Saint Peters, MO: MP Press.

Chapter 9

USING THE TELEPHONE FOR CONDUCTING A THERAPEUTIC RELATIONSHIP

Denise E. Saunders and Debra S. Osborn

INTRODUCTION

The telephone has been used for the delivery of counseling services for many decades. Perhaps most widely known and recognized were the crisis hotlines of the late sixties and seventies (Lester, 2002). Many of these remain in use and offer effective services for those in need all over the world. Using the telephone in the therapeutic relationship grew in acceptance among counselors and clients with the advent of these hotlines and has expanded to the use of contracted counseling delivered exclusively over the phone for individuals, couples, and groups. Historically, practitioners utilized this technology primarily for initial contact with clients, follow-up and in-between session contact. Today, telephone counseling has been adapted to assist clients with numerous counseling and clinical needs in a variety of settings (Rosenfield, 2003) and as a modality to provide support for behavioral health interventions (Boucher et al., 1999; Stead, Perera, & Lancaster, 2009). Technological advances and client desire for counseling services offered via telephone have contributed to the feasibility and increase in the use of this modality for direct service delivery.

DEFINING TELEPHONE COUNSELING

A variety of terms have been used to refer to the use of the telephone in counseling and therapy services. Among those in the literature are telehealth, telemedicine, telephone-based counseling, telephonic counseling, telephone counseling and telecounseling. The terms telehealth and telemedicine are used more frequently in referring to medical environments where physicians and other health service providers utilize the telephone for patient care and management and health information dissemination delivered through telecommunication technology, including videoconferencing. Telehealth and telemedicine are umbrella terms encompassing physical and mental health services delivered via electronic transmission of communication. Telephonic refers directly to the technologies used for service delivery, i.e., the telephone (Maheu, Pulier, Wilhelm, McMenamin, & Brown-Connolly, 2005).

The use of multiple terms and references to similar yet different aspects of telephone technology can be confusing and overwhelming to readers. For this reason a brief definition of telephone counseling may be helpful. For purposes of the discussion in this chapter the term "telephone counseling" will be used and refers to the use of the telephone for contracted counseling and therapy services between a counselor or mental health practitioner and a client (or clients in the case of couples or groups).

THE STATE OF TELEPHONE COUNSELING IN PRACTICE

Evidence-Based Findings

Having been in existence for multiple decades, telephone counseling has seen the benefits of research studies examining both process and outcome variables. Although the research is still limited in scope, it does provide support for the effectiveness and use of this modality for work with clients. Studies using control and comparison groups have repeatedly found significant positive results for those in telephone counseling. Specifically, gains have been found for those suffering from depressive symptoms (Himelhoch et al., 2013; Miller & Weissman, 2002; Mohr, Vella, Hart, Heckman, & Simon, 2008; and Stiles-Sheilds, Kwasny, Cai, & Mohr, 2014), anxiety (Olthuis, Watt, Mackinnon, & Steward, 2014); general mental health (Carmody et al., 2013; Leach & Christensen, 2005), and quality of life and social support (Napolitano, Babyak, Tapson, Davis, & Blumenthal, 2002).

The telephone provides clients with the perception of distance and safety in the therapeutic process allowing them to more quickly share their concerns (Day & Schnieder, 2002). Studies investigating client experience using telephone counseling found that clients viewed telephone counseling as an effective and satisfactory experience that improved their lives (Reese, Conoley, & Brossart, 2006). Clients reported that immediate feedback, convenience, anonymity, inhibition reduction and feeling empowered and in control,

were important features contributing to satisfaction and effectiveness of the experience (Coman, Burrows, & Evans, 2015; Reese et al., 2006). These studies provide support for the effective use of telephone counseling and suggest overall satisfaction and comfort using the telephone for counseling services.

Benefits of Use

Telephone counseling provides several benefits, including accessibility, client control and anonymity (Coman, Burrows, & Evans, 2015). Many individuals in the United States and around the world have access to a telephone. Increasing use and availability of mobile phones has contributed to affordable, global phone access. Clients and counselors report that convenience and ease of use are appealing aspects of telephone counseling (Djadali & Malone, 2003; Reese et al., 2006), as well as the cost-effective nature of the modality (Brenes, Ingram, & Danhauer, 2011). With increasing globalization of our society, many individuals travel extensively for work. The availability and convenience of counseling sessions via telephone is desirable given the increasing demands of everyday life. Individuals in disadvantaged regions of the world are gaining access to mobile phones in part due to their cost-effective nature where other forms of communication such as the Internet are not available. Wide spread mobile phone accessibility in these regions can be used to provide supportive therapies for clients who might not otherwise have access to services.

An important advantage of telephone counseling is client control and anonymity. The perceived anonymity of the relationship provides clients with a feeling of greater control in the therapeutic relationship (Coman et al., 2015; Reese et al., 2006). One could easily choose to end the counseling communication by simply ending the call. This sense of control in the therapeutic process leads to feelings of comfort using the modality and client disclosure of difficult material more quickly in the counseling process. This serves to "jump start" the process and further motivate clients in doing the work of the counseling. Despite this, it is important to establish a contract to address how to handle problems that could stem from increased client control in the counseling process.

Although at a distance, being able to hear a client's voice over the phone can serve as an important counseling tool. Awareness of voice tone, pace, inflection and silence are all cues to aid the counselor. In the absence of visual cues, counselors may find that they rely more heavily on these characteristics. Counselors are afforded the flexibility to use the telephone as the sole means of therapeutic communication or as an adjunct to face-to-face counseling. Clients receiving counseling in a more traditional face-to-face environment may perceive the use of the phone for adjunct support as an added benefit to their counseling work, further enhancing the counseling relationship.

Limitations of Use

Potential limitations of telephone counseling include limited nonverbal communication and a reduction in the number of exercises that are dependent on visual cues, such as referring to a picture or using a whiteboard (Coman et al., 2015). Critics argue that without visual cues counselors will be unable to develop a strong therapeutic relationship or that important clinical data will be overlooked. Although it is true that some material may be missing when one cannot see the client visually, those same cues may easily be "heard" over the phone as the counselor further develops skill and comfort in listening in a different counseling environment. Telephone counselors may find it useful to engage in more directive counseling work with clients, following up with questions, summarizing more frequently and using inquiry to further clarify

client's communication (Rosenfield, 2013). In comparing e-therapy to telephone therapy, Lester (2006) draws attention to potential problem areas when conducting phone counseling that need further investigation: the less formal nature of communication, management of transference and countertransference and the effects of anonymity. Counselors are encouraged to be mindful of the impact of these changes in the counseling environment and their potential impact on the development of the therapeutic relationship.

Telephone counseling may not be suitable for everyone. Those who are not comfortable using the phone or do not articulate well verbally may feel more comfortable engaging in counseling via a different modality. Consideration of cultural and or socioeconomic issues and concerns when using telephone counseling may present limitations such as how different groups and cultures use the telephone for communication. Language barriers may be present that require alternative modalities for communication to support and enhance both client and counselor understanding. Due to the informal nature of phone communication, clients may not recognize the potential for interruption or reduction in privacy from animals, noise on a busy street, others in the room or other distractions during the counseling session. It is important to discuss such issues prior to beginning telephone counseling so that clients and counselors are aware of the potential for disruptions during phone sessions and work together to minimize them.

In a 2008 meta-analysis of telephone counseling, Mohr, Vella, Hart, Hecman and Simon argue that although research consistently provides evidence of benefit of use, there is little empirical support identifying which clients are most appropriate for and would benefit most from telephone counseling. In an earlier meta-analytic study of effective phone interventions, Leach and Christensen (2005) surmised that a clear structure for phone sessions coupled with homework between sessions was more likely to yield positive outcomes. As telephone counseling continues to grow as an option for distance work with clients, it will be important to better identify those who are best suited to the modality to ensure that client needs in the United States and around the world are being met in beneficial and cost-effective ways.

ETHICAL CONSIDERATIONS

Professional organizations are responding to client and practitioner interest in providing counseling through distance modalities by developing appropriate guidelines and standards for the provision of these services. The American Counseling Association's most recent revision of their Code of Ethics includes a new section entitled "Distance Counseling, Technology and Social Media" for the use of technology in counseling including telephone contact (American Counseling Association, 2014). The National Board for Certified Counselors (NBCC, 2012) created a policy statement on "the provision of distance professional services" to outline standards for delivery of counseling services via different technological venues, including telephone counseling. The United Kingdom has often been at the forefront of distance services such as telephone counseling. The British Association of Counselling and Psychotherapy's *Guidelines for Telephone Counselling and Psychotherapy* is an example of that (Payne, Casemore, Neat, & Chambers, 2006). These guidelines focus entirely on the use of the telephone in a counseling or therapeutic relationship and include case illustrations and suggested reading for further information on this counseling topic. Issues highlighted in these various resources include security, privacy and confidentiality, client verification, evaluating service effectiveness and issues of access, among others. One topic that has received considerable attention is security and confidentiality.

SECURITY AND CONFIDENTIALITY

Just as counselors work to maintain a high degree of security and confidentiality in face-to-face work with clients, so too must practitioners work toward a similar environment when engaging in telephone counseling. There are numerous phone technologies in existence today. In the United States alone, it is estimated that 90% of adults have a mobile phone (Pew Internet Project, 2014). It has become commonplace for households to eliminate home phone lines, opting for the convenience of mobile phones for all telephone communication. Despite their convenience, we must be cautious regarding their use and fully inform our clients regarding potential threats to the security of the communication.

Until recently, landline phones were thought to be the most secure form of telephone communication. Today, most mobile phones operate on digital signals for transmission of communication, reducing the opportunity for hackers to break into and access the communication. As technology has advanced in the area of telecommunication, sending a more rapid digital signal provides a higher degree of security. Despite these advances, one cannot guarantee complete security using these technologies. It is the counselor's responsibility to thoroughly explain potential breeches to confidentiality and work to minimize the risk of these prior to beginning telephone counseling with clients. Information regarding confidentiality, security and privacy issues should be included in the informed consent document of the counseling practice or setting. As part of this informed consent, counselors will want to help clients understand that mobile phone records that are not password-protected on their devices could allow others to access their phone logs and contact lists.

Encryption affords the highest level of security. This technology is a form of secure transmission that scrambles the communication making it more difficult for hackers to decipher what is being sent. There are several vendors who provide software for the encryption of telephone communication and some mobile phone models that will do this at a distance if the phone is lost. Voice over Internet Protocol (VoIP) technologies have led to an increase in telephone communication via the Internet. Caution should be maintained when using VoIP and clarification from individual vendors on security issues is advised. VoIP remains an evolving technology, with ongoing advancements in sound quality, security and transmission.

PRACTICAL APPLICATIONS

Effective telephone counseling utilizes structure as a tool in the counseling process. Brief therapy models work well in this modality. Many cognitive behavioral tools and techniques are easily adapted to the modality and support the need for structure in the process. Establishing a contract with clients for telephone counseling services helps to eliminate confusion and uncertainty about how services will be delivered and what clients can expect. The contract would include specifics about number of sessions, length of sessions, understanding of how telephone counseling will occur and fees involved. This information could be discussed when initial contact is made via a website or phone consultation and included in the client terms of agreement or informed consent. Rosenfield (2013) offers further advisement regarding development of contracts with clients and structuring of sessions in her book, *Telephone Counselling: A Handbook for Practitioners.*

Telephone counseling may not be appropriate for all clients or counselors. Some clients may prefer to work with counselors in a different modality or present with high-risk behaviors or other issues that may be better

addressed through an alternative counseling modality. It is ethically appropriate for counselors to provide clients with referrals when issues presented fall outside of their scope of practice or boundaries of competence. This helps ensure that clients and counselors make informed choices about services being offered. Newly trained counselors and practitioners are advised to work in a face-to-face environment before offering telephone counseling to clients (Rosenfield, 2013). This allows for development of counseling skill and expertise and counselor comfort in managing the dynamics of the counseling process in this modality.

Logistics of telephone counseling are often dependent on the individual setting or practice providing the service. Some settings may offer telephone counseling services for a specified number of sessions, whereas individuals offering this service may be more comfortable with an open-ended number of sessions. Most counselors will initiate calls to their clients at the scheduled appointment time to a predetermined number. Costs involved in using the telephone to provide counseling services have dropped considerably with the advent of mobile phone plans that cover long distance and specific plans for international coverage. Mental health providers will need to contact individual insurance panels they provide service for to inquire about third party reimbursement for telephone counseling.

CASE STUDIES

May

May lost her husband six years ago to cancer. She has been living by herself in their home since his death. Her health has declined, limiting her physical mobility. She was told she would need a hip replacement – however, at 81, May doesn't feel the costs and recuperation are worth it. She no longer drives and is dependent on friends or a shuttle service for transportation. Her two children live out of the area and visit infrequently. Lately, she has felt depressed, spends the day looking out of her front window and has limited social contact outside the growing number of visits to healthcare providers. May decided to schedule a telephone counseling session after being encouraged by her primary care physician to work with a counselor on their staff for telephone counseling.

Initial Session

May and the counselor discussed her feelings of loss, not only for loved ones, but also the impact of losses she experienced due to physical ailments. May was pleased that the counselor understood her and found it helpful to talk with someone outside her circle of friends and family. After asking questions about telephone counseling and determining that she felt at ease communicating with the counselor over the phone, May expressed interest in continuing work with the counselor and agreed to schedule sessions weekly for the next month.

The Fourth Session

Over the course of that month, May found herself appreciating her days more. She and the counselor further explored her feelings of loss. By the third contact, May had felt comfortable sharing with the counselor her disappointment that her children were not more involved in her life. This was difficult for her, as she felt selfish acknowledging this. The counselor assisted her in getting involved with a local organization that knitted baby blankets for the local hospital neonatal unit. She now expressed a willingness to consider medication and surgery options to improve her physical mobility as her doctor felt she was a good candidate for surgery. May felt the telephone counseling experience had been beneficial in many ways and she was appreciative of her physician's initial referral. She requested on-going contact with the counselor and they agreed to continue with weekly sessions.

Jonathan

Jonathan is a 32-year-old male in a committed relationship of five years with two young children. He recently returned home from a deployment overseas while serving in his country's armed services. Since returning home, he has felt tense and anxious and has been having difficulty sleeping. Jonathan called in sick to work four days out of the past two weeks. Since he was currently unable to work effectively and his tension was causing problems in his relationships both at work and at home, his supervisor encouraged him to access the counseling service available to him via the phone. He was initially resistant as he didn't want to share what he had been experiencing with anyone and had been trying to manage the worries on his own; however, after investigating the services he was eligible for, he decided to try telephone counseling. He was pleased that he could access this in the evening after his usual work hours and the children's bedtimes.

Initial Session

After registering for the service and setting up an appointment, Jonathan contacted the counselor as instructed for the scheduled appointment. He felt uncertain about what to expect and how the relationship would develop. His counselor sensed his worry and quickly put him at ease by sharing more about telephone counseling and how the two might work together. As they talked, Jonathan became less anxious. He shared openly his frustrations with not having better managed his feelings. The counselor heard what Jonathan was communicating and helped to normalize his thoughts and feelings. As the relationship developed, Jonathan's reluctance to share diminished and he began talking about his experiences. He soon became aware of past experiences and connections to his emotions and more recent irritability with his family. Jonathan felt comfortable with this modality of counseling and enjoyed the convenience of it. He requested additional calls, which the counselor was able to provide working around his family and work schedule.

Three Months Later

Jonathan and his counselor worked together for three months varying session frequency dependent on Jonathan's schedule. To his surprise, he was comfortable engaging in telephone counseling and enjoyed the anonymity of the modality. During his counseling sessions, Jonathan began to acknowledge how difficult it was for him to have been exposed to circumstances that threatened his life during his recent deployment. He worked with his counselor to further develop stress management techniques to help manage his daily life stress and enhance his resilience for challenges that he might face in the future.

CONCLUSION

With the impact of the global workplace, advancements in technology and lifestyle changes, telephone counselors will continue to be a growing part of the provision of mental health counseling and therapy services. As telephone counseling and other distance modalities are given greater favor in the provision of counseling services, there will be a need to further explore the process of telephone counseling and its unique contributions to the counseling/therapeutic relationship. Counselor training programs will be called upon to include instruction on distance modalities available for counseling, ethical and legal concerns in using these modalities, and

research findings that support the use of telephone and other technologies in counseling. Expanded use of telephone counseling will necessitate practitioners' understanding of client suitability for this modality through research and professional practice. Given society's increasing use of technology in all facets of daily living, client desire for provision of counseling services via distance modalities is likely to increase. In part due to its widespread availability and client familiarity, it is certain that the telephone will continue to have a prominent role in this movement.

REFERENCES

American Counseling Association. (2014). *ACA code of ethics.* Alexandria, VA: Author.

Boucher, J., Schaumann, J., Pronk, N., Priest, B., Ett, T., & Gray, C. (1999). The effectiveness of telephone-based counseling for weight management. *Diabetes Spectrum, 12*(2), 121–123.

Brenes, G. A., Ingram, C. W., & Danhauer, S. C. (2011). Benefits and challenges of conducting psychotherapy by telephone. *Professional Psychology: Research and Practice, 42*, 543–549.

Coman, G. J., Burrows, G. D., & Evans, B. J. (2015). Telephone counseling in Australia: Applications and consideration for use. *British Journal of Guidance & Counselling, 29*, 247–258.

Carmody, T. P., Duncan, C. L., Huggins, J., Solkowitz, S. N., Lee, S. K., Reyes, N., Mozgai, S., & Simon, J. A. (2013). Telephone-delivered cognitive-behavioral therapy for pain management among older military veterans: A randomized trial. *Psychological Services, 10*, 265–275.

Day, S. X., & Schneider, P. (2002). Psychotherapy using distance technology: A comparison of face-to-face, video and audio treatment. *Journal of Counseling Psychology, 49*, 499–503.

Djadali, Y., & Malone, J. (2003). Distance career counseling: A technology-assisted model for delivering career counseling services. In G. Walz & C. Kirkman (Eds.), *CyberBytes: Highlighting compelling issues of technology in counseling.* Greensboro, NC: CAPS Publications.

Himelhoch, S., Medoff, D., Maxfield, J., Dihmes, S., Dixon, L., Robinson, C., Potts, W., & Mohr, D. C. (2013). Telephone based cognitive behavioral therapy targeting major depression among urban dwelling, low income people living with HIV/AIDS: Result of a randomized controlled trial. *AIDS Behavior, 17,* 2756–2764.

Leach, L. S., & Christensen, H. (2005). A systematic review of telephone-based interventions for mental disorders. *Journal of Telemedicine and Telecare, 12,* 122–129.

Lester, D. (2002). *Crisis intervention and counseling by telephone* (2nd ed.). Springfield, IL: Charles C Thomas.

Lester, D. (2006). E-therapy: Caveats from experience with telephone therapy. *Psychological Reports, 99,* 894–906.

Maheu, M. M., Pulier, M. L., Wilhelm, F. H., McMenamin, J. P., & Brown-Connolly, N. E. (2005). *The mental health professional and the new technologies: A Handbook for practice today.* Mahwah, NJ: Lawrence Erlbaum.

Miller, L., & Weissman, M. (2002). Interpersonal psychotherapy delivered over the telephone to recurrent depressives. *Depression and Anxiety, 16,* 114–117.

Mohr, D. C., Vella, L., Hart, S., Heckman, T., & Simon, G. (2008). The effect of telephone-administered psychotherapy on symptoms of depression and attrition: A meta-analysis. *Clinical Psychology: Science and Practice, 15,* 243–253.

Napolitano, M. A., Babyak, M. A., Palmer, S., Tapson, V., Davis, R. D., & Blumenthal, J. A. (2002). Effects of a telephone-based psychosocial intervention for patients awaiting lung transplantation. *CHEST, 122,* 1176–1184.

National Board for Certified Counselors. (2012). *National board for certified counselors (NBCC) policy regarding the provision of distance professional services.* Accessed April 15, 2015]. Available from: http://www.nbcc.org/Assets/Ethics/NBCCPolicyRegardingPracticeofDistanceCounselingBoard.pdf.

Olthuis, J. V., Watt, & M. C., Mackinnon, S. P., & Steward, S. H. (2014). Telephone-delivered cognitive behavioral therapy for high anxiety sensitivity: A randomized controlled trial. *Journal of Consulting and Clinical Psychology, 82,* 1005–1022.

Payne, L., Casemore, R., Neat, P., & Chambers, M. (2006). *Guidelines for telephone counselling and psychotherapy.* Lutterworth, UK: BACP.

Pew Internet Project. (2014). *Mobile technology fact sheet.* Washington, DC. Retrieved from The PEW Research Center website: http://pewinternet.org/fact-sheets/mobile-technology-fact-sheet.

Reese, R. J., Conoley, C. W., & Brossart, D. F. (2006). The attractiveness of telephone counseling: An empirical investigation of client perceptions. *Journal of Counseling and Development, 84,* 54–60.

Rosenfield, M. (2003). Telephone counselling and psychotherapy in practice. In S. Goss & K. Anthony (Eds). *Technology in counselling and psychotherapy: A practitioner's guide.* New York: Palgrave Macmillan.

Rosenfield, M. (2013). *Telephone counseling: A handbook for practitioners.* London: Palgrave MacMillan.

Stead, L., Perera, R., & Lancaster, T. (2009). Telephone counseling for smoking cessation (review). *The Cochran Library, Issue 3.* Wiley.

Stiles-Sheilds, C., Kwasny, M. J., Cai, X., & Mohr, D. C. (2014). Therapeutic alliance in face-to-face and telephone-administered cognitive behavioral therapy. *Journal of Consulting and Clinical Psychology, 82,* 349–354.

Chapter 10

THERAPEUTIC ALLIANCE IN VIDEOCONFERENCING-BASED PSYCHOTHERAPY

Susan Simpson, Lisa Richardson and Corinne Reid

INTRODUCTION

Videoconferencing is rapidly becoming a common method for the delivery of psychotherapy and a range of other mental health services. A range of client groups are likely to benefit as these services become increasingly available, in particular those living in remote and rural areas and those who are unable to travel due to disability, age, incarceration, work and family commitments. Recent reviews report a profusion of emerging evidence suggesting that videoconferencing outcomes are equivalent to in-person settings (e.g., Backhaus et al., 2012; Boydell et al., 2014; Gros et al., 2012; Hilty et al., 2013; Lozano, Birks, Kloezeman, Cha, Morland, & Tuerk, 2015; Richardson, Frueh, Grubaugh, Egede, & Elhai, 2009; Simpson, 2009). These positive findings are tempered by the fact that many studies in this area have methodological shortcomings and small sample sizes. However, these limitations are often countered in the strongest studies by the use of mixed methodologies, drawing on both qualitative and quantitative methods and providing a rich source of naturalistic data from which we can develop a better understanding of outcomes (e.g., Richardson, 2011). While generalisability remains limited by the heterogeneity of client groups, measures, therapeutic models

and technologies, the majority of early and contemporary studies consistently report high levels of client satisfaction (Mair & Whitten, 2000; Richardson et al., 2009).

In spite of these promising findings, studies suggest that mental health clinicians often view videoconferencing-based psychotherapy (VT) as the 'poor cousin' of in-person services (Wray & Rees, 2003). In particular, those who are inexperienced in VT remain skeptical regarding both the effectiveness of clinical outcomes and potential for developing a sound therapeutic alliance via this modality (Rees & Haythornthwaite, 2004; Baer, Cukor, & Coyle, 1997; Steel, Cox, & Garry, 2011). It appears that the perception that rapport will be experienced as 'artificial' leads many to question the potential of VT as a modality for communicating warmth, empathy and sensitivity (Rees & Stone, 2005).

The purpose of this chapter is to explore the research which has explicitly examined therapeutic alliance (TA) in VT and to explore preliminary findings regarding the important factors associated with development of rapport via this mode of treatment delivery. Although TA has been defined in many ways, Bordin has delineated the concept in terms of the degree to which three main components are met: therapist and client concur on the therapeutic goals, therapist and client reach agreement on the actual therapeutic tasks, and the affective bond or attachment between therapist and client (Bordin, 1979). Others have also emphasised the importance of the central role of a collaborative connection between therapist and client (Horvath & Symonds, 1991; Martin, Garske, & Davis, 2000). The importance of the alliance is underpinned by consistent findings that TA alongside therapist effects, appears to be the strongest single predictor of successful therapy outcomes more generally (Wampold, 2001; Tichenor & Hill, 1989; Safran & Wallner, 1991; Hatcher, Barends, Hansell, & Gutfreund, 1995). In fact, TA ratings in the early phase of treatment have also reliably been found to predict both attrition and outcome (Horvath, Del Re, Flückiger, & Symonds, 2010). A meta-analysis of 201 studies found that TA accounted for approximately 8% of variance in treatment outcomes across a wide range of therapeutic models (Horvath et al., 2011). TA rated by adult clients and observers has been shown to be more strongly correlated with clinical outcomes than therapist ratings (Horvath, 2001; Horvath & Symonds, 1991), with the reverse being the case for child and adolescent clients (Shirk & Karver, 2003).

WHAT DO WE KNOW ABOUT THERAPEUTIC ALLIANCE IN VIDEO THERAPY?

A recent review of the literature identified 23 articles that specifically measured TA either as a primary or secondary outcome measure in research trials that utilised VT as the mode of treatment delivery (Simpson & Reid, 2014). A range of technologies were employed, including IP (Internet Protocol) and ISDN (Integrated Services Digital Network) based videoconferencing, closed circuit television, and some proprietary systems. The

consensus across studies was that both therapists and clients consistently rated moderate to high levels of TA throughout therapy. For some, TA increased over the course of therapy (Yuen et al., 2013; Richardson, 2011), while others indicated high TA throughout therapy (Krumm-Heller Roe, 2006; Bouchard et al., 2004; Bouchard, 2004; Day & Schneider, 2002; Ertelt et al., 2011; Germain, Marchand, Bouchard, Guay, & Drouin, 2010; Glueckauf et al., 2002; Goetter et al., 2013; Greene et al., 2010; Himle et al, 2006; Manchanda & McLaren, 1998; Simpson, Bell, Knox, & Mitchell, 2005; Simpson, Deans, & Brebner, 2001; Simpson & Slowey, 2011; Wade, Wolfe, Brown, & Pestian, 2005; Yuen et al., 2013). In spite of significant variations between technologies, and quality of video and sound, preliminary data suggest that the mode of delivering VT does not appear to reduce TA, with even less reliable forms of videoconferencing (e.g., low bandwidth ISDN) eliciting high levels of TA and satisfaction (Simpson, 2001; Simpson, Morrow, Jones, Ferguson, & Brebner, 2002; Stubbings, 2012; Yuen et al., 2013). It is interesting to note that client-rated TA does not appear to be influenced by initial anxieties or beliefs associated with VT and that even those with initial negative expectations tend to overcome this and develop a connection with their therapist (Germain et al., 2010). Similarly, in spite of initial concerns, therapists generally rate moderate to high satisfaction with videoconferencing technology once they have begun incorporating it into their practice (Austen & McGrath, 2006; Foster & Whitworth, 2005; Grealish, Hunter, Glaze, & Potter, 2005; Ruskin et al., 2004; Starling & Foley, 2006; Whitten & Mackert, 2005; Wagnild, Leenknecht, & Zauher, 2006).

Only two studies indicated a higher TA rated by clients in the in-person condition, both of which were conducted in group settings. One of these investigated the TA in the context of six sessions of issue-specific family counseling with 22 teenagers diagnosed with epilepsy and their parents and found that TA was moderately high to very high across all three treatment modalities (in-person, home-based VT and home-based speaker phone). Parents reported good TA across modalities, whereas teenagers reported lower TA in the home VT-based condition. The authors speculated that the lower rating may have been associated with the teens neuropsychological deficits, including problems with concentration, memory and attention that may have interfered with their ability to process and interpret information via VT (Glueckauf et al., 2002). Similarly, the other study found that 125 male veterans with Post Traumatic Stress Disorder (PTSD) and moderate to severe anger problems attending 12 sessions of group anger management rated high levels of TA across in-person and VT conditions (Greene et al., 2010). However, the ratings within the VT condition were more variable and significantly lower than those for the in-person group, though mean ratings of TA within conditions did not mediate clinical outcomes, which were roughly equivalent across modalities. The authors hypothesised that the duration and intense nature of the group therapy may be more taxing than individual therapy for VT participants and that other patient-specific factors such as experience with technology and treatment history may have interfered with their comfort with the technology. Group treatment may place additional demands on participants due to the need to regularly shift focus (when different group members are speaking), deal with numerous distractions and to balance VT etiquette with multiple relationships and interpersonal interactions. Those with PTSD may experience additional demands associated with using videoconferencing technology due to hyper-arousal and increased distractability and startle response (Greene et al., 2010). In contrast, a similar study that compared in-person group therapy with group VT reported equivalent

TA across conditions. Although most expressed a preference for in-person therapy, 90% indicated they were satisfied with VT and particularly the reduced requirement to travel (Porcari et al., 2009). Conservatively, what is clear is that in a choice of VT or no treatment, VT wins hands down and is experienced as a very acceptable form of treatment to clients in terms of the ability to build and maintain a therapeutic alliance.

BOND AND PRESENCE

Bond and presence are key to our understanding of the microprocesses that underpin TA. Both concepts have been explored in preliminary studies that have investigated TA within VT (e.g., Bouchard et al., 2000; Bouchard et al., 2004; Bouchard et al., 2007; Krumm-Heller Roe, 2006) and may cast some light onto the actual "embodied" experience of being a participant in VT, both from client and therapist perspectives. Therapeutic bond represents the degree of attachment between therapist and client and is a key aspect of TA, as measured on several alliance questionnaires including the Working Alliance Inventory (Horvath & Leslie, 1994), the Agnew Relationship Measure (Agnew-Davies et al., 1998), and the Group Therapy Alliance Scale (Pinsof & Catherall, 1986). Those studies which have specifically explored bond have reported high levels from the outset of VT (Bouchard et al., 2007; Bouchard et al., 2000; Bouchard et al., 2004; Krumm-Heller Roe, 2006). A study which investigated TA in a sample of 11 participants with agoraphobia with panic disorder, reported an initial mean bond score of 26 (maximum possible score was 28) which was maintained throughout the remaining 12 sessions of Cognitive Behavioural Therapy (CBT) (Bouchard et al., 2004). It was suggested that the "P in P" (i.e., Picture-in-Picture – a small image of oneself in the corner of the screen) function that enables the therapist to adjust their style by monitoring their own behaviour and responses via a small box on the screen may have facilitated therapist self-insight and continual feedback on the way in which they presented themselves to their clients (Bouchard et al., 2004). Similarly, Richardson (2011) reported a significant increase in bond of over the course of 15 sessions of CBT for eight clients with mixed anxiety and depression. Ratings indicated that the most important factor influencing the intial development of bond appeared to be warmth and a friendly therapeutic style, with a sense of being understood and supported as essential to deepening the bond as therapy progressed. Bond ratings were consistently high throughout treatment. In a study by Ertelt et al. (2011), high bond ratings were also reported over 20 sessions of CBT for bulimic disorders, with both therapist and client ratings improving even further over time. Of key importance, these authors concur that therapists who are trained and experienced in VT are indeed able to convey warmth and empathy and that this modality of treatment may in fact facilitate the emotional connection between therapist and client (Richardson, 2011).

A key factor in the development of therapeutic bond within VT is the ability of the therapist to demonstrate *empathy* in ways that circumvent technological limitations (Elliott, 1999; Farber, 2002). Empathy has been shown to reliably predict treatment outcome in a meta-analysis of 57 studies and requires conscious attention by the therapist to their clients' experience with a view to meeting emotional needs for understanding and connection (Elliott, Bohart, Watson, & Greenberg, 2011). This requires an ability to listen attentively, to regularly check out their understanding to ensure they are accurately attuned, to provide validation and acknowledgment of the clients' experience and to convey empathy through verbal and non-verbal gestures. It appears that in VT, therapists may rely more

heavily on verbal gestures than in in-person therapy and that the technology can in fact facilitate communication as a result of conversations being slowed down, turn-taking being more deliberate and heightened awareness of facial and bodily gestures (facilitated by a good visual image), as well as signs of emotional expression (Himle et al., 2006; Richardson, 2011; Simpson, 2009).

Another factor which appears to contribute to TA in VT is presence, as defined by the experience and "felt-sense" that one is in the *presence* of the other person at the remote site. In one study, social presence, as indicated by feeling present *with* the therapist and *absorbed in* the therapeutic process was found to predict 20% of therapeutic bond (Bouchard et al., 2007). Several studies have indicated that both clients and therapists develop a sense of connection and often feel as if they are in the same room, in spite of the fact that they can be hundreds of kilometres apart. Indeed, clients have frequently described becoming deeply involved in the therapeutic communication and dynamics early in therapy with minimal if any distraction by the technology (Bouchard et al., 2004; Goetter et al., 2013; Himle et al., 2006; Porcari et al., 2009; Sadowski, 2002).

Preliminary research suggests that some clients may prefer VT over in-person therapy, due to an enhanced sense of control and the perception that VT can equalise the power balance between therapist and client (Allen, Roman, Cox, & Cardwell, 1996; Kavanagh & Yellowlees, 1995; Simpson, Bell, Knox, Mitchell, 2005; Simpson, Deans, & Brebner, 2001). Some have argued that in VT, the client has greater personal space within a more neutral therapeutic territory than in in-person settings (Omodei & McLennan, 2000). Those with eating disorders have described VT as less "pressured" and "intimidating" than in-person contact, which may be of particular importance when dealing with shame-related issues (e.g., sexual abuse, body-image disorders) (Simpson, 2005; Simpson, Bell, &

Britton, 2006). Some clients also describe reduced self-consciousness (Manchanda & McLaren, 1998; Richardson, 2011; Simpson & Slowey, 2011), which appears to be associated with reduced emotional inhibition and greater engagement (Allen et al., 1996; Himle 2006; McLaren et al., 1995; McLaren & Ball, 1997; Onor & Misan, 2005; Thomas, Miller, Hartshorn, Speck, & Walker, 2005). Anecdotal reports suggest that the unique qualities of VT may therefore lend itself to enhanced engagement, alliance and clinical outcomes for certain client populations and may in some cases be the superior treatment option (Mitchell et al., 2003; Simpson et al., 2005; Simpson et al., 2003). Aside from those with shame-based clinical issues, VT may also lend itself to the treatment of those clients who with a high need for control as well as those with avoidant coping styles such as in Agoraphobia, Social Phobia and Avoidant Personality Disorder, either as the sole treatment modality or as a precursor to in-person sessions (Bouchard et al., 2004; Richardson, 2011; Simpson et al., 2005; Yuen et al., 2013). The space and distance associated with VT, alongside the safety and confidentiality of the therapeutic setting, may enable the client experience of being 'held' whilst experimenting with relating and connecting to another person (i.e., their therapist) without the fear of their space or thought processes being invaded. The increased sense of control and reduced experience of being "scrutinised" may also facilitate the exploration and discussion of hitherto hidden aspects of the self and the growth of personal identity in therapy (Krumm-Heller Roe, 2006; Simpson & Slowey, 2011).

THERAPIST AND CLIENT FACTORS ASSOCIATED WITH THE QUALITY OF THERAPEUTIC ALLIANCE

There is some evidence that therapist characteristics may either enhance or detract from

the development of TA. It is not uncommon for therapists to feel uncomfortable with the concept of changing their practice to communicate via videoconferencing, especially in the first session or two (Germain, Marchand, Bouchard, Guay, & Drouin, 2010). In particular, therapist anxiety can lead to a tendency to be critical or tense, which in turn appears to be linked to client reactivity (Germain et al., 2010; Ackerman & Hilsenroth, 2001). In addition, therapist rated TA can be biased by negative pretreatment expectations of VT (Rees & Stone, 2005). This appears to be linked to anxieties and expectations that rapport will be compromised via videoconferencing, that clients will be dissatisfied and that it will be more difficult to respond to emergencies (Gibson, O'Donnell, Coulson, & Kakepetum-Schultz, 2011; Hopp et al., 2006; Whitten & Kuwahara, 2004; Mitchell, Simpson, Ferguson, & Smith, 2003). Many clinicians describe fears that the use of technology will increase their workload and expectations that the technology will fail, be of poor quality or too difficult to operate (Simms, Gibson, & O'Donnell, 2011). Indeed, there is a general lack of awareness that specialist high-quality training on the use of VT and other technology-based therapies does exist and is readily available (e.g., Online Therapy Institute offer a specialist programme at http://onlinetherapy institute.com/using-video conferencing-to-con duct-online-therapy/ and at http://www.kate anthony.net/consultancy/). Evidence suggests that therapist self-confidence and frequency of VT uptake are positively associated with their level of training and experience (Gibson et al., 2011; Whitten & Kuwarahara, 2004).

There is some evidence that therapists often take the time to better prepare for VT sessions (compared with in-person sessions), which may lead to enhanced clinical outcomes (Richardson, 2011; Simpson et al., 2001). Therapists tend to adjust their usual communication style by making three main accommodations when working therapeutically via VT

(Bischoff et al., 2004; Manchanda & McLaren, 1998): (1) Nonverbal responses become more deliberate and explicit, by slightly exaggerating voice inflections, tone and mannerisms, including gestures of encouragement and support; (2) Asking more questions or making more detailed reflections, in order to seek clarification of their clients' facial expressions and gestures; (3) Offering a preliminary in-person session to facilitate rapport and to introduce the mechanisms for VT. In addition, therapists who are competent in VT tend to display more signs of clinical flexibility, rapport building skills and creativity (Tuerk et al., 2010). If used judiciously, the PinP function can provide real-time feedback that allows the therapist to adjust their style and they way they present themselves to their clients in order to enhance rapport. However, this must be balanced with ensuring that the self-image remains small enough to minimise distraction of attention away from the dialogue and flow of communication with the client. One way of ensuring this is to keep the PinP on for the first few minutes of the session and then to switch it off. Although it can also be usefully used at the client's end to address specific clinical issues (e.g., body image distortion, avoidant coping) (Mitchell, Myers, Swan-Kremeier, & Wonderlich, 2003; Simpson et al., 2005), it can also increase distress and self-consciousness if not monitored carefully and should therefore mostly be switched off unless there is a specific requirement of therapeutic task that calls for it to be left on.

Evidence suggests that clients tend to be more active in VT encounters than in in-person settings, as shown by an increase in verbal communication, higher levels of initiative, spontaneity, trust and disinhibition and increased confidence to ask questions (Day & Schneider, 2002, Tachakra & Rajani, 2002). Authors speculate that clients tend to take more responsibility for the interaction in a VT setting and that this may be due to an enhanced sense of safety associated with the distance and technology, that enhances their ability to be open (Day & Schneider, 2002). Even those factors associated with poor TA in an in-person setting (such as a defensive attitude, or poor psychological preparedness) have not been found to interfere with alliance in VT (Germain et al., 2010).

LIMITATIONS

Generalisability of findings is limited due to methodological shortcomings associated with the preliminary nature of studies in this area. Many of the studies that have been referred to in this chapter are pilot studies with small sample sizes, with less robust methodological designs. Studies in this area tend to be carried out by those who are telehealth "champions" and are therefore already committed to advancing the field. Research studies in this area are difficult to integrate due to the fact that they are focused on a wide range of clinical populations and have utilised a variety of measures of TA and several types of videoconferencing technology (Simpson & Reid, 2014).

RECOMMENDATIONS FOR ENHANCING RAPPORT IN VIDEO THERAPY

Based largely on our own clinical experience in VT, we propose the following recommendations for practitioners who are working or planning to set up a VT clinic. These recommendations are based on enhancing the therapeutic environment with a view to maximising the potential for TA.

Which Videoconferencing Platform Should I Use?

- Choice of videoconferencing platform depends on cost and the function for which it is required (Jones, Leonard, & Birmingham, 2006; Ronzio, Tuerk, & Shore, 2015). Using a system for peer consultation or training may require quite different features to a system used solely for therapeutic interactions or clinical assessments.

- Skype is not an option. Microsoft owns Skype and they can and do access data from your communications, leading to issues of confidentiality and privacy. By consenting to Skype's Terms and Conditions, you give permission to Microsoft to retain all your information for as long as is required. Skype is not HIPAA compliant (The USA's Health Insurance Portability and Accountability Act) and although encrypted it does not meet the USA's Federal Information Processing Standard FIPS140 (Dear, 2015).
- Other inexpensive and HIPAA compliant options that have successfully been used for therapeutic purposes, include VSee and Facetime. For a comparison of platforms, see http:/www.telemental-healthcomparisons.com/ and Ronzio, Tuerk, & Shore 2015 for detailed review.

Setting Up the Videoconferencing Room

The size and layout of the room is very important and influences the user's perception of the system. Negative attitudes towards VT can be influenced by the experience of the working environment rather than on the quality of the interaction for both the client and the clinician. There are some factors that need to be considered about the environment in which VT takes place and these include:

- Both the local and remote rooms should appear as close as possible to a normal office or consulting room, arranged and decorated to create a pleasant ambiance.
- As in an in-person therapy setting, it is important to minimise interruptions and the

possibility that voices will be overheard by others – as disruptions can interfere with confidentiality and sense of safety. Headphones can be used if there is a risk of being overheard to reduce the problem to just one half of the conversation. Always use a "do not disturb" sign.

- The appearance and décor of the room and the background behind the therapist should be plain and uncluttered so as to avoid distraction from visual images on the screen. Some organisations insist on a midrange blue-coloured background, which facilitates better visual image quality of skin tone (Martin, 2004; Jones et al., 2011).
- Lighting in the room should be warm/diffuse (i.e., not fluorescent). Whilst it should be light enough to see each person's face, if it is too bright (e.g., direct sunlight), this can "wash out" colour and reduce the ability to discriminate nuances in facial expressions. Cameras generally cannot adequately capture views with a wide range in contrast.
- Do not set up a camera facing either a window or a door. Too much backlight from a window will silhouette the appearance of the individual on camera, making it difficult to see their face. Background movement seen through a window or glass pane in a door will be distracting.
- Avoid hallways, windows to other rooms, mirrors or reflective glass. Make sure other people (or pets) are not visible to the client. Clients have a right to confidentiality.
- The client's chair should be close to and directly facing the camera and screen. If they are more comfortable sitting further away, use the "zoom" control to ensure a close image allows a perspective of facial expressions and upper torso (or whole body in the case of exposure

and response prevention).

- Avoid placing furniture between the camera and client (e.g., large desks) as this can increase the perception of distance between therapist and client. Once the room has been set up, the camera view can be preset to allow this same view to be easily accessible on future visits (Loranzo et al., 2015).
- When using VT with clients who are based at home, assist them in setting up their space in order to best utilise the sessions. This will include adequate bandwidth so as to avoid the line frequently dropping out, being situated close to a wireless router to increase speed of connection, switching other devices off the network so that connection quality is not compromised by competition for the bandwidth (Loranzo et al., 2015).

Audio Connections

- It is good practice to ask explicitly at the start of each session whether one can be heard clearly enough, given variations in connection quality.
- Place microphone on a firm, flat surface as close as possible to participants to enhance audio quality and minimise background noise.
- Participants should speak clearly at a normal rate and volume and be aware of allowing others to finish before they start speaking. Clinicians need to be mindful not to interrupt – which can be difficult when we feel tempted to point out critical in-session moments, observations, reflections, behaviours, etc.
- In systems that use lower bandwidths such as ISDN 128 Kbps, sound is often not conveyed in both directions simultaneously. Therefore if individuals at both locations are talking at the same time, the incoming sound will cut out. The clinician must consciously adapt their style of interviewing to accommodate this by avoiding verbal gestures (such as 'mm' and 'uh-hu') when the client is talking and instead use non-verbal gestures such as nodding of the head. This is not a problem at higher bandwidths (Jones et al., 2011).
- In the case of an echo due to microphones detecting and retransmitting remote-site sound coming through the speakers, volume should be turned down (at both sites), or by placing the speaker and microphone further apart, using headset microphones, or by switching the microphone on and off at the power source. It can be useful to check on the quality of sound at the client's end in the early stage of therapy sessions in order to ensure that this is optimal and that confidentiality is not compromised by the possibility that they will be overheard by others due to the volume being up too high.
- As in in-person settings, it is essential to avoid interruptions and maintain privacy through ensuring that mobile phones are switched off or to silent mode before the session. If you must have your phone on, set it to vibrate and keep it away from the microphone.
- Minimise background noise such as typing on a computer, rustling papers, or writing on a hard surface. Sometimes using the mute button can be helpful during breaks in an interaction, but be aware that it can be perceived to be suspicious by the other person if it is used too often. Clients can also be taught to use their mute button when required in order to reinforce their right to protect their confidentiality and enhance TA (Lozano et al., 2015).
- The clinician should be careful to mute the microphone at the end of the session to avoid inadvertent breaches of confidentiality.

Visual Connection

- Positioning of camera relative to the screen is an important visual and therapeutic consideration as well as a technical etiquette one. A camera placed below the screen gives the remote viewer the sense that they are being 'looked down on.' Looking at the screen and not the camera lens can give the impression of avoidant or unnatural eye contact and that one is being 'observed' not 'engaged' with.
- Use the picture-in-picture (PinP) option in order to monitor the way you appear to the far end site. Always try to see yourself from the client's point of view. The default mode at the client site should be 'off' to minimise distraction and distress but can be switched back on when required for specific clinical work.
- Typically, to improve the impression of eye contact, and reduce the angle between eye, camera, and screen, most services position the camera on top of the screen and it is helpful for users to sit as far away from the camera as is practical (approximately 2–4m). The video-window in which the client's image is shown should be as close to the camera location as the screen will allow. Additionally, when using the PinP function, the practitioner's own image should be placed immediately adjacent to the client's image so that their line of vision does not appear to flicker away.
- Face the camera/screen when speaking – don't talk while turning your head or moving out of shot.
- Use typical gestures as you would when talking in-person and maintain good-posture and congruent body language, but remember if you are an "expansive gesticulator," the camera may not catch all of that in the frame.
- The camera gaze angle should be checked before sessions begin and adjusted to

ensure that good eye contact, and therefore effective communication, can be achieved. It can also be useful to move the gaze between the lens and monitor, according to whether they are speaking or listening.
- The camera frame should be large enough to capture a head and shoulders view for most interactions; however, from personal experience, clients also like to be able to see some of what you are doing on a desk (i.e., writing).
- When using IP-based videoconferencing, learning to manipulate the camera to zoom and pan is an important skill to master. An important aspect of VT is that the clinician can use discrete zooming in on unusual and difficult-to-see physical movements or changes, which can in turn provide valuable information and facilitate understanding during the session. For those using laptop- or PC-based videoconferencing software, ensure that all settings are correct prior to the start of the session. At the start of the session, ensure that you have a clear image of the client and that their image of the therapist is adequate.
- Your appearance matters on camera. Your clothing choice is important – what looks great in real life may not look ideal digitally. Be mindful not to wear brightly patterned/striped/checked or reflective (especially bright white) clothing as this may interfere with the focus of the camera. Avoid reds and oranges, which have a tendency to glow and sometimes "bleed" on camera. Many webcams tend to oversaturate red which can magnify the problem. Avoid noisy or 'jangly' jewelery.
- Avoid fidgeting with pens, glasses, etc. Avoid unnecessary movements such as rocking in a chair or moving side to side. Movements you make that may seem slight can be magnified on camera.

- Tipping the bows of your spectacles slightly off your ears may reduce glare off the lenses. Also note what is being reflected in your glasses. Is it something you don't want the person on the other end to see?
- If the person being filmed needs to move out of the camera frame, it is helpful to attempt to move the camera to follow them; however, this can become distracting in the context of a great deal of movement (e.g., frequent moving as means of pain management), so it may be a better solution to take a wide-angled approach.
- Check with the client or person setting up the remote site that they have a clear and large image of the therapist in order to allow observation of the therapists' facial expressions and nonverbal gestures to convey empathy, attunement and warmth.

Be Prepared

- As in in-person settings, it is essential for clinicians to be on time and prepared.
- Pretest the video conference equipment to make sure the audio and visual quality is adequate.
- Arrange a backup plan for technology failure (i.e., to call the client on the landline telephone) or psychiatric crisis (i.e., "in the event of acute suicidal risk, I will advise a local mental health case worker or family etc. . . .") worked out before the session gets underway. Have all the relevant phone numbers of the client, the support services and the IT support with you to enact the emergency plans.
- Advance preparation of sessions gives a better impression that the therapist is "present" and can give their undivided attention to the client without needing to rush off and collect paperwork.
- The technology environment provides a different context to the therapeutic

process and therefore requires different skills and awareness of the professional relationship. Fortunately, evidence suggests that telemental health usually requires little to no additional clinician preparation time than a traditional consultation (Aas, 2003) and typically does not require significant modifications to adult protocols (Singh et al., 2007). However, therapists are advised to rehearse using the equipment in advance of seeing their clients by becoming familiar with the controls, 'zooming' in and out, initiating and disconnecting calls and practicing the PinP function.

- TA can be enhanced by preparing in advance of the first VT encounter. For those seeing clients at a remote site (e.g., a mental health or general practice clinic), this might include establishing a rapport and communication with staff at the remote site, visiting the remote site in-person in order to establish a protocol and view the VT room that clients will be using. This visit can also be used to set up emergency procedures, set up a system for collecting outcome measures and to clarify the logistics of turning on equipment, making calls, adjusting camera views and even to meet clients and demonstrate the equipment if so desired (Simpson, Rochford, Livingstone, English, & Austin, 2014). However, VT is now widely available and increasingly used for private clients as well as via large health services. For some, an introductory telephone call or email to make contact with clients can facilitate the development of rapport and reduce anxiety in preparation for subsequent VT sessions.

Therapeutic communication via VT

- There is some evidence that therapist anxiety can interfere with therapeutic sensitivity by increasing overreactivity in sessions (Ackerman & Hilsenroth, 2001; Germain et al., 2010). Clinicians should therefore take the time to familiarise themselves with the technology and practice using the controls before using it for therapeutic purposes. In addition, clinicians are advised to familiarise themselves with professional guidelines on the use of technology in mental health and pay close attention to ethical and legal guidance.

- Therapist behaviours can enhance TA, including making nonverbal responses more deliberate and explicit, by slightly exaggerating voice inflections, tone and mannerisms, including gestures of encouragement and support; asking more questions or making more detailed reflections, in order to seek clarification of their clients' facial expressions and gestures; offering a preliminary in-person session to facilitate rapport and to introduce the mechanisms for VT (Bischoff et al., 2004; Manchanda & McLaren, 1998). Focusing on clinical flexibility and tapping in to their own creativity can also enhance TA (Tuerk et al., 2010). Be aware that facial and hand gestures are the most effective way of conveying warmth and empathy, especially as the client is usually unable to see their therapist's whole body posture. This can be exaggerated to slightly more than one might show in an in-person setting (Loranzo et al., 2015).
- Ensure that a normal voice is used during VT encounters as in an in-person setting and avoid the urge to increase volume in order to compensate for perceived distance.
- Loranzo et al., (2015) suggest that the first session is essential in building rapport. Initially, a connection can be made with the client through greeting them warmly, then proceeding to introduce

yourself as you would in an in-person setting. Clients can be asked about the experience of travelling to the appointment and checking-in at the remote clinic. The therapist can also ask the client about their position in the room, what else they can see in the room and their level of comfort in order to gain a sense of their environment, as well as to convey interest in their experience and enhance TA.

- The therapist should let the client know about the quality of their sound/picture connection and enquire about the sound and image of the therapist on the screen at the remote site. The therapist can scan their room to show the client where they are situated and to alleviate any concerns that there may be someone else present in the background.
- Clients can be asked about previous experience and comfort with using this type of technology and it can help to orient them to the equipment and remote control so that they have the ability to use the "zoom" function and control camera direction if they are interested in this. This can increase confidence in using the equipment and enhance the communication and rapport. It is suggested that orientation to the equipment be used as a tool to enhance the TA, rather than simply a practical task to be completed.
- Discussion should include informing the client about what they should do if the call drops, whom they can contact and where to find a landline telephone (if this is part of the plan).
- Clients should be given the opportunity to discuss any concerns or anxieties about VT and provide self-disclosure about their own concerns and experiences in order to normalise this. They can also inform clients that research strongly suggests that initial anxieties are

usually allayed after only a short time in VT and that confidence and ease of communication usually increase with experience. The specific advantages of VT can also be explored, both from a general standpoint (based on the research) and from the client's own perspective.

- Informed consent should also be discussed in detail, so that clients understand the implications of sessions being conducted via videoconferencing, and limits associated with confidentiality (Loranzo et al., 2015).

- Therapeutic boundaries should be adhered to throughout VT in order to maintain the professional nature of the interactions and to avoid overlap with more informal types of social media interchange. The following measures are suggested in order to assist with maintaining boundaries (Drum & Littleton, 2014). Arranging sessions to take place within business hours (where possible) can help to differentiate them from other everyday communications and interactions. Sessions should be scheduled so as to maximise consistency, predictability and structure where possible. Be mindful of and flexible around cultural variations – not all cultures place the same importance on structure and punctuality. Familiarise yourself with relevant cultural guidance and expectations when working with those from other cultures (e.g., rules associated with making eye contact, seating height, etc.). Ensure that VT sessions take place in a private setting (at both ends) with minimal background noise. Dress professionally. Take measures to protect the confidentiality of clients, their families and others in their home environment. Use professional language in verbal and written communication to minimise boundary confusion with that of social interactions. Ensure therapist is competent in providing VT services and

has the skills and knowledge necessary to carry out this work by attending relevant training and continuing professional development courses.

CONCLUSION

VT is rapidly establishing itself as a commonly used modality of mental health treatment delivery. TA in VT is increasingly a priority focus as we move beyond the question of *whether* to use VT and instead focus on *how best* to use VT. There are notably several confounding factors associated with interpreting and combining the studies that have been conducted in this area, including the wide range of diagnostic groups, therapeutic treatment models, and technologies used. Nevertheless, preliminary evidence suggests that not only are clinical outcomes roughly equivalent to those in in-person settings, but that TA also appears equivalent. In general, clients rate a high level of TA even from the early stages of therapy, even when technology is low quality. Therapists also adjust to the technology relatively early, with TA ratings increasing over the course of treatment. Therapists appear to accommodate their communication style to work with the technology, thereby facilitating the expression of warmth and empathy. Evidence suggests that they are more likely to ask questions in order to clarify client behaviours and assist with interpretation of client facial expressions and gestures (Bischoff et al., 2004).

Moreover research findings and anecdotal accounts suggest that both clients and therapists perceive a strong social and physical presence within VT, often forgetting that they are not in the same room (Bouchard et al., 2004; Goetter et al., 2013). There is a suggestion that it is in fact the ability of the therapist to connect and to create a warm and empathic therapeutic environment that enables the therapy to bypass any technological barriers (Simpson, Guerrini, & Rochford, 2015). Indeed, it appears to be that the actual 'barriers' themselves may in fact facilitate rapport by providing additional space and an 'equalising' influence on the therapeutic relationship (Richardson, Reid, & Dziurawiec, 2015). Clients often describe feeling less intimidated and scrutinised, thereby facilitating discussion of shame-based difficulties. It is hypothesised that particular client groups may even benefit more from VT than in-person treatment, particularly in the early stages of therapy, such as those who are avoidant of close relationships, those who have body-image difficulties or high levels of self-consciousness and those with a high need for control or personal space. It will be important for future studies to investigate this further and to determine whether VT lends itself to working with particular diagnostic groups and, most importantly, under what circumstances engagement and rapport may be enhanced by the technology. This research will be undertaken in a broader social context in which smartphone video-technology is becoming a familiar part of daily life for young people. As these "digital natives" grow up and become the clients of the future, the demand for technology aided service is likely to increase as will their expectation of "fluency" in the use of these technologies on the part of service providers (Reid, Campbell, Locke, & Charlesworth, 2015). Future research in this area is needed to provide guidance regarding what will provide the strongest basis for training for therapists in this growing field.

REFERENCES

Ackerman, S. J., & Hilsenroth, M. J. (2001). A review of therapist characteristics and techniques negatively impacting the therapeutic alliance. *Psychotherapy: Theory, Research, Practice, Training, 38*: 171–185. DOI: 10.1037/0033-3204.38.2.171.

Agnew-Davies, R., Stiles, W. B., Hardy, G. E., Barkham, M., & Shapiro, D. A. (1998). Alliance structure assessed by the Agnew Relationship Measure (ARM). *British Journal of Clinical Psychology, 37*: 155–172. DOI: 10.1111/j.2044-8260.1998.tb01291.x.

Allen, A., Roman, L., Cox, R., & Cardwell, B. (1996). Home health visits using a cable television network: User satisfaction. *Journal of Telemedicine and Telecare, 2*, 92–94. DOI: 10.1258/1357633961929439.

Austen, S., & McGrath, M. (2006). Attitudes to the use of videoconferencing in general and specialist psychiatric services. *Journal of Telemedicine and Telecare, 12*: 146–150. DOI: 10.1258/135763306776738594.

Backhaus, A., Agha, Z., Maglione M.L., Repp, A., Ross, R., Zuest, D., Rice-Thorp, N.M., Lohr, J., & Thorp, S.R. (2012). Videoconferencing psychotherapy: A systematic review. *Psychological Services, 9*: 111–131. doi: 10.1037/a0027924.

Bischoff, R. J., Hollist, C. S., Smith, C. W., & Flack, P. (2004). Addressing the mental health needs of the rural underserved: findings from a multiple case study of a behavioral telehealth project. *Contemporary Family Therapy, 26*: 179–198.

Bordin, E. S. (1979). The generalizability of the psychoanalytic concept of the working alliance. *Psychotherapy: Theory, Research & Practice, 16*: 252–260. DOI: 10.1037/h0085885.

Bouchard, S. (2004). How to create a therapeutic bond in telehealth: The contribution of telepresence and emotions. Oral presentation at the 7th annual meeting of the Canadian Society of Telehealth, Québec, October 3–5, 2004.

Bouchard, S., Paquin, B., Payeur, R., Allard, M., Rivard, V., Fournier, T., Renaud, P., & Lapierre, J. (2004). Delivering cognitive-behavior therapy for panic disorder with agoraphobia in videoconference. *Telemedicine Journal and E-Health, 10*: 13–25. DOI: 10.1089/153056204773644535.

Bouchard S, Payeur R, Rivard, V. Allard, M., Paquin, B., Renaud, P. & Goyer, L. (2000). Cognitive behavior therapy for panic disorder with agoraphobia in videoconference: preliminary results. *CyberPsychology & Behavior 2000, 3*: 999–1007. doi:10 .1089/109493100452264.

Bouchard S, Robillard G, Marchand A, Renaud P, Riva G, (Eds.) (2007). Presence and the bond between patients and their psychotherapists in the cognitive-behavior therapy of panic disorder with agoraphobia delivered in videoconference. Proceedings of 10th International Workshop on Presence, Barcelona, Spain.

Day, S. X., & Schneider, P. L. (2002). Psychotherapy using distance technology: A comparison of face-to-face, video, and audio treatment. *Journal of Counseling Psychology, 49*: 499–503. DOI: 10.1037//0022 -0167.49.4.499.

Dear, B. (2015) A therapist and coach guide to encryption. *Therapeutic Innovations in Light of Technology, 5*(2), 24–30.

Drum, K. B., & Littleton, H. L. (2014). Therapeutic Boundaries in Telepsychology: unique issues and best practice recommendations. *Prof Psychol Res Pr 45*(5), 309–315. DOI:10.1037/a0036127.

Elliot, R. (1999). Client change interview protocol. Qualitative Interview Protocol ed. Network for Research on Experiential Psychotherapies website. Available at URL: http://experiential-researchers.org/ instruments.html.

Elliott, R., Bohart, A. C., Watson, J. C., & Greenberg, L. S. (2011). Empathy. *Psychotherapy (Chicago, Ill.), 48*: 43–49. doi: 10.1037 /a0022187.

Ertelt, T. W., Crosby, R. D., Marino, J. M., Mitchell, J. E., Lancaster, K., & Crow, S. J. (2011). Therapeutic factors affecting the cognitive behavioral treatment of bulimia nervosa via telemedicine versus face-to-face delivery. *International Journal of Eating Disorders, 44*: 687–691. DOI: 10.1002/eat .20874.

Foster, P., Whitworth, J. (2005). The role of nurses in telemedicine and child abuse. *Computers, Informatics, Nursing, 23*:127–131. DOI: 10.1097/00024665-200505000-00007.

Germain, V., Marchand, A., Bouchard, S., Guay, S., & Drouin, M. S. (2010). Assessment of the therapeutic alliance in face-to-face or videoconference treatment for posttraumatic stress disorder. *Cyberpsychology, Behavior and Social Networking, 13*: 29–35. DOI: 10.1089/cpb.2009.0139.

Gibson, K., O'Donnell, S., Coulson, H., & Kakepetum-Schultz, T. (2011). Mental health professionals' perspectives of telemental health with remote and rural First Nations communities. *Journal of Telemedicine and Telecare, 17*:263–7. doi: 10.1258/jtt .2011.101011.

Glueckauf, R. L., Fritz, S. P., Ecklund-Johnson, E. P., Liss, H. J., Dages, P., & Carney, P. (2002). Videoconferencing-based family counseling for rural teenagers with epilepsy: Phase 1 findings. *Rehabilitation Psychology, 47*: 49–72. DOI: 10.1037/0090 -5550.47.1.49.

Goetter, E. M., Herbert, J. D., Forman, E. M., Yuen, E. K., Gershkovich, M., Glassman, L. H., Rabin, S. J., & Goldstein, S. P. (2013). Delivering exposure and ritual prevention for obsessive-compulsive disorder via videoconference: Clinical considerations and recommendations. *Journal of Obsessive-Compulsive and Related Disorders, 2*: 137–143. doi:10.1016/j.jocrd.2013.01.003.

Grealish, A., Hunter, A., Glaze, R., & Potter, L. (2005). Telemedicine in a child and adolescent mental health service: Participants' acceptance and utilization. *Journal of Telemedicine and Telecare, 11* Suppl 1: 53–5. doi: 10.1258/1357633054461921.

Greene, C. J., Morland, L. A., MacDonald, A., Frueh, B. C., Grubbs, K. M., & Rosen, C. S. (2010). How does tele-mental health affect group therapy process? Secondary analysis of a noninferiority trial. *Journal of*

Consulting and Clinical Psychology, 78: 746–750. doi: 10.1037/a0020158.

Hatcher, R. L., Barends, A., Hansell, J., & Gutfreund, M. J. (1995). Patients' and therapists' shared and unique views of the therapeutic alliance: An investigation using confirmatory factor analysis in a nested design. *Journal of Consulting and Clinical Psychology, 63*: 636–643. DOI: 10.1037/0022-006X.63.4.636.

Hilty, D. M., Ferrer, D. C., Parish, M. B., Johnston, B., Callahan, E. J., & Yellowlees, P. M. (2013). The effectiveness of telemental health: A 2013 review. *Telemedicine and e-Health, 19*(6), 444–454. DOI: 10.1089/tmj.2013.0075.

Himle, J. A., Fischer, D. J., Muroff, J. R., Van Etten, M. L., Lokers, L. M., Abelson, J. L., & Hanna, G. L. (2006). Videoconferencing-based cognitive-behavioral therapy for obsessive-compulsive disorder. *Behaviour Research and Therapy, 44*: 1821–1829. doi:10.1016/j.brat.2005.12.010.

Hopp, F., Whitten, P., Subramanian, U., Woodbridge, P., Mackert, M., & Lowery, J. (2006). Perspectives from the Veterans Health Administration about opportunities and barriers in telemedicine. *Journal of Telemedicine and Telecare, 12*:404–9. doi: 10.1258/135763306779378717.

Horvath, A. O. (2001). The alliance. *Psychotherapy, 38*(4):365–72. http://dx.doi.org/10.1037/0033-3204.38.4.365.

Horvath, A. O., & Symonds, D. B. (1991). Relation between working alliance and outcome in psychotherapy: A meta-analysis. *Journal of Counseling Psychology, 38*:139–49. doi.org/10.1037/0022-0167.38.2.139.

Horvath, A. G., & Leslie, S. (1994). *The working alliance: Theory, research, and practice.* New York: John Wiley.

Horvath, A. O., Del Re, A., Flückiger, C., & Symonds, D. (2011). Alliance in individual psychotherapy. *Psychotherapy* (Chicago, Ill.), *48*: 9–16. doi: 10.1037/a0022186.

Jones, R. M., Leonard, S., & Birmingham, L.

(2006). Setting up a telepsychiatry service. *Psychiatric Bulletin, 30*:464–467. DOI: 10.1192/pb.30.12.464

Kavanagh, S. J., & Yellowlees, P. M. (1995). Telemedicine: Clinical applications in mental health. *Australian Family Physician, 24*:1242.

Krumm-Heller Roe, I. (2006). Therapeutic alliance in psychotherapy conducted through videoconferencing (PhD). Santa Barbara, CA: Fielding Graduate University.

Lozano, B. E., Birks, A. H., Kloezeman, K., Cha, N., Morland, L. A., & Tuerk, P. W. (2015). Therapeutic alliance in clinical videoconferencing: Optimizing the communication context. In P. W. Tuerk & P. Shore (Eds.), *Clinical Videoconferencing in telehealth: Program development and practice.* Switzerland: Springer, pp. 221–251. doi: 10.1007/978-3-319-08765-8_10.

Manchanda, M., & McLaren, P. (1998). Cognitive behaviour therapy via interactive video. *Journal of Telemedicine and Telecare, 4* (Suppl1): 53–55. doi: 10.1258/1357633981931452.

Mair, F., & Whitten, P. (2000). Systematic review of studies of patient satisfaction with telemedicine. *British Medical Journal* (Clinical Research Ed.), *320*: 1517–1520. doi: http://dx.doi.org/10.1136/bmj.320.7248.1517.

Martin, C. (2004). *Corrections telemedicine services program.* Sacramento, CA: Office of Telemedicine Services.

Martin, D. J., Garske, J. P., & Davis, M. (2000). Relation of the therapeutic alliance with outcome and other variables: A meta-analytic review. *Journal of Consulting and Clinical Psychology, 68*: 438–450. doi. apa.org/journals/cou/38/2/139.pdf.

McLaren, P., & Ball, C. J. (1997). Interpersonal communications and telemedicine: Hypotheses and methods. *Journal of Telemedicine & Telecare, 3* (Suppl. 1), 5–7.

McLaren, P., Ball, C. J., Summerfield, A. B., Watson, J. P., & Lipsedge, M. (1995). An evaluation of the use of interactive television in an acute psychiatric service. *Journal of Telemedicine & Telecare, 1*, 79–85.

Mitchell, D., Simpson, S., Ferguson, J., & Smith, F. (2003). NHS staff attitudes to the use of videoconferencing to deliver clinical services. Poster presentation. In: *Telemed 2003*. London, Royal Society of Medicine.

Mitchell, J. E., Myers, T., Swan-Kremeier, L., & Wonderlich, S. (2003). Psychotherapy for bulimia nervosa delivered via telemedicine. *European Eating Disorders Review, 11*: 222–230. DOI: 10.1002/erv.517.

Onor, M. L., & Misan, S. (2005). The clinical interview and the doctor-patient relationship in telemedicine. *Telemedicine and e-Health, 11*(1), 102–105. doi:10.1089/tm .2005.11.102.

Omodei, M., & McLennan, J. (1998). The more I see you? Face-to-face, video and telephone counselling compared. A programme of research investigating the emerging technology of videophone for counselling. *Australian Journal of Psychology, 50*(1) (suppl.), 109. doi: 10.1080/00049 539808258786.

Pinsof, W. M., & Catherall, D. R. (1986). The integrative psychotherapy alliance: Family, couple, and individual therapy scales. *Journal of Marital and Family Therapy, 12*: 137–151. doi: 10.1111/j.1752-0606.1986. tb01631.x.

Porcari, C. E., Amdur, R. L., Koch, E. I., Richard, D. C., Favorite, T., Martis, B., & Liberzon, I. (2009). Assessment of post-traumatic stress disorder in veterans by videoconferencing and by face-to-face methods. *Journal of Telemedicine and Telecare, 15*: 89–94. doi: 10.1258/jtt.2008.080612.

Rees, C. S., & Haythornthwaite, S. (2004). Telepsychology and videoconferencing: Issues, opportunities and guidelines for psychologists. *Australian Psychologist, 39*: 212–219. DOI:10.1080/000500604123312 95108.

Rees, C. S., & Stone, S. (2005).Therapeutic alliance in face-to-face versus video-conferenced psychotherapy. *Professional Psychology, Research and Practice, 36*: 649. DOI: 10.1037/0735-7028.36.6.649.

Reid, Campbell, Locke, & Charlesworth. (2015). Australian men's hockey team: Virtually there. Telepsychology in Olympic sport. *Australian Psychologist.*

Richardson, L. (2011). *'Can you see what i am saying?': An action-research, mixed methods evaluation of telepsychology in rural Western Australia.* Perth, Australia: Murdoch University.

Richardson, L. K., Frueh, B., Grubaugh, A. L., Egede, L., & Elhai, J. D. (2009). Current directions in videoconferencing telemental health research. *Clinical Psychology: Science and Practice, 16*: 323–338. doi: 10.1111 /j.1468-2850.2009.01170.x.

Richardson, L. K., Reid, C., & Dziurawiec, S. (2015). "Going the extra mile": Satisfaction and alliance findings from an evaluation of videoconferencing telepsychology in rural Western Australia. *The Australian Psychologist.*

Ronzio, J. L., Tuerk, P. W., & Shore, P. (2015). Technologies and clinical videoconferencing infrastructures: A guide to selecting appropriate systems. In P. W. Tuerk & P. Shore (Eds.), *Clinical videoconferencing in telehealth: Program development and practice.* Switzerland: Springer, pp. 3–23. 10.1007/ 978-3-319-08765-8_1.

Ruskin, P. E., Silver-Aylaian, M., Kling, M. A., Reed, S. A., Bradham, D. D. & Hebel, J. R. (2004). Treatment outcomes in depression: Comparison of remote treatment through telepsychiatry to in-person treatment. *American Journal of Psychiatry, 161*: 1471–1476. doi: 10.1176/appi.ajp.161.8.1471.

Sadowski, W. (2002). Presence in virtual environments. In K. M. Stanney (Ed.), *Handbook of virtual environments: Design, implementation and applications.* Mahwah, NJ: IEA, pp. 791–806.

Safran, J. D., & Wallner, L. K. (1991). The relative predictive validity of two therapeutic alliance measures in cognitive therapy. *Psychological Assessment: A Journal of Consulting and Clinical Psychology, 3*: 188–195. doi: 10.1037/1040-3590.3.2.188.

Shirk, S. R., & Karver, M. (2003). Prediction of treatment outcome from relationship variables in child and adolescent therapy: A meta-analytic review. *Journal of Consulting Clinical Psychology, 71*(3): 452–64.

Simms, D.C., Gibson, K., & O'Donnell, S. (2011). To use or not to use: Clinicians' perceptions of telemental health. *Canadian Psychology, 52*:41–51.

Simpson, S. (2001). The provision of a tele-psychology service to Shetland: Client and therapist satisfaction and the ability to develop a therapeutic alliance. *Journal of Telemedicine & Telecare, 7*(Suppl. 1): 34–36. doi:10.1258/1357633011936633.

Simpson, S. (2005). Videoconferencing and technological advances in the treatment of eating disorders. In P. Swain (Ed.), *Eating disorders: New research.* New York: Nova Biomedical, pp. 99–115.

Simpson, S. (2009). Psychotherapy via video-conferencing: A review. *British Journal of Guidance and Counselling, 37*(3): 271–286. doi:10.1080/03069880902957007.

Simpson, S. (2010). The use of alternative technology for conducting a therapeutic relationship on videoconferencing. In K. Anthony, D. M. Nagel, & S. Goss S. (Eds.), *The use of technology in mental health: Applications, ethics and practice.* Springfield, IL: Charles C Thomas, pp. 94–103.

Simpson S., Bell L., & Britton P. (2006). Does video therapy work? A single case series of bulimic disorders. *European Eating Disorders Review, 14*: 226–241.

Simpson, S., Bell, L., Knox, J., & Mitchell, D. (2005). Therapy via video-conferencing: A route to client empowerment? *Clinical Psychology and Psychotherapy, 12*: 156–165. doi:10.1002/cpp.436

Simpson, S., Deans, G., & Brebner, E. (2001).

The delivery of a tele-psychology service to Shetland. *Clinical Psychology & Psychotherapy, 8*(2): 130–135.

Simpson, S., Guerrini, L., & Rochford, S. (2015). Videoconferencing psychotherapy in a university psychology clinic setting: A pilot project. *Australian Psychologist.*

Simpson, S., Knox, J., Mitchell, D., Ferguson, J., Brebner, J., & Brebner, E. (2003). A multidisciplinary approach to the treatment of eating disorders via videoconferencing in northeast Scotland. *Journal of Telemedicine and Telecare, 9*: 37–38. doi: 10.1258/135763303322196286.

Simpson, S., Morrow, E., Jones, M., Ferguson, J., & Brebner, E. (2002). Tele-hypnosis – the provision of specialized therapeutic treatments via teleconferencing. *Journal of Telemedicine and Telecare, 8*(Suppl. 2)78–79. DOI:10.1258/135763302320302136.

Simpson, S. G., & Slowey, L. (2011). Video therapy for atypical eating disorder and obesity: A case study. *Clinical Practice and Epidemiology in Mental Health, 7*, 38–43. doi: 10.2174/1745017901107010038.

Simpson, S., & Reid, C. (2014). Therapeutic alliance in videoconferencing psychotherapy: A review. *Australian Journal of Rural Health, 22*(6): 280–299. doi:10.1111/ajr.12149.

Simpson, S., Rochford, S., Livingstone, A., English, S., & Austin, C. (2014). Tele-web psychology in rural south Australia: The logistics of setting up a remote university clinic staffed by clinical psychologists in training. *Australian Psychologist, 49*(4): 193–199. doi:10.1111/ap.12049.

Simpson, S. G., & Slowey, L. (2011). Video therapy for atypical eating disorder and obesity: A case study. *Clinical Practice and Epidemiology in Mental Health, 7*: 38–43. doi: 10.2174/1745017901107010038.

Starling, J., & Foley, S. (2006). From pilot to permanent service: Ten years of pediatric telepsychiatry. *Journal of Telemedicine and Telecare, 12*: S80–S82. doi: 10.1258/135763306779380147

Steel, K., Cox, D., & Garry, H. (2011). Therapeutic videoconferencing interventions for the treatment of long-term conditions. *Journal of Telemedicine and Telecare, 17*: 109–17. doi: 10.1258/jtt.2010.100318.

Stubbings, D. R. (2012). *The effectiveness of videoconference-based cognitive-behavioural therapy* (PhD). Perth, Australia: Curtin University.

Tachakra, S., & Rajani, R. (2002). Social presence in telemedicine. *Journal of Telemedicine and Telecare, 8*: 226–230. doi: 10.1258/1357633302320272202.

Thomas, C. R., Miller, G., Hartshorn, J. C., Speck, N. C., & Walker, G. (2005). Telepsychiatry program for rural victims of domestic violence. *Telemedicine and e-Health, 11*: 567–573. doi: 10.1089/tmj.2005.11.567.

Tichenor, V., & Hill, C. E. (1989). A comparison of six measures of working alliance. *Psychotherapy: Theory, Research, Practice, Training, 26*: 195–199. doi: 10.1037/h0085419.

Tuerk, P. W., Yoder, M., Ruggiero, K. J., Gros, D. F., & Acierno R. (2010). A pilot study of prolonged exposure therapy for posttraumatic stress disorder delivered via telehealth technology. *Journal of Traumatic Stress, 23*: 116–123. DOI: 10.1002/jts.20494.

Wade, S. L., Wolfe, C., Brown, T. M., & Pestian, J. P. (2005). Putting the pieces together: Preliminary efficacy of a web-based family intervention for children with traumatic brain injury. *Journal of Pediatric Psychology, 30*: 437–442. doi: 10.1093/jpepsy/jsi067.

Wagnild, G., Leenknecht, C., & Zauher, J. (2006). Psychiatrists' satisfaction with telepsychiatry. *Telemedicine Journal and E-Health, 12*: 546–551. doi:10.1089/tmj.2006.12.546.

Wampold, B. E. (2001). *The great psychotherapy debate: Models, methods, and findings.* Mahwah, NJ: Lawrence Erlbaum.

Whitten, P. S., & Mackert, M. S. (2005). Addressing telehealth's foremost barrier: Provider as initial gatekeeper. *International Journal of Technology Assessment in Health Care, 21*: 517–521. doi: 10.1017/S0266462305050725.

Whitten, P., & Kuwahara, E. (2004). A multiphase telepsychiatry programme in Michigan: Organizational factors affecting utilization and user perception. *Journal of Telemedicine and Telecare, 10*: 254–61. doi: 10.1258/1357633042026378.

Wray, B. T., & Rees, C. S. (2003). Is there a role for videoconferencing in cognitive-behavioural therapy? 11th Australian Association for Cognitive and Behaviour Therapy State Conference, Perth, Australia, 2003.

Yuen, E. K., Herbert, J. D., Forman, E. M., Goetter, E. M., Juarascio, A. S., Rabin, S., Goodwin, C., & Bouchard, S. (2013). Acceptance based behavior therapy for social anxiety disorder through videoconferencing. *Journal of Anxiety Disorders, 27*: 389–397. doi:10.1016/j.janxdis.2013.03.002.

Chapter 11

USING VIRTUAL REALITY IMMERSION THERAPEUTICALLY

Giuseppe Riva and Claudia Repetto

INTRODUCTION

How is it possible to change a client? Even if this question has many different answers according to the specific psychotherapeutic approach, in general, change comes through an intense focus on a particular instance or experience (Wolfe, 2002; Inghilleri et al., 2015). By exploring it as much as possible, the client can relive all of the significant elements associated with it (i.e., conceptual, emotional, motivational and behavioral) and make them available for a reorganization of his or her perspective.

Within this general model we have, for example, the insight-based approach of psychoanalysis, the schema-reorganization goals of cognitive therapy, or the enhancement of experience awareness in experiential therapies. What are the differences between them? According to Safran and Greenberg (1991), behind the specific therapeutic approach, we can find two different models of change: bottom-up and top-down.

These two models of change are focused on two different cognitive systems, one for information transmission (top-down) and one for conscious experience (bottom-up), both of which may process sensory input. The existence of two different cognitive systems is clearly shown by the distinction between verbal knowledge and task performance: people learn to control dynamic systems without being able to specify the nature of the relations within the system and they can sometimes describe the rules by which the system operates without being able to put them into practice.

Even if many therapeutic approaches are based on just one of the two change models, a therapist usually requires both. Some clients seem to operate primarily by means of top-down information processing, which may then prepare the way for corrective emotional experiences. For others the appropriate access point is the intensification of their emotional experience and their awareness of it. Finally, different clients who initially engage the therapeutic work only through top-down processing may be able later in the therapy to make use of bottom-up emotional processing. A possible way to address this issue is through use of advanced technologies. In particular, using a novel technology – Virtual Reality (VR) – it is now possible to create synthetic experiences that allow both bottom-up and top-down interventions (Riva et al., 2014).

A VR system is the combination of the hardware and software that enables developers to create synthetic life-like experiences.

The hardware components receive input from user-controlled devices and convey multisensory output to create the illusion of a virtual world. The software component of a VR system manages the hardware that makes up the VR system. The virtual world may be a model of a real-world object, such as a house, or an abstract world that does not exist in a real sense but is understood by humans, such as a chemical molecule or a representation of a set of data, or it might be a completely imaginary world.

According to the hardware and software included in a VR system, it is possible to distinguish between (Riva, 2014):

- *Fully Immersive VR:* the user appears to be fully inserted in the computer generated environment. This illusion is produced by providing immersive output devices (e.g., head mounted display, force feedback robotic arms, etc.) and a system of head/body tracking to guarantee the exact correspondence and coordination of users' movements with the feedback of the environment.
- *CAVE:* This is a small room where a computer-generated world is projected on the walls. This solution is particularly suitable for collective VR experiences because it allows different people to share the same experience at the same time.
- *Augmented:* the user's view of the world is supplemented with virtual objects, usually to provide information about the real environment.
- *Desktop VR:* uses subjective immersion on a standard PC screen. The feeling of immersion can be improved through stereoscopic vision.

VR IN CLINICAL PSYCHOLOGY

Several VR applications for the understanding, assessment and treatment of mental health problems have been developed in the last 15 years (Riva, 2005; Wiederhold & Riva, 2014).

Typically, in VR Exposure (VRE) therapy, the client learns to manipulate problematic situations related to his/her difficulties by working both on its experiential/emotional and cognitive/behavioral aspects. For this reason, common applications of VR in this area include the treatment of anxiety disorders (Emmelkamp, 2005; Parsons & Rizzo, 2008), simple phobias (Krijn et al., 2007; Opris et al., 2012; Rothbaum et al., 2006), panic disorders (Botella et al., 2007; Quero et al, 2014; Vincelli et al., 2003), posttraumatic stress disorder (Gerardi et al., 2008; Rothbaum et al., 2001) and stress management (Villani et al., 2007; Serino et al., 2014).

Indeed, VRE has been proposed as a medium for exposure therapy (Gorini & Riva, 2008) that is safer, less embarrassing and less costly than reproducing the real world situations. The rationale is simple: in VR the client is intentionally confronted with the feared stimuli while allowing the anxiety to attenuate. Avoiding a dreaded situation reinforces a phobia and each successive exposure to it reduces the anxiety through the processes of habituation and extinction.

VRE offers a number of advantages over *in vivo* or imaginal exposure. Firstly, VRE can be administered in traditional therapeutic settings. This means VRE may be more convenient, controlled and cost-effective than *in vivo* exposure. Secondly, it can also isolate fear components more efficiently than *in vivo* exposure. For instance, in treating fear of flying, if landing is the most fearful part of the experience, landing can be repeated as often as necessary without having to wait for the airplane to take-off. Finally, the immersive nature of VRE provides a real-like experience that may be more emotionally engaging than imaginal exposure.

However, it seems likely that VR can be more than a tool to provide exposure and desensitisation (Riva, 2005, 2014). As noted by Glantz et al. (1997), "VR technology may create enough capabilities to profoundly influence the shape of therapy" (p. 92). In fact, the key characteristics of virtual environments for most clinical applications are the high level of control of the interaction with the tool and the enriched experience provided to the client (Schultheis & Rizzo, 2001).

On the one hand, it can be described as an advanced form of human-computer interface that allows the user to interact with and become immersed in a computer-generated environment in a naturalistic fashion. On the other hand, VR can also be considered as an advanced imaginal system: a medium that is as effective as reality in inducing emotional responses. This is achieved through its ability to induce a feeling of "presence" in the computer-generated world experienced by the user (Riva et al., 2007).

These features transform VR in an "empowering environment," a special, sheltered setting where clients can start to explore and act without feeling actually threatened (Botella et al., 2007). Nothing the client fears can "really" happen to them in VR. With such assurance, they can more freely explore, experiment, feel, live and experience feelings and/or thoughts. VR thus becomes a very useful intermediate step between the therapist's office and the real world (Botella et al., 2004).

Emerging applications of VR in psychotherapy include sexual disorders (Optale, 2003; Optale et al., 1998), pain management (Garrett et al., 2014; Hoffman, 2004; Hoffman et al., 2008; Keefe et al., 2012; Triberti et al., 2014), addictions (Bordnick et al., 2005; Bordnick et al., 2008; Gatti et al., 2008; Lee et al., 2007), persecutory delusions (Fornells-Ambrojo et al., 2008, 2015), stress management (Villani et al., 2007; Serino et al., 2014) and eating disorders and obesity (Riva et al., 2006; Riva et al., 2003; Ferrer-Garcia et al., 2013). In fact, immersive VR can be considered an "embodied technology" for its effects on body perceptions (Lambrey & Berthoz, 2003; Riva, 2008; Vidal et al., 2003; Vidal et al., 2004). VR users become aware of their bodies during navigation: e.g., their head movements alter what they see. The sensorimotor coordination of the moving head with visual displays produces a much higher level of sensorimotor feedback and first person perspective (egocentric reference frame).

For example, through the use of immersive VR, it is possible to induce a controlled sensory rearrangement that facilitates the update of the biased body image. This allows the differentiation and integration of new information, leading to a new sense of cohesiveness and consistency in how the self represents the body. The results of this approach are very promising. As shown by different experimental research, VR is effective in producing fast changes in body experience (Murray & Gordon, 2001; Riva, 1998) and in body dissatisfaction (Riva et al., 1998; Riva et al., 2000; Riva et al., 2002; Perpina et al., 2003; Riva et al., 2004; Riva et al., 2006; Ferrer-Garcia et al., 2013) that may improve long-term outcomes of the cognitive behavioural approach to eating disorders and obesity.

Apparently, a similar approach may be used in other pathologies. Lambrey and Berthoz (2003) showed that subjects use conflicting visual and nonvisual information differently according to individual "perceptive styles" (bottom-up processes) and that these "perceptive styles" are made more observable by the subjects changing their perceptive strategy, i.e., reweighting (top-down processes).

Viaud-Delmon and colleagues (Viaud–Delmon et al., 2000; Viaud-Delmon et al., 2002) showed that subjects with high trait anxiety, such as people with symptoms of panic and agoraphobia, have a strong dependence on a particular reference frame in which the sensory information are interpreted and in which they would remain anchored. A VR experience aimed at modifying the sensory reference frame may be useful in speeding up the process of change. Future studies are needed both to identify specific perceptive styles in different pathologies and to define the best protocols for changing them.

Future VR clinical applications will also include online virtual worlds (such as Second Life, There or Active Worlds): computer-based simulated environments characterized by the simultaneous presence of multiple users within the same simulated space, who inhabit and interact via avatars (Gorini et al., 2007). Online virtual worlds can be considered as 3-D social networks, where people can collaboratively create and edit objects, besides meeting each other and interacting with existing objects (Gorini et al., 2008). Over the last few years the number of virtual worlds' users has dramatically increased and today Second Life, the largest 3-D on line digital world, counts about 12 million subscribers.

VR IN CLINICAL PRACTICE: FROM THEORY TO PRACTICE

Although it is indisputable that VR has come of age for clinical and research applications, the majority of them are still in the laboratory or investigation stage. In a review, Riva (2005) identified four major issues that limit the use of VR in psychotherapy:

- the lack of standardisation in VR hardware and software and the limited possibility of tailoring the virtual environments (VEs) to the specific requirements of the clinical or the experimental setting;
- the low availability of standardised protocols that can be shared by the community of researchers;
- the high costs (up to 200,000 US$) required for designing and testing a clinical VR application;
- some VEs in use today not being user-friendly, as expensive technical support

or continual maintenance are often required.

To address these challenges, we have designed and developed NeuroVR (http://www.neurovr.org), a cost-free virtual reality platform based on open-source software, that allows nonexpert users to easily modify a virtual environment (VE) and to visualise it using either an immersive or nonimmersive system.

The NeuroVR platform is implemented using open-source components that provide advanced features; this includes an interactive rendering system based on OpenGL, which allows for high quality images. The NeuroVR Editor is realised by customising the user interface of Blender, an integrated suite of 3D creation tools available on all major operating systems; this implies that the program can be distributed even with the complete source code. Thanks to these features, clinicians and researchers have the freedom to run, copy, distribute, study, change and improve the Neuro VR Editor software, so that the whole VR community benefits.

THE NEUROVR EDITOR

The majority of existing VEs for psychotherapy are proprietary and have closed source code, meaning they cannot be tailored from the ground up to fit specific needs of different clinical applications (Riva, 2005). NeuroVR addresses these issues by providing the clinical professional with a cost-free VE editor, which allows nonexpert users to easily modify a virtual scene to best suit the needs of the clinical setting.

USING THE NEUROVR EDITOR

The psychological stimuli/stressors appropriate for any given scenario (see Figure 11.1) can be chosen from a rich database of 2D

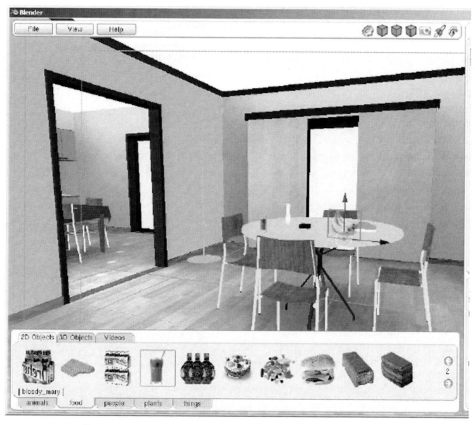

Figure 11.1. A screenshot taken from the NeuroVR Editor.

and 3D objects and easily placed into the pre-designed virtual scenario by using an icon-based interface (no programming skills are required). In addition to static objects, the NeuroVR Editor allows the user to combine a video with the 3D background to create the appearance of partial transparency (known as alpha compositing).

The editing of the scene is performed in real time and effects of changes can be checked from different views (frontal, lateral and top). Currently, the NeuroVR library includes different pre-designed virtual scenes, representing typical real-life situations, e.g., the supermarket, the apartment, the park. These VEs have been designed, developed and assessed in the past ten years by a multidisciplinary research team in several clinical trials, which have involved over 400 clients (Riva et al., 2004, 2011). On the basis of this experience, only the most effective VEs have been selected for inclusion in the NeuroVR library.

An interesting feature of the Neuro VR Editor is the possibility to add new objects to the database. This feature allows the therapist to enhance the client's feeling of familiarity and intimacy with the virtual scene by using photos of objects/people that are part of the client's daily life, thereby improving the efficacy of the exposure (Riva et al., 2004, 2011).

THE NEUROVR PLAYER

The second main component of NeuroVR is the Player, which allows the user to navigate and interact with the VEs created using the NeuroVR Editor. When running simulations, the system offers a set of standard features that contribute to increase the realism of the simulated scene. These include collision detection to control movements in the environment, realistic walk-style motion, advanced lighting techniques for enhanced image quality and streaming of video textures using alpha channel for transparency. The NeuroVR player can be configured for two basic visualisation modalities: immersive and nonimmersive. The immersive modality allows the scene to be visualised using a head-mounted display, either in stereoscopic or in mono-mode; compatibility with head-tracking sensor is also provided. In the nonimmersive modality, the virtual environment can be displayed using a desktop monitor or a wall projector. The user can interact with the virtual environment using either keyboard commands, a mouse, or a joypad, depending on the hardware configuration chosen.

CONCLUSION

Clients are not all the same. Some clients seem to operate primarily by means of top-down information processing (from cognition to emotions), which may then prime the way for corrective emotional experiences. For others, the appropriate access point is the intensification of their emotional experience and their awareness of it (from emotions to cognitions). Nevertheless, psychotherapeutic approaches usually do not target both paths for change, even if having a dual approach could improve the long-term efficacy of the treatment. The use of Virtual Reality (VR), an experiential technology that puts the client inside a life-like synthetic world, can be a so-lution for this issue.

The key characteristics of virtual environments for most clinical applications are the high level of control of the interaction with the tool and the enriched experience provided to the client (Schultheis & Rizzo, 2001). For these features, VR is described as a "simulation technology" with and within which people can interact. In summary, VR provides a new human-computer interaction paradigm in which users are no longer simply external observers of images on a computer screen but are active participants within a computer-generated, three-dimensional virtual world (Riva, 1997).

Even if the potential impact of VR in clinical psychology is high – as shown by the many articles discussing VR applications for simple phobias (Krijn et al., 2007; Opris et al., 2012; Rothbaum et al., 2006), panic disorders (Botella et al., 2007; Quero et al, 2014; Vincelli et al., 2003), posttraumatic stress disorder (Gerardi et al., 2008; Rothbaum et al., 2001), sexual disorders (Optale, 2003; Optale et al., 1998), pain management (Garrett et al., 2014; Hoffman, 2004; Hoffman et al., 2008; Keefe et al., 2012; Triberti et al., 2014), addictions (Bordnick et al., 2005; Bordnick et al., 2008; Gatti et al., 2008; Lee et al., 2007), persecutory delusions (Fornells-Ambrojo et al., 2008, 2015), stress management (Villani et al., 2007; Serino et al., 2014) and eating disorders and obesity (Riva et al., 2006; Riva et al., 2003; Ferrer-Garcia et al., 2013 – the majority of the existing clinical VR applications are still in the laboratory or investigation stage.

To address the challenges outlined in this chapter, we have designed and developed NeuroVR (http://www.neurovr.org), a cost-free virtual reality platform based on open-source software that allows nonexpert users to test VR use in clinical practice using either an immersive or nonimmersive system (Riva et al., 2011). Currently, the NeuroVR library includes different predesigned virtual worlds that can be easily adapted for targeting different clinical applications: from phobias to eating disorders.

However, to exploit the full potential of VR tools, the development of future clinical applications will require multidisciplinary teams of engineers, computer programmers, and therapists working in concert to treat specific problems. Hopefully, by bringing this community of experts together, further interest from clinicians and granting agencies will be stimulated. In particular, information on VR technology must be made available to the health care community in a format that is easy-to-understand and which invites participation.

Acknowledgment

The present work was supported by the Italian MIUR FIRB programme (Project "IVT2010 – Immersive Virtual. Telepresence (IVT) for Experiential Assessment and Rehabilitation – RBIN 04BC5C) and by the European Union IST Programme (Project "INTREPID – A Virtual Reality Intelligent Multi-sensor Wearable System for Phobias' Treatment" – IST-2002- 507464).

REFERENCES

Bordnick, P. S., Graap, K. M., Copp, H. L., Brooks, J., & Ferrer, M. (2005). Virtual reality cue reactivity assessment in cigarette smokers. *Cyberpsychology and Behavior, 8*(5), 487–492.

Bordnick, P. S., Traylor, A., Copp, H. L., Graap, K. M., Carter, B., Ferrer, M., & Walton, A. P. (2008). Assessing reactivity to virtual reality alcohol based cues. *Addictive Behaviors, 33*(6), 743–756.

Botella, C., García-Palacios, A., Villa, H., Baños, R. M., Quero, M., Alcañiz, M., & Riva, G. (2007). Virtual reality exposure in the treatment of panic disorder and agoraphobia: A controlled study. *Clinical Psy-*

chology and Psychotherapy, 14(3), 164–175.

Botella, C., Quero, S., Baños, R. M., Perpiña, C., Garcia Palacios, A., & Riva, G. (2004). Virtual reality and psychotherapy. *Studies in Health Technology and Informatics, 99,* 37–54.

Emmelkamp, P. M. (2005). Technological innovations in clinical assessment and psychotherapy. *Psychotherapy and Psychosomatics, 74*(6), 336–343.

Ferrer-Garcia, M., Gutiérrez-Maldonado, J., & Riva, G. (2013). Virtual reality based treatments in eating disorders and obesity: A review. *Journal of Contemporary Psychotherapy, 43*(4), 207–221.

Fornells-Ambrojo, M., Barker, C., Swapp, D., Slater, M., Antley, A., & Freeman, D. (2008). Virtual reality and persecutory delusions: Safety and feasibility. *Schizophrenia Research, 104*(1–3), 228–236.

Fornells-Ambrojo, M., Freeman, D., Slater, M., Swapp, D., Antley, A., & Barker, C. (2015). How do people with persecutory delusions evaluate threat in a controlled social environment? A qualitative study using virtual reality. *Behavioural and cognitive psychotherapy, 43*(01), 89–107.

Garrett, B., Taverner, T., Masinde, W., Gromala, D., Shaw, C., & Negraeff, M. (2014). A rapid evidence assessment of immersive virtual reality as an adjunct therapy in acute pain management in clinical practice. *The Clinical Journal of Pain, 30*(12), 1089–1098.

Gatti, E., Massari, R., Sacchelli, C., Lops, T., Gatti, R., & Riva, G. (2008). Why do you drink? Virtual reality as an experiential medium for the assessment of alcohol-dependent individuals. *Studies in Health Technology and Informatics, 132,* 132–137.

Gerardi, M., Rothbaum, B. O., Ressler, K., Heekin, M., & Rizzo, A. (2008). Virtual reality exposure therapy using a virtual Iraq: Case report. *Journal of Traumatic Stress, 21*(2), 209–213.

Glantz, K., Durlach, N. I., Barnett, R. C., &

Aviles, W. A. (1997). Virtual reality (VR) and psychotherapy: Opportunities and challenges. *Presence, Teleoperators, and Virtual Environments, 6*(1), 87–105.

Gorini, A., Gaggioli, A., & Riva, G. (2007). Virtual worlds, real healing. *Science, 318* (5856), 1549.

Gorini, A., Gaggioli, A., Vigna, C., & Riva, G. (2008). A second life for eHealth: Prospects for the use of 3-D virtual worlds in clinical psychology. *Journal of Medical Internet Research, 10*(3), e21.

Gorini, A., & Riva, G. (2008). Virtual reality in anxiety disorders: The past and the future. *Expert Review of Neurotherapeutics, 8*(2), 215–233.

Hoffman, H. G. (2004). Virtual-reality therapy: Clients can get relief from pain or overcome their phobias by immersing themselves in computer-generated worlds. *Scientific American, 291*(2), 58–65.

Hoffman, H. G., Patterson, D. R., Seibel, E., Soltani, M., Jewett-Leahy, L., & Sharar, S. R. (2008). Virtual reality pain control during burn wound debridement in the hydrotank. *Clinical Journal of Pain, 24*(4), 299–304.

Inghilleri, P., Riva, G., & Riva, E. (Eds.). (2015). *Enabling positive change. flow and complexity in daily experience.* Berlin: De Gruyter Open. Online: http://www.degruyter.com/view/product/449663.

Keefe, F. J., Huling, D. A., Coggins, M. J., Keefe, D. F., Rosenthal, M. Z., Herr, N. R., & Hoffman, H. G. (2012). Virtual reality for persistent pain: A new direction for behavioral pain management. *PAIN®, 153*(11), 2163–2166.

Krijn, M., Emmelkamp, P. M., Olafsson, R. P., Schuemie, M. J., & van der Mast, C. A. (2007). Do self-statements enhance the effectiveness of virtual reality exposure therapy? A comparative evaluation in acrophobia. *Cyberpsychology and Behavior, 10*(3), 362–370.

Lambrey, S., & Berthoz, A. (2003). Combination of conflicting visual and non-visual information for estimating actively performed body turns in virtual reality. *International Journal of Psychophysiology, 50*(1–2), 101–115.

Lee, J. H., Kwon, H., Choi, J., & Yang, B. H. (2007). Cue-exposure therapy to decrease alcohol craving in virtual environment. *Cyberpsychology and Behavior, 10*(5), 617–623.

Murray, C. D., & Gordon, M. S. (2001). Changes in bodily awareness induced by immersive virtual reality. *Cyberpsychology and Behavior, 4*(3), 365–371.

Optale, G. (2003). Male sexual dysfunctions and multimedia immersion therapy. *Cyberpsychology and Behavior, 6*(3), 289–294.

Optale, G., Chierichetti, F., Munari, A., Nasta, A., Pianon, C., Viggiano, G., & Ferlin, G. (1998). Brain PET confirms the effectiveness of VR treatment of impotence. *International Journal of Impotence Research, 10*(Suppl 1), 45.

Opriş, D., Pintea, S., García-Palacios, A., Botella, C., Szamosközi, Ş., & David, D. (2012). Virtual reality exposure therapy in anxiety disorders: A quantitative meta-analysis. *Depression and Anxiety, 29*(2), 85–93.

Parsons, T. D., & Rizzo, A. A. (2008). Affective outcomes of virtual reality exposure therapy for anxiety and specific phobias: A meta-analysis. *Journal of Behavior Therapy and Experimental Psychiatry, 39*, 250–261.

Perpiña, C., Botella, C., & Baños, R. M. (2003). Virtual reality in eating disorders. *European Eating Disorders Review, 11*(3), 261–278.

Quero, S., Pérez-Ara, M. Á., Bretón-López, J., García-Palacios, A., Baños, R. M., & Botella, C. (2014). Acceptability of virtual reality interoceptive exposure for the treatment of panic disorder with agoraphobia. *British Journal of Guidance & Counselling, 42*(2), 123–137.

Riva, G. (Ed.) (1997). *Virtual reality in neuropsychophysiology: Cognitive, clinical and methodological issues in assessment and reha-*

bilitation. Amsterdam: IOS Press.

Riva, G. (1998). Modifications of body image induced by virtual reality. *Perceptual and Motor Skills, 86*(1), 163–170.

Riva, G. (2005). Virtual reality in psychotherapy: Review. *Cyberpsychology and Behavior, 8*(3), 220–240.

Riva, G. (2008). From virtual to real body: Virtual reality as embodied technology. *Journal of Cybertherapy and Rehabilitation, 1*(1), 7–22.

Riva, G. (2014). Medical clinical uses of virtual worlds. In M. Grimshaw (Ed.), *The Oxford handbook of virtuality.* New York, Oxford University Press (2014), pp. 649–665

Riva, G., Bacchetta, M., Baruffi, M., Rinaldi, S., & Molinari, E. (1998). Experiential cognitive therapy in anorexia nervosa. *Eating and Weight Disorders, 3*(3), 141–150.

Riva, G., Bacchetta, M., Baruffi, M., Cirillo, G., & Molinari, E. (2000). Virtual reality environment for body image modification: A multidimensional therapy for the treatment of body image in obesity and related pathologies. *Cyberpsychology and Behavior, 3*(3), 421–431.

Riva, G., Bacchetta, M., Baruffi, M., & Molinari, E. (2002). Virtual-reality-based multidimensional therapy for the treatment of body image disturbances in binge eating disorders: A preliminary controlled study. *IEEE Transactions on Information Technology in Biomedicine, 6*(3), 224–234.

Riva, G., Bacchetta, M., Cesa, G., Conti, S., Castelnuovo, G., Mantovani, F., & Molinari, E. (2006). Is severe obesity a form of addiction? Rationale, clinical approach and controlled clinical trial. *Cyberpsychology and Behavior, 9*(4), 457–479.

Riva, G., Bacchetta, M., Cesa, G., Conti, S., & Molinari, E. (2003). Six-month follow-up of in-client experiential-cognitive therapy for binge eating disorders. *Cyberpsychology and Behavior, 6*(3), 251–258.

Riva, G., Bacchetta, M., Cesa, G., Conti, S., & Molinari, E. (2004). The use of VR in the treatment of eating disorders. *Studies in Health Technology and Informatics, 99*, 121–163.

Riva, G., Botella, C., Légeron, P., & Optale, G. (Eds.). (2004). *Cybertherapy: Internet and virtual reality as assessment and rehabilitation tools for clinical psychology and neuroscience.* Amsterdam: IOS Press.

Riva, G., Gaggioli, A., Grassi, A., Raspelli, S., Cipresso, P., Pallavicini, F., & Donvito, G. (2011). NeuroVR 2 – A free virtual reality platform for the assessment and treatment in behavioral health care. In *MMVR* (pp. 493–495).

Riva, G., Mantovani, F., Capideville, C. S., Preziosa, A., Morganti, F., Villani, D., Gaggioli, A., Botella, C., & Alcañiz, M. (2007). Affective interactions using virtual reality: The link between presence and emotions. *Cyberpsychology and Behavior, 10*(1), 45–56.

Riva, G., Waterworth, J. A., & Murray, D. (Eds.). (2014). *Interacting with presence: HCI and the sense of presence in computer-mediated environments.* Berlin: De Gruyter Open – Online: www.presence-research.com.

Rothbaum, B. O., Anderson, P., Zimand, E., Hodges, L., Lang, D., & Wilson, J. (2006). Virtual reality exposure therapy and standard (in vivo) exposure therapy in the treatment of fear of flying. *Behavior Therapy, 37*(1), 80–90.

Rothbaum, B. O., Hodges, L. F., Ready, D., Graap, K., & Alarcon, R. D. (2001). Virtual reality exposure therapy for Vietnam veterans with posttraumatic stress disorder. *Journal of Clinical Psychiatry, 62*(8), 617–622.

Safran, J. D., & Greenberg, L. S. (1991). *Emotion, psychotherapy and change.* New York: The Guilford Press.

Schultheis, M. T., & Rizzo, A. A. (2001). The application of virtual reality technology in rehabilitation. *Rehabilitation Psychology, 46*(3), 296–311.

Serino, S., Triberti, S., Villani, D., Cipresso, P., Gaggioli, A., & Riva, G. (2014). Toward a validation of cyber-interventions for stress disorders based on stress inoculation training: A systematic review. *Virtual Reality, 18*(1), 73–87.

Triberti, S., Repetto, C., & Riva, G. (2014). Psychological factors influencing the effectiveness of virtual reality-based analgesia: A systematic review. *Cyberpsychology, Behavior, and Social Networking, 17*(6), 335–345.

Viaud-Delmon, I., Berthoz, A., & Jouvent, R. (2002). Multisensory integration for spatial orientation in trait anxiety subjects: Absence of visual dependence. *European Psychiatry, 17*(4), 194–199.

Viaud-Delmon, I., Ivanenko, Y. P., Berthoz, A., & Jouvent, R. (2000). Adaptation as a sensorial profile in trait anxiety: A study with virtual reality. *Journal of Anxiety Disorders, 14*(6), 583–601.

Vidal, M., Amorim, M. A., & Berthoz, A. (2004). Navigating in a virtual three-dimensional maze: How do egocentric and allocentric reference frames interact? *Cognitive Brain Research, 19*(3), 244–258.

Vidal, M., Lipshits, M., McIntyre, J., & Berthoz, A. (2003). Gravity and spatial orientation in virtual 3D-mazes. *Journal of Vestibular Research, 13*(4–6), 273–286.

Villani, D., Riva, F., & Riva, G. (2007). New technologies for relaxation: The role of presence. *International Journal of Stress Management, 14*(3), 260–274.

Vincelli, F., Anolli, L., Bouchard, S., Wiederhold, B. K., Zurloni, V., & Riva, G. (2003). Experiential cognitive therapy in the treatment of panic disorders with agoraphobia: A controlled study. *Cyberpsychology and Behavior, 6*(3), 312–318.

Wiederhold, B. K., & Riva, G. (Eds.). (2014). *Annual review of cybertherapy and telemedicine 2014: Positive change: Connecting the virtual and the real* (Vol. 199). Amsterdam: IOS Press.

Wolfe, B. E. (2002). The role of lived experience in self- and relational observation: A commentary on Horowitz. *Journal of Psychotherapy Integration, 12*(2), 147–153.

Chapter 12

THE USE OF COMPUTER-AIDED COGNITIVE BEHAVIOURAL THERAPY (CCBT) IN THERAPEUTIC SETTINGS

Kate Cavanagh and Rebecca Grist

INTRODUCTION

The use of computer technologies is widespread in the psychological therapies. From practice portals offering screening tools and appointment bookings, to patient record systems, peer support networks and psychoeducation hubs. The idea of a therapeutic practice without the assistance of some computing technology is becoming alien. However, the role of the computer as the therapist, delivering a portion or the entirety of treatment, remains controversial.

Since the 1960s researchers have attempted to identify the replicable ingredients of effective therapeutic encounters both in terms of specific techniques and nonspecific contextual and interpersonal factors. Attempts to translate these features into computer-delivered behavioural health interventions have met with varying success (see Barazzone, Cavanagh, & Richards, 2012 and Cavanagh et al., 2003a for a review). Most recently, technological advances have permitted the development of relatively sophisticated computer systems designed to replicate ingredients of cognitive behaviour therapy (CBT) for a growing range of mental health problems. In contrast to previous waves of development in computer-aided therapy which have largely remained in the lab, computer-aided cognitive behavioural therapy (CCBT) has made its way from the research clinic to the mainstream of patient care in the UK (National Institute for Clinical Excellence, 2006; 2009; 2011) and elsewhere (see Marks & Cavanagh, 2009 for a global perspective).

This chapter defines what CCBT is (and what it is not) and describes, with examples, some of the CCBT packages available. It goes on to explore the evidence base for CCBT and its impact on improving mental health for clients through self-help. The ethical considerations of offering CCBT are outlined. Finally, the future of CCBT, as a method of extending the reach of CBT and increasing access to evidence based psychological therapies, particularly using the example of the NHS in the UK, is discussed.

DEFINING COMPUTER-AIDED COGNITIVE BEHAVIOURAL THERAPY

Psychotherapeutic software can reduce client-practitioner contact time, can meaningfully and effectively deliver the training elements of the psychotherapeutic intervention and can transmit positive nonspecific ingredients of therapy such as empathy and motivation in the absence of human interaction (Cavanagh et al., 2003b); moreover, computer-aided psychotherapy uses patient input to make some computations and treatment decisions and thus is interactive and responsive (Marks et al., 1998). By extension, computer-aided cognitive behavioural therapy (CCBT) does this attuned to the cognitive behavioural therapy (CBT) method. Therefore, within the focus of this chapter, this definition excludes computer systems that only improve access or bridge distance via communication technologies (e.g., telephone therapy, email therapy). It also excludes non-responsive technologies such as psychoeducation websites or e-workbooks which are not interactive. It also excludes virtual reality systems which, while retaining CBT outcomes for many problems, do not make treatment decisions.

As technological advances have permitted, CCBT software has been developed for a range of platforms. Initially, much CCBT was accessed on non-networked personal computers and transferred by loading software from removable discs such as CD-ROMS and DVDs. Much of this software is now historical and has been translated into Internet delivered programmes. Good Days Ahead, a CCBT programme for depression, began in CD – ROM format (Wright et al., 2005); however, by 2009 had been converted into an Internet-based programme. More recently, networked software can be accessed on intranets and the Internet. As well as access on personal computers, software is also accessible via interactive voice response technology over the phone (e.g., BT Steps for obsessive compulsive disorder). Due to the ever-increasing pervasiveness of mobile technology, interventions are also progressively being developed and accessed on mobile or tablet devices. MyCompass is a self-guided programme for mild to moderate depression, anxiety and stress which has been developed for delivery via mobile phone and the Internet (Proudfoot et al., 2013).

WHAT CCBT PACKAGES ARE AVAILABLE?

It is impossible to say how many CCBT interventions are in existence. However, reviews have identified at least 100 therapy packages, many of which are cognitive behavioural in therapeutic orientation (Grist & Cavanagh, 2013; Hedman, Ljótsson, & Lindefors, 2012; Marks, Cavanagh, & Gega., 2007). These packages cover mental health problems as diverse as anxiety disorders (generalized anxiety disorder, panic disorder, specific phobias, posttraumatic stress disorder and obsessive compulsive disorder), stress, severe health anxiety, depression, eating disorders, schizophrenia, insomnia, alcohol and drug misuse and childhood anxiety and depression. These packages also target health and functional disorders such as chronic pain, tinnitus, headache, sexual difficulties, fatigue and irritable bowel syndrome. The efficacy of CCBT has been tested in relation to at least 25 different clinical disorders (Hedman et al., 2012).

The evidence base for individual programs ranges from uncontrolled proof of concept studies to large randomised controlled trials of therapeutic efficacy and practice-based evidence of effectiveness. Some programs have been taken to market, some are "under development" and some remain locked away in the filing cabinet of lost-innovations.

How many evidence-based CCBT packages are available might be easier to quantify, although the number of packages falling into this category will obviously vary depending on what criteria for "good-enough" evidence is set. Health technology assessment bodies typically view the randomised controlled trial (RCT) as the "gold-standard" of research evidence, although not all RCTs are designed to answer important questions and many other types of study design may give powerful information about the value of healthcare technologies. Through systematic review, 29 CCBT packages for common mental health disorders have been identified that have demonstrated effectiveness in at least one RCT (Grist & Cavanagh, 2013). Examples of these packages include Fearfighter and Panic Online for panic disorder, The Anxiety Program for generalized anxiety disorder, and The Shyness Program for social phobia. For depression, evidenced CCBT programs include Beating the Blues, MoodGYM, The Sadness Program, and Color Your Life.

The next section describes, in a little more detail, two CCBT programs for common mental health problems that are commercially available to healthcare providers and individuals seeking treatment.

Beating the Blues

Beating the Blues is an interactive, multimedia CCBT package for depression and anxiety accessed on a personal computer (PC) either within a healthcare setting or elsewhere via the Internet. Following an "Introduction to Therapy" presentation of 15 minutes, Beating the Blues comprises an eight-session program (each session lasting about one hour). Sessions are usually accessed weekly and there are individualised "homework" assignments to complete between sessions.

The first interactive session introduces and socialises to the CBT model focusing on problem definition and pleasurable activities with behavioural activation as the first homework exercise. Session two introduces the role of automatic thoughts in depression and anxiety and guides the user to begin one of two parallel behavioural programs (activity scheduling or problem solving). Session three explores thinking errors.

Session four guides the user through challenging unhelpful thinking and introduces a second behavioural method. Session five introduces the idea of core beliefs and the downward arrow technique. Sessions six and seven explore helpful and unhelpful attributional styles and guide the user to work on sleep management, graded exposure, or task breakdown in order to manage their own specific problems. Session eight focuses on longer-term goals, action planning and relapse prevention.

Beating the Blues utilises a range of multimedia capabilities. The user is guided through the programme by a narrator (who is a well-known medical doctor) and features a series of filmed case studies of fictional patients who are used to model both the symptoms of anxiety and depression and their treatment by CBT, as well as animations, voice-overs and interactive modules. Users can work at their own pace and repeat elements of the program if they want to. Session summaries, homework guides and clinical progress reports are generated during each session. The program is readily usable by patients with no previous computer experience.

The standard delivery model for Beating the Blues is such that clinical supervision and responsibility rest with the primary care doctor or other appropriately qualified professional (such as a nurse or clinical psychologist), to whom reports (including warnings of suicide or other risk) are automatically delivered by the computer program. If accessed in a healthcare setting, a paraprofessional worker typically supports the practical aspects of using the program such as session bookings, logging on and any technical difficulties. If accessed at home, technical support may be given by email or telephone, along with therapeutic support and progress monitoring depending on local implementation, policy and practice.

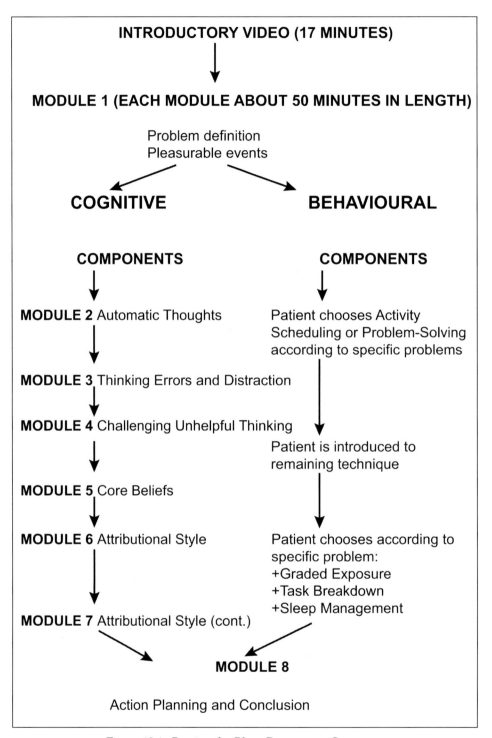

Figure 12.1. Beating the Blues Programme Structure.

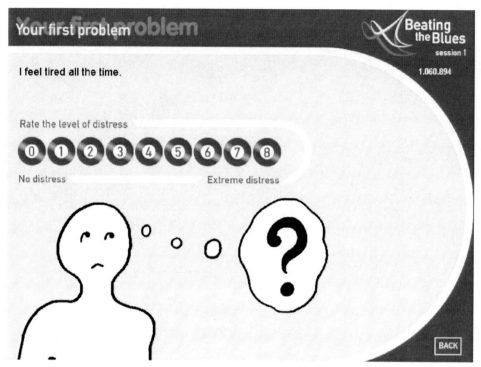

Figure 12.2. Screenshot from Beating the Blues.

FearFighter

Fearfighter is a CCBT package for phobia and panic disorder. The program is delivered through the Internet and can be accessed from any computer linked to the web. Fearfighter guides patients through nine steps. It explains the exposure therapy rationale with case examples and helps patients to identify their triggers and goals in a step-by-step personalized program, with homework diary, feedback on progress and troubleshooting advice.

Patients are also given coping strategies before doing exposure, in order to better learn to cope with the anxiety-provoking situation without escaping from it. Patients using the programme are supported by a suitably qualified support worker, who has access to the Patient Progress Monitoring System (PPMS) that comes with the programme. On the PPMS, support workers can monitor login history, step progression, and clinical measures of their patients. Brief support is given by means of scheduled support calls prearranged with the patients. No more than one hour of telephone support in total is usually required per patient. Fearfighter has been sold to, and is in use by, many Primary Care Trusts around the UK and has now become available for private patients globally.

EVIDENCE OF OUTCOMES

Over the past decade, a growing body of evidence has demonstrated the efficacy, effectiveness, acceptability and cost-effectiveness of CCBT (e.g., Andersson et al., 2015; Andrews, Cuijpers, Craske, McEvoy, & Titov., 2010; Arnberg, Linton, Hultcrantz, Heintz, & Jonsson., 2014; Cuijpers et al., 2009; Kaltenthaler

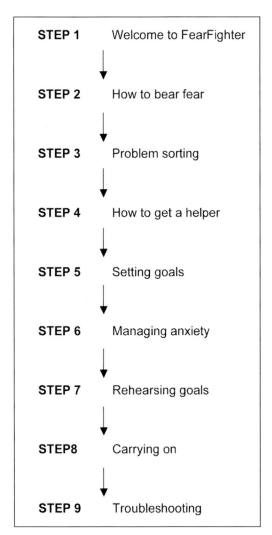

STEP 1	Welcome to FearFighter
STEP 2	How to bear fear
STEP 3	Problem sorting
STEP 4	How to get a helper
STEP 5	Setting goals
STEP 6	Managing anxiety
STEP 7	Rehearsing goals
STEP8	Carrying on
STEP 9	Troubleshooting

Figure 12.3. Program structure for FearFighter.

et al., 2008ab; Nordgren et al., 2014). Evidence is also beginning to emerge pertaining to the long-term benefits and cost effectiveness of CCBT at three (Andersson et al., 2013) and four-year follow-up (Hedman et al., 2014). Large, randomised, controlled trials in realistic healthcare settings have indicated benefits beyond waitlist control and usual care for a number of CCBT programs including Beating the Blues (Proudfoot et al., 2004) and Fearfighter (e.g., Marks et al., 2004). Subsequent practice-based evidence has supported the generalizability of these findings (Cavanagh et al., 2006; Kenwright et al., 2001; Learmonth et al., 2008) and the acceptability (Cavanagh et al., 2009) of CCBT programs in mainstream practice. As well as these UK-based trials, evidence from studies conducted in Australia, Sweden, the Netherlands and the United States suggests CCBT can be implemented successfully in routine primary care (de Graaf, Hollon, & Huijpers., 2010; Hedman, Ljótsson et al., 2014; Newby, Mewton, Williams, & Andrews., 2014; Whiteside et al., 2014). Evidence is also accumulating suggesting outcomes between CCBT and equivalent face-to-face therapy are similar (Andersson, Cuijpers, Carlbring, Riper, & Hedman., 2014; Andersson et al., 2013; Wagner, Horn, & Maercker., 2014). Evidence for CCBT coupled with that for other self-help CBT methods such as bibliotherapy (e.g., Farrand & Woodford., 2013; Gellatly et al., 2007) have potentiated enthusiasm for access to "low-intensity" CBT, where self-help CBT resources are facilitated or supported by paraprofessional workers (Department of Health, 2007; National Institute for Clinical Excellence, 2009, 2011).

The National Institute for Clinical Excellence (NICE) provide advice on which treatments should be made available on the NHS in England and Wales as well as providing evidence-based guidelines on how conditions should be treated. The most recent National Institute for Clinical Excellence guideline for depression (National Institute for Clinical Excellence, 2009) have advocated a "class effect" for CCBT for depression, echoing sentiments expressed during their consultations, "that any competently created CCBT package will be effective" (http://www.nice.org.uk/media/88D/7A /TA97CommentsTable.pdf).

The NICE guidelines (National Institute for Clinical Excellence, 2009) do not recommend any specific CCBT program as a treatment choice, but indicate some features of

CCBT requisite for the treatment of persistent subthreshold and mild to moderate depression, including CBT features (explanation of the CBT model, encourage tasks between sessions and use thought-challenging and active monitoring of behaviour, thought patterns and outcomes), support features (supported by a trained practitioner who offers limited facilitation and reviews progress and outcome) and service features (treatment program to typically last 9–12 weeks, including follow-up).

However, given the wide range of outcomes for CCBT packages in research trials, claiming a class effect seems premature. We would not champion the pharmaceutical industry if it argued that any "competently created" antidepressant should be recommended to healthcare professionals without a body of high-quality supporting evidence for that specific antidepressant. Neither can we do this for CCBT. For the time being, CCBT packages need to demonstrate their value by research rather than judgment and practice-based evidence for each individual program in context is needed to demonstrate effectiveness. In the future, dismantling studies may help us to learn more about the key elements of CCBT that drive outcome, whether these differ from what works in face-to-face therapies and how we might enhance package outcomes by replicating more of what works and eliminating what is unnecessary or distracting. This will add to a framework for anticipating which CCBT programs will or will not be helpful therapeutically.

ETHICAL CONSIDERATIONS

In addition to the standard ethical considerations needed for any psychotherapeutic encounter, any resource saving technology is bound to carry dilemmas of its own.

Users are typically both screened and assessed for the suitability of CCBT programs and finding a balance between brevity and sufficiency is a clinical challenge. It would be paradoxical for a low-intensity service to routinely invest several hours of senior practitioner time in assessing a patient's needs. Equally, it may be unhelpful to triage someone with multiple and complex needs to a CCBT service. A balance must be found.

Risk assessment and risk monitoring need to be part of a programme of care, whether this is a feature of the computer program or a task for human workers managing the program. For example, following initial risk screening by a health professional, the Beating the Blues program assesses risk at each session with the user. The results of this are fed back to a supporting practitioner and, if risk is high, the user can be advised to stop using the program and seek face-to-face help.

Subjective distress and problem ratings are also assessed on a session-by-session basis in Beating the Blues. This allows the user and their supporting practitioner to see if any improvement is being made and to note if any deterioration is present. It is up to local protocols to activate alternative help or a treatment review when appropriate.

CCBT programs raise issues of confidentiality and specifically the storage of data and, in the case of web-based products, the transfer of digital information. In developing CCBT software, consideration to appropriate levels of data access and data protection must be employed. Entry to the clients' therapeutic sessions should be password protected, the password being generated and held solely by the client. Healthcare professionals holding clinical responsibility for client well-being may wish to have access to progress information regarding mood and problem monitoring, as well as risk information. The parameters of this data access must be made clear to the client. Data entered by the client should be encrypted and retained within the program database for later retrieval by the client but not, without permission, their clinician. The confidential features of psychotherapeutic software may be viewed as an advantage by some clients who wish to work through their problems privately.

Ethical benefits of CCBT include that they may overcome some human foibles and threats to confidentiality. They will never discuss users' difficulties outside of work and will never breach boundaries of therapy by developing an inappropriate relationship with the user. Computers will never forget what your answers to questions are and will never be shocked. The content of CCBT programs can be updated to reflect the best evidence for therapy more quickly than human practitioners can be systematically trained.

CCBT programs raise a number of ethical questions and may solve some others. The mass implementation of a CCBT offer in healthcare organisations will no doubt bring further ethical issues to light.

THE IMPLEMENTATION OF CCBT IN THE UK NATIONAL HEALTH SERVICE

Currently, the UK remains the only nation to implement specific recommendations for when and how to implement CCBT in primary care (National Institute for Clinical Excellence, 2011). From a global perspective, large scale adoption of CCBT in routine care services remains to be fully realised. Consequently, recent reviews have sought to address the concerns of clinicians and encourage the upscaling of CCBT for depression and anxiety disorders into routine practice in other developed counties (Andrews & Williams, 2014) as well as low and medium income countries (Watts & Andrews, 2014).

In the UK, the National Institute for Clinical Excellence (NICE) has recommended CCBT programs as treatment options for common mental health problems (including a range of programs for depression and Fearfighter for panic and phobia) in its guidance to the National Health Service (National Institute for Clinical Excellence, 2006; 2009). Commissioning guidance advises NHS Trusts to conduct local needs assessment, purchase software licences, ensure any necessary computing hardware is in place, ensure staff are trained to support CCBT and referral pathways are in place.

In addition, radical health service initiatives under the major, UK–wide policy known as Improving Access to Psychological Therapies (IAPT) incorporate access to CCBT for depression and anxiety as a routine care option for service-users with mild-moderate difficulties, along with other "low intensity" resources (Department of Health, 2007, 2008).

By 2012, the IAPT initiative was part way through roll out and the Department of Health released its three-year report. At this stage, more than 1.1 million people had been treated in IAPT services and more than 680,000 people had completed a course of treatment (Department of Health, 2012). Furthermore, nearly 4,000 new practitioners had been trained to deliver NICE recommended treatments within these services. Through the final three years of roll-out to March 2015, the initiative aims to expand these services, train a further 2,000 additional practitioners and transform services for children and young people (CYP), which includes the exploration of whether CCBT can successfully be delivered in these CYP services (Department of Health, 2012). CCBT programs will have to evolve to meet the needs of these developing services.

CONCLUSION

CCBT is becoming a hands-on early option for effective self-help for a growing number of mental health problems including anxiety and depression. A number of programs are building a promising evidence base and professionals and healthcare systems are exploring cost-effective ways to employ this new approach to benefit sufferers. While many people will continue to choose face-to-face therapy, others may prefer emerging computer-aided options that could reduce overlong waiting lists, increase convenience and confidentiality and reduce the impact of stigma.

REFERENCES

Andersson, E., Hedman, E., Ljótsson, B., Wikström, M., Elveling, E., Lindefors, N., Rück, C. (2015). Cost-effectiveness of internet-based cognitive behavior therapy for obsessive-compulsive disorder: Results from a randomized controlled trial. *Journal of Obsessive-Compulsive and Related Disorders, 4,* 47–53.

Andersson, G., Hesser, H., Veilord, A., Svedling, L., Andersson, F., Sleman, O., Carlbring, P. (2013). Randomised controlled non-inferiority trial with 3-year follow-up of internet-delivered versus face-to-face group cognitive behavioural therapy for depression. *Journal of Affective Disorders, 151*(3), 986–994.

Andersson, G., Cuijpers, P., Carlbring, P., Riper, H., & Hedman, E. (2014). Guided Internet-based vs. face-to-face cognitive behavior therapy for psychiatric and somatic disorders: a systematic review and meta-analysis. *World Psychiatry, 13,* 288–295.

Andrews, G., Cuijpers, P., Craske, M. G., McEvoy, P., & Titov, N. (2010). Computer therapy for the anxiety and depressive disorders is effective, acceptable and practical health care: A meta-analysis. *PloS One, 5*(10), e13196.

Andrews, G., & Williams, A. D. (2014). Upscaling clinician assisted internet cognitive behavioural therapy (iCBT) for depression: A model for dissemination into primary care. *Clinical Psychology Review.* In press.

Arnberg, F. K., Linton, S. J., Hultcrantz, M., Heintz, E., & Jonsson, U. (2014). Internet-delivered psychological treatments for mood and anxiety disorders: a systematic review of their efficacy, safety, and cost-effectiveness. *PloS One, 9*(5), e98118.

Barazzone, N., Cavanagh, K., & Richards, D. A. (2012). Computerized cognitive behavioural therapy and the therapeutic alliance: A qualitative enquiry. *British Journal of Clinical Psychology, 51*(4), 396–417.

Cavanagh, K., Shapiro, D., Van den Berg, S., Swain, S., Barkham, M., & Proudfoot, J. (2006). Effectiveness of CCBT in routine primary care. *British Journal of Clinical Psychology, 45*(4), 499–514.

Cavanagh, K, Shapiro, D. A., Van den Berg, S., Swain, S., Barkham, M., & Proudfoot, J. (2009). The acceptability of computer-aided cognitive behavioural therapy: A pragmatic study. *Cognitive Behaviour Therapy, 38*(4), 235–246.

Cavanagh, K., Shapiro, D., & Zack, J. (2003a). Computer plays therapist: The challenges and opportunities of psychotherapeutic software. In S. Goss & K. Anthony (Eds.), *Technology in counselling and psychotherapy: A practitioners' guide.* Basingstoke, UK: Palgrave/Macmillan.

Cavanagh, K., Zack, J. S., Shapiro, D. A., & Wright, J. H. (2003b). Computer programs for psychotherapy. In S. Goss & K. Anthony (Eds.), *Technology in counselling and psychotherapy: A practitioner's guide.* Basingstoke, UK: Palgrave/MacMillan.

Cuijpers, P., Marks, I. M., van Straten, A., Cavanagh, K., Gega, L., & Andersson, G. (2009). Computer-aided psychotherapy for anxiety disorders: A meta-analytic review. *Cognitive Behaviour Therapy, 38*(2), 66–82.

De Graaf, L. E., Hollon, S. D., & Huibers, M. J. H. (2010). Predicting outcome in computerized cognitive behavioral therapy for depression in primary care: A randomized trial. *Journal of Consulting and Clinical Psychology, 78*(2), 184–189.

Department of Health. (2007). *Improving access to psychological therapies (IAPT) programme: Computerised cognitive behavioural therapy (cCBT) implementation guidance.* London: Department of Health.

Department of Health. (2008). *Improving access to psychological therapies (IAPT) implementation plan: National guidelines for regional delivery.* London: Department of Health.

Department of Health. (2012). *IAPT three-year report: The first million patients.* London: Department of Health

Farrand, P., & Woodford, J. (2013). Impact of support on the effectiveness of written cognitive behavioural self-help: A systematic review and meta-analysis of randomised controlled trials. *Clinical Psychology Review, 33*(1), 182–95.

Gellatly, J., Bower, P., Hennessy, S., Richards, D., Gilbody, S., & Lovell, K. (2007). What makes self-help interventions effective in the management of depressive symptoms? Meta-analysis and meta regression. *Psychological Medicine, 37,* 1217–1228.

Grist, R., & Cavanagh, K. (2013). Computerised cognitive behavioural therapy for common mental health disorders: What works, for whom under what circumstances? A systematic review and meta-analysis. *Journal of Contemporary Psychotherapy, 43*(4), 243–251.

Hedman, E., El Alaoui, S., Lindefors, N., Andersson, E., Rück, C., Ghaderi, A., Ljótsson, B. (2014). Clinical effectiveness and cost-effectiveness of Internet- vs. group-based cognitive behavior therapy for social anxiety disorder: 4-year follow-up of a randomized trial. *Behaviour Research and Therapy, 59,* 20–9.

Hedman, E., Ljótsson, B., Kaldo, V., Hesser, H., El Alaoui, S., Kraepelien, M., Lindefors, N. (2014). Effectiveness of Internet-based cognitive behaviour therapy for depression in routine psychiatric care. *Journal of Affective Disorders, 155,* 49–58.

Hedman, E., Ljótsson, B., & Lindefors, N. (2012). Cognitive behavior therapy via the Internet: A systematic review of applications, clinical efficacy and cost-effectiveness. *Expert Review of Pharmacoeconomics & Outcomes Research, 12*(6), 745–764.

Kaltenhaler, E., Sutcliffe, P., Parry, G., Beverly, C., & Ferriter, M. (2008a). The acceptability to patients of computerized cognitive behavioural therapy for depression: A systematic review. *Psychological Medicine, 38,* 1521–1530.

Kaltenhaler, E., Parry, G., Beverly, C., & Ferriter, M. (2008b). Computerised cognitive-behavioural therapy for depression: Systematic review. *British Journal of Psychiatry, 193*(3), 181–184.

Kenwright, M., Liness, S., & Marks, I. (2001). Reducing demands on clinicians by offering computer-aided self-help for phobia/panic: Feasibility study. *British Journal of Psychiatry, 179,* 456–459.

Learmonth, D., Trosh, J., Rai, S., Sewell, J., & Cavanagh, K. (2008). The role of computer-aided psychotherapy within an NHS CBT specialist service. *Counselling and Psychotherapy Research, 8*(2), 117–123.

Marks, I. M., & Cavanagh, K. (2009). Computer-aided psychotherapy: State of the art and state of the science. *Annual Review of Clinical Psychology, 5,* 121–141.

Marks, I. M., Cavanagh, K., & Gega, L. (2007). *Hands-on help: Computer-aided psychotherapy.* Hove: Psychology Press.

Marks, I. M., Kenwright, M., McDonough, M., Whittaker, M., & Mataix-Cols, D. (2004). Saving clinicians' time by delegating routine aspects of therapy to a computer: A RCT in phobia/panic disorder. *Psychological Medicine, 34,* 9–18.

Marks, I. M., Shaw, S., & Parkin, R. (1998). Computer-aided treatments of mental health problems. *Clinical Psychology: Science and Practice, 5*(2), 151–170.

National Institute for Clinical Excellence. (2006). *Guidance on the use of computerised cognitive behavioural therapy for anxiety and depression.* Technology Appraisal no. 97. London: NICE.

National Institute for Clinical Excellence. (2009). *Depression: Management of depression in primary and secondary care – NICE guidance*, CG90. London: NICE.

National Institute for Clinical Excellence. (2011). *Common mental health disorders: Identification and pathways to care – NICE clinical guideline 123.* London: NICE.

Newby, J. M., Mewton, L., Williams, A. D., & Andrews, G. (2014). Effectiveness of transdiagnostic Internet cognitive behavioural treatment for mixed anxiety and depression in primary care. *Journal of Affective Disorders, 165,* 45–52.

Nordgren, L. B., Hedman, E., Etienne, J., Bodin, J., Kadowaki, A., Eriksson, S., Carlbring, P. (2014). Effectiveness and cost-effectiveness of individually tailored Internet-delivered cognitive behavior therapy for anxiety disorders in a primary care population: A randomized controlled trial. *Behaviour Research and Therapy, 59,* 1–11.

Proudfoot, J., Ryden, C., Everitt, B., Shapiro, D., Goldberg, D., Mann, A., Tylee, A., Marks, I., & Gray, J. (2004). Clinical efficacy of computerised cognitive behavioral therapy for anxiety and depression in primary care. *British Journal of Psychiatry, 185*(1), 46–54

Proudfoot, J. G., Clarke, J., Birch, M. R., Whitton, A. E., Parker, G., Manicavasagar, V., Hadzi-Pavlovic, D. (2013). Impact of a mobile phone and web program on symptom and functional outcomes for people with mild-to-moderate depression, anxiety and stress: A randomised controlled trial. *BMC Psychiatry, 13,* 312.

Proudfoot, J. G., Ryden, C., Everitt, B., Shapiro, D. a, Goldberg, D., Mann, A., Gray, J. A. (2004). Clinical efficacy of computerised cognitive-behavioural therapy for anxiety and depression in primary care: randomised controlled trial. *The British Journal of Psychiatry: The Journal of Mental Science, 185,* 46–54.

Wagner, B., Horn, A. B., & Maercker, A. (2014). Internet-based versus face-to-face cognitive-behavioral intervention for depression: A randomized controlled non-inferiority trial. *Journal of Affective Disorders, 152–154,* 113–121.

Watts, S. E., & Andrews, G. (2014). Internet access is NOT restricted globally to high income countries: so why are evidenced based prevention and treatment programs for mental disorders so rare? *Asian Journal of Psychiatry, 10,* 71–4.

Wright, J. H., Wright, A. S., Albano, A. M., Basco, M. R., Goldsmith, L. J., Raffield, T., & Otto, M. W. (2005). Computer-assisted cognitive therapy for depression: maintaining efficacy while reducing therapist time. *The American Journal of Psychiatry, 162*(6), 1158–64.

Whiteshide, U., Richards, J., Steinfeld, B., Simon, G., Caka, S., Tachibana, C., Ludman, E. (2014). Online Cognitive Behavioral Therapy for Depressed Primary Care Patients: A Pilot Feasibility Project. *The Permanente Journal, 18*(2), 21–27.

Chapter 13

THE ROLE OF GAMING IN MENTAL HEALTH

Mark Matthews and David Coyle

INTRODUCTION

Many adolescents experience difficulties in engaging directly with traditional face-to-face therapeutic approaches (BMA, 2006). Recent research suggests that computer assisted mental health interventions may provide one potential way of working more successfully with adolescent clients (Matthews et al., 2008). Research also suggests that the choice of technology is a key factor in the success of computer-assisted interventions. For example, it is suggested: "a quality therapeutic process will actively engage the client's participation, by involving their interests, strengths and ideas. Similarly, technologies are most likely to prove effective if they are designed to be client-centred" (Coyle et al., 2007a).

Whilst much attention in recent years has focused on the negative effects of computer games, a review of literature and an initial pilot study (Coyle et al., 2005) have provided strong initial indications that appropriately designed games may have potential to assist in clinical interventions. Therapeutic games offer the opportunity to engage with adolescents through a medium with which they are comfortable. Surveys on the use of computer games consistently find that the majority of adolescents play computer games regularly. A US-focused survey found that 97% of 12–17-year-olds report playing computer games

(Lenhart et al., 2008). Further surveys in the US and the UK indicate that under-16's rank computer gaming as their number one entertainment form (Gentile & Walsh, 2002; Pratchett, 2005).

This chapter focuses on the use of computer games to improve mental health and includes a review of previous research into the use of computer games to support therapy. Over the past fifteen years there has been an increasing number of research studies investigating the potential of computer games to aid in the treatment of mental illness. However, we still have a very limited understanding of the use of computer games in mental health care (Ceranoglu, 2010). Initial evidence suggests the medium has promise to help in the development of a therapeutic alliance, as a nonconfrontational method of conducting psychotherapy (Coyle et al., 2009) and as a vehicle for Psychoeducation (Fleming et al., 2012). But the broader potential for the use of therapeutic computer games is unclear. Are games just a useful icebreaker or can they assist in other ways? Can they, for instance, assist in improving client engagement and even serve as a stand-alone intervention? We focus on two prominent therapeutic computer games. The first, Personal Investigator, designed for us was in clinical settings with a therapist, and the second, SPARX, was created as a stand-alone intervention for adolescent depression. The chapter ends by taking a more speculative perspective on future directions for therapeutic gaming.

ETHICAL CONCERNS

Before discussing ongoing research on therapeutic computer games, it is important to note that many Mental Health Care (MHC) researchers and practitioners are skeptical of the benefits, not just of games, but also of technology in general. Caspar (2004) cites fears such as damage to the client-therapist relationship, ethical and security issues and worries that the current skills of therapists may become obsolete. Others fear that technology in and of itself has a damaging impact on the mental health of society, suggesting dangers such as increased isolation due to excessive time spent online (Caspar, 2004).

In the case of computer games, much literature in recent years has focused on the negative effects of computer games. Risks such as addiction and increased aggressiveness and violence have been suggested (Gentile et al. 2004). However, while these fears must be considered, there are initial indications that the positive potential of therapeutic games may be substantial and MHC researchers have begun to show an increased interest in the use of suitably designed games (Griffiths, 1997; Parkin, 2000). It is important to note that technology-based interventions do not generally seek to replace existing methods. Rather, they seek to offer new and complementary options. Rather than detracting from critical therapeutic factors such as the client-therapist relationship, games, when appropriately designed and used in appropriate circumstances, may offer a way of improving such factors, complementing face-to-face work or providing an alternative when face-to-face support is not available.

PREVIOUS USES OF COMPUTER GAMES

Research on computer games in MHC settings has been limited. Some early research was conducted in the 1980s and early 1990s. Several researchers from a psychology/psychotherapy background developed their own games (Clark & Schoech, 1984; Griffiths, 1997; Hyland et al., 1993; Oakley, 1994; Resnick & Sherer, 1994), while others examined the potential of off-the-shelf commercial games (Gardner, 1991; Hyland et al., 1993). Increases in the costs, development time and technical expertise involved in developing modern games were key factors in the decline of this work. Research on the use of biofeedback-based games for the treatment of anxiety disorders and attention problems has received more recent attention (Pope & Paisson, 2001). Some suggested benefits from research into therapeutic computer games are:

- Games can successfully engage clients previously difficult to engage by other means;
- Clients were more cooperative with their therapists with whom they developed effective therapeutic relationships.
- Session attendance rates greatly improved and the stigma felt in attending therapy was reduced (Clark & Schoech, 1984; Hyland et al., 1993);
- Games can help adolescents develop "more self-confidence, a sense of mastery, more willingness to accept responsibility" (Hyland et al., 1993);
- Games can help children displace their aggression, develop problem solving skills and deal with negative and positive outcomes in the game (Gardner, 1991).

It is important to note that these findings must be viewed with a large degree of caution. Research in the area has been largely uncoordinated and the difficulties surrounding clinical evaluations mean that trials typically had limited user numbers. Substantially more work has been conducted in educational and other health care areas, with suggested benefits including increased motivation; increased self-esteem; increased health care knowledge and self-efficacy; improved problem-solving and discussion skills; and improved storytelling skills (Bers, 2001; Gee, 2003; HopeLab, 2006). The degree to which such benefits are transferable to MHC settings remains an open question.

PERSONAL INVESTIGATOR (PI)

PI is a 3D computer game that incorporates Solution Focused Therapy (SFT), a goal-oriented, strengths-based intervention model. It is the first time this intervention approach has been integrated into a 3D game. The game uses a detective metaphor. Players visit a Detective Academy and play the role of a "personal investigator" hunting for the clues that will help them solve a personal problem. Players are given a detective notebook, where they are asked to record their thoughts and ideas. Five solution-focused conversational strategies are mapped into five distinct game areas. The player meets a master detective in each area who talks with the player in an informal way and asks the player to answer questions in their notebook. Three of the dialogues incorporate videos of adolescents describing how they overcame personal problems using the strategies described. To complete the game and "graduate," the academy players must complete the tasks set by each master detective. Upon completing the game, they receive a printout of their notebook (further details of PI can be found in Coyle et al., 2005; Coyle et al., 2011; Matthews et al., 2006; Matthews et al., 2008).

The first character the player meets is the principal of the Detective Academy, whose job is to guide players through the goal-setting stage of therapy. He gives the player their detective notebook, which appears at the bottom of the screen and tells them "this book will be a mirror to your mind, it is where you can write all your ideas and hunches as you go along." The player is asked to identify a problem to work on and asked to describe this problem as a solution they would like to achieve. From this point on, the game attempts to focus the player's attention on achieving this solution.

Goal-setting can be a difficult step to complete in regular therapeutic sessions. When using PI, the goal-setting process is incorporated within the game. Achieving the client's solution becomes the objective of the game.

Inside the Detective Academy, there are four distinct areas to be explored, with four master detective characters, each corresponding to the four remaining aspects of SFT:

- **Recognizing exceptions:** the player meets Damini, a forensic scientist who specializes in spotting hidden evidence. This section aims to help the player recognize times when their problem is less

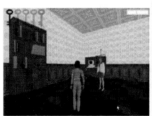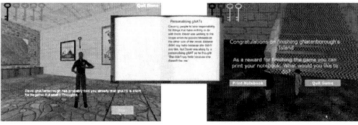

Figure 13.1. Screenshots from Personal Investigator.

acute with a view to repeating them more often.

- **Coping:** in this area, the player meets Inspector Clueso. He helps players recognize ways they currently have of dealing with their problem and explores how they might have successfully overcome problems in the past.
- **Identifying resources:** the player meets Detective Spade, a New York cop. He helps the player identify "Backup," family and friends whose support they can draw on in future times of need. He also discusses other resources, such as their own strengths, which the player can use.
- **Miracle question:** in this area, the player meets Siobhán, an artist, who helps people visualise their life without their current problems. This dialogue is based on the SFT miracle question. By imagining a future without their problems, clients are motivated to seek a solution.

Having met all the other characters and collected the four keys, the player can then open the final door to graduate from the Detective Academy. The player meets the principal again, who congratulates the player and rewards their effort with a printout of their notebook.

USING PERSONAL INVESTIGATOR IN CLINICAL SESSIONS

In clinical sessions, the therapist and adolescent sit together at a computer, but the adolescent has full control of the keyboard and mouse. The adolescent chooses a username and logs into the game. The game creates an individual account for each adolescent, automatically saving their progress and allowing them to return to saved games at a later date. The adolescent has full control over the game; they play at their own pace and choose their own path through the world. Throughout the game the therapist is a partner in the exploration of the game world and is no longer an interlocutor. If the adolescent asks for help, the therapist can elaborate on the subjects brought up by the game or answer more specific questions from the adolescent in relation to their situation.

A multi-site evaluation has been conducted in which eight therapists used PI with a total of 22 adolescent clients. Approximately equal numbers of male and female clients, experiencing a broad range of difficulties and ranging in age from 10 to 16, used the game. Each therapist agreed that PI had a positive impact in the majority of sessions in which it was used. They also agreed that PI complemented their traditional ways of working and all but one stated that they would like to continue using PI with further clients. All eight therapists agreed that while PI is useful as an icebreaker, it is also more than this. It helped therapists engage constructively with their clients. It helped with the development of the client-therapist relationship and it also helped in structuring sessions.

A key finding to emerge was the importance of the therapist's role in using the game effectively. The real benefit of games such as PI is that they can help to raise issues in a client-centred way and create a context for more detailed discussions between the therapist and client. Games can serve as a therapeutic tool, but the work jointly undertaken by the therapist and client remains important. This factor is highlighted in the rules one therapist established for using PI with clients. The therapist described the initial discussion she had with clients prior to using PI as follows:

> Prior to commencing the game we have a discussion about the game – and I gauge the interest level. If they are very interested I outline some important things to remember. I describe it as a thinking game. I talk about needing to take time to

think before we write down our answers [in the game notebook]. So rule no 1 is the therapist or child reads out the question – and we have a talk about it before we write anything down. Once we have decided we type it and only then press next. Rule 2 – if we are going too fast and not taking our time, we may need to stop the game completely and work from a page instead. (This is a good strategy for assisting in patience in the game).

Alongside acknowledging therapists' largely positive opinions of PI, it is important to note several concerns raised by the group. These concerns focused on three main issues: difficulties some clients experienced reading and writing in the game notebook, some adolescents engage with the game but not with the therapeutic issues raised and some adolescents engage with the game but not with the therapist, using the game as another way of avoiding discussion with the therapist.

CASE MATERIAL

This case study describes the opinions of the therapist who has used PI most often. He states: "The notable benefit has to be removing the impact of face-to-face grilling, which for young people who want to oppose adults has to be a plus."

In all, this therapist used PI with seven clients and stated that the game was "helpful" in two cases and "very helpful" in five. The therapist strongly agreed that PI provided benefits as an icebreaker, as an aid to the therapeutic relationship and to client engagement. He expressed the opinion that PI had the ability to help clients take ownership of the therapeutic process: "The cognitive goal of PI is to enable and encourage the client towards ownership of the problem. Talking therapy alone can take up to 3 or 4 times longer to reach the same small part of understanding

that PI can bring out in 1 session."

One of the issues also addressed in feedback was the importance of the therapist's role in using PI effectively. For example, he stated: "Skillful use of the introduction of PI into a session just makes for better and better interventions that students/clients can handle at their own pace. Any tool in a therapists 'toolkit' that can open a dialogue of any sort can only be of benefit if used with skill."

The therapist described the way in which he used PI to complement some of his other day-to-day techniques. For example, if he felt that a client had a moment of significant understanding while playing PI, he moved away from the computer and addressed this issue in more detail:

"Playing PI created some nice 'Aha moments'. . . . Moving away from the PC at these points, using reflection flowcharts, mind maps, etc. helped to solidify the new learning and turn what was once a block or problem into a manageable challenge that can be dealt with one piece at a time."

What is significant here was that this therapist had integrated the game with his traditional working methods and had begun to use PI as a context for, and complement to, other forms of therapeutic work. As such, PI became part of this therapist's overall therapeutic toolkit, rather than a stand-alone game used in isolation.

SPARX

SPARX was developed for adolescents with depression (Fleming et al., 2012). Unlike PI, it is designed as a self-help stand-alone treatment; there is no therapist involvement. Similar to many online therapeutic interventions, it incorporates elements of Cognitive Behavioral Therapy (CBT) into the program. Adolescent participants complete seven modules over four to seven weeks.

SPARX is a 3D fantasy game where the

player, an adolescent with depression, plays the role of a character trying to rid the world of GNATS (Gloomy Negative Automatic Thoughts). Players can customize their characters and the gameplay is a mix of interactive dialogues and in-game activities. The game structure is similar to PI. Players make their way through seven levels, each focusing on a distinct aspect of therapy. At the beginning of each level, players meet a guide who explains what challenges they will face in the level, asks questions about the young person's challenges in real life and assesses their mood. Players use a paper notebook alongside the game that includes summaries of each module and provides space for players to add their own content.

SPARX has been evaluated in two studies comparing that provided evidence that the game can be an effective tool for helping adolescents with depression (Fleming et al., 2012, Merry et al., 2012). The game was compared to treatment as usual comprising primarily face-to-face counseling delivered by trained counselors and clinical psychologists.

The first study, a randomized comparison of SPARX to a waitlist control for young people excluded from education (N=20) showed that the computerized CBT intervention was more effective that the waitlist control (Fleming et al., 2012). The intervention lasted five weeks, with assessments at baseline, five weeks and 10 weeks. The results showed significant differences between SPARX and the waiting list groups on depression ratings and remission, and these gains were maintained at 10-week follow-up. No differences were found on other self-rating scales.

In the second study, a randomized control noninferiority trial (RCT), 187 adolescent participants, adolescents aged 12-19, were randomized to two conditions (Merry et al., 2012). Ninety-four adolescents were allocated to SPARX and 93 to treatment as usual. The results indicated that SPARX was not inferior to treatment as usual for these participants;

there was an average reduction in depression and other factors and these results were maintained after three months.

While both studies provide evidence that SPARX can help with adolescent depression, the first study had a larger effect on participant depression, indicating possibly that the game was more effective with adolescents excluded from mainstream education (Li et al., 2014).

Seeking to understand the impact of various design elements, Cheek et al. (2014) explored adolescent experiences with the game via interviews. They found that participants valued interventions that maintained their privacy and supported a range of choices. Young people reported that they found the following elements most useful: (1) the ability to personalize the visual appearance of their character, (2) the narrative dimension of the program, (3) interactions with the "guide" character, (4) the optional journaling, and (5) the use of encouraging feedback (Cheek et al., 2014).

Evidence indicates that SPARX is an effective method for reducing adolescent depression and improving quality of life. A randomized control trial is the gold standard for clinical evidence. Few computer game interventions have been evaluated using this method. Since SPARX is designed to be played as a stand-alone intervention, it could be used as an intervention for adolescents on waiting lists or in a maintenance phase of therapy, similar to other computerized cognitive behavioral therapy programs.

CONSIDERATIONS

Although findings from the research studies related to both PI and SPARX is encouraging, and aligned with what similar studies have found (Li et al., 2014), we really do not have a firm understanding of why computer games might have positive therapeutic effects, in what contexts and for which individuals. Even in the evaluation of SPARX that used the same outcome measure, there was a large variance in the effect size for both studies (Sally et al., 2012; Fleming et al., 2012). Further research on the benefits of video game use in psychotherapy, including patient characteristics and the role of the therapist that may moderate outcomes, is needed. Bearing this in mind, the following are some considerations practicing clinicians might take into account when deciding to use games with clients.

It is worth remembering that computer games are simply a digital medium for play, albeit with unique characteristics not present in traditional games, such as the ability to play over geographic distance or the possibility of adding motion graphics to better support the game fantasy. As a medium, however, computer games are multifaceted and can range from cinematic adventures with budgets on a par with a Hollywood movie to simple text-based interactions. Where in the past user interaction was limited to pushing a joystick one way or the other and pressing a button, players can now use a wide range of inputs including facial expressions, physical activity and voice controls. Although biofeedback has a long legacy in psychotherapy, it is now becoming more convenient to use as part of treatment. Games are highly varied regarding both the overall time they take to play and the average time per game during each session.

There is the potential for computer games to have a positive therapeutic impact and offer individuals support in various ways: (1) by encouraging positive mental health and socialization in a general audience, (2) by providing a means in clinical situations through which therapists can engage clients, (3) by acting as a prescribed self-help program that keeps clients motivated and engaged throughout a tailored program.

Like any therapeutic tool, each game should be considered on its own merits and with a particular focus on the therapeutic goal. Individual preference, as in any treatment tool, should play a central role and having a clear idea of the desired therapeutic outcome will help guide the decision-making process. Deciding in advance the reason for including a computer game as part of treatment is perhaps the most critical step. Based on our current knowledge, computer games would seem to offer a range of potential to engage clients in less confrontational face-to-face therapy and also serve as effective stand-alone interventions for treating some illnesses.

While more detailed studies are now required to confirm these initial findings, there are strong initial grounds to suggest that games such as PI offer therapeutic benefits. Along-side use in clinical sessions, there is the potential for games to impact adolescent mental health in many new ways. Between sessions, games like SPARX may help to encourage clients to complete homework activities and reflect on issues raised in sessions or even serve as an intervention when face-to-face treatment is not an option.

THE FUTURE

As computer games allow for more subtle interactions and appeal to a wider, more diverse, audience, the potential for positive impact on mental health will increase. Games that encourage greater physical activity or socialization are just the beginning.

In the future, it is reasonable to assume we will have a better understanding of the therapeutic dimension of computer games that will support a more precise use of this medium in clinical interventions. It is not difficult to imagine digital games forming part of face-to-face therapy (they already play a significant role in treatment for phobia via exposure therapy), stand-alone treatments for people on waiting list or in a maintenance phase, or individual or collective "homework" activities to improve mental health (e.g., exercise or cognitive training games).

Games may also provide a way to reduce

the stigma often associated with accessing mental health information and services. Reach Out Central (ROC) is an example of one such game. It is an online game incorporating a CBT approach, designed for young people aged 16 to 25. The game allows players to play through life situations and is designed to help develop a range of skills from general life management skills to dealing with negative feelings or depression.

In the near future, alongside using existing games, it is likely that greater opportunities will exist for MHC professionals to become more directly involved in designing their own therapeutic games. For example, PlayWrite is a tool, developed by the authors of this chapter, which allows therapists to easily create character-based games similar to PI. Using PlayWrite, it is possible to tailor games to suit particular therapeutic approaches, particular mental health difficulties, or the needs of specific groups or individual clients. To date, 10 games have been designed by MHC professionals to treat a range of issues (Coyle et al., 2007b).

In the long term, research in this area should explore the potential of new and diverse forms of computer games, the merits of which have begun to be seen in other areas. The Nintendo Wii console allows for new forms of physical interaction with games. For example, Wii Fit Yoga, which appeals to a wider audience than traditional games, takes the player calmly through a tailored yoga routine. In West Virginia, 103 high schools incorporated computer games with a physical element to them (Exergames) into physical education classes, to help tackle obesity by offering students an alternative to traditional physical education activities. In the future, Exergames could assist in the treatment of depression. A new generation of daily training games (often called "brain games"), designed to help increase a wide variety of mental skills, have also become popular. The most successful of these games is the Brain Age series (Brain Training in Europe) based on the research of Dr. Ryuta Kawashima. Mind Habits is an online "brain game" based on social intelligence research at McGill University. It is designed to give you a rating on how stressed or focused you are and to help you improve this rating.

Extrapolating further, we can imagine games being prescribed routinely to help diagnosis and treat various mental diseases. Research evidence in related fields provides encouraging evidence that this is viable. Dandeneau et al. (2004) found that attentional bias for rejection can be measured and modified using simple tasks and a computer game. In their study, participants with chronic low self-esteem who played a simple game, where they were asked to click on the one smiling face from a 4x4 grid of images of people, showed noticeable improvements relative to control participants who did not play the game. Similar results have been found in addiction studies. Schoenmaker et al. (2010) evaluated an attentional bias modification training task with alcohol-dependent patients (alongside cognitive behavioral therapy) and found that the task helped participants disengage from alcohol-related cues. There have been similar positive gains found in attentional bias training in mild depression, but not for more severe forms of the illness (Baert et al., 2010). Tasks like cognitive bias modification and others that involve modifying cognitive patterns or behavioral responses would seem well suited to use as part of a game since they are often highly structured and repetitive tasks that show therapeutic benefits with practice. As we learn more about the potential of such games, we should expect to see them play a role in clinical interventions.

CONCLUSION

Research into the therapeutic potential of computer games is in its infancy. More robust research studies like that of SPARX are needed to assess the therapeutic impact of computer games in various settings with a range of individuals with mental illness. Yet, the popularity of video games among youth make them a very suitable candidate for engaging children and adolescents more readily in psychotherapy. The potentially unique value of video games in psychotherapy will serve to expand the conceptualization of such therapy for youth. Yet, how video game use may influence different stages of psychotherapy remain to be explored.

Moreover, research that seeks to understand the therapeutic effect of elements of computer games will lead to a more nuanced understanding of their impact (i.e., if and why they have a therapeutic effect) and in turn enable a more purposeful therapeutic game design. The two games described in this chapter are essentially game-based versions of therapeutic approaches. There may be potential for more innovative uses of computer games. What is now needed is a greater concerted exploration of the potential of various computer games, in order to identify how they can best be applied to support positive mental health.

REFERENCES

Baert, S., De Raedt, R., Schacht, R., et al. (2010). Attentional bias training in depression: Therapeutic effects depend on depression severity. *Journal of Behavior Therapy and Experimental Psychiatry, 41*(3), 265–274.

Bers, M. (2001). Identity construction environments: Developing personal and moral values through the design of a virtual city. *Journal of the Learning Sciences, 10*(4), 365–415.

BMA. (2006). *Child and adolescent mental health – A guide for healthcare professionals.* London: Board of Science of the British Medical Association.

Caspar, F. (2004). Technological developments and applications in clinical psychology: Introduction. *Journal of Clinical Psychiatry, 60*(3), 221–238.

Ceranoglu, T. A. (2010). Video games in psychotherapy. *Review of General Psychology, 14*(2).

Cheek, C., Bridgman, H., & Fleming, T. et al. (2014). Views of young people in rural Australia on SPARX, a fantasy world developed for New Zealand youth with depression. *JMIR Serious Games, 2*(1).

Clark, B., & Schoech, D. (1984). A computer-assisted therapeutic game for adolescents: Initial development and comments. In M. D. Schwartz (Ed.), *Using computers in clinical practice: Psychotherapy and mental health applications.* New York: Haworth Press.

Coyle, D., Matthews, M., Sharry, J., Nisbet, A., & Doherty, G. (2005). Personal Investigator: A therapeutic 3D game for adolescent psychotherapy. *International Journal of Interactive Technology and Smart Education, 2*(2), 73–88.

Coyle, D., Doherty, G., Sharry, J., & Matthews, M. (2007a). Computers in talk-based mental health care. *Interacting with Computers, 19*(4), 545–562 [online].

Coyle, D., Sharry, J., & Doherty, G. (2007b). PlayWrite – publishing and playing 3D computer games in adolescent mental health interventions. XXIV World Congress – International Association for Suicide Prevention, Killarney, Ireland, 28 August–1 September.

Coyle, D., Doherty, G., & Sharry, J. (2009). An evaluation of a solution focused computer game in adolescent interventions. *Clinical Child Psychology and Psychiatry, 14*(3), 345–360, 1359–1045.

Coyle, D., McGlade, N., Doherty, G., & O'Reilly, G. (2011). Exploratory Evaluations of a Computer Game Supporting Cognitive Behavioural Therapy for Adolescents. ACM CHI 2011, pp. 2937–2946.

Fleming, T., Dixon, R., Frampton, C. et al. (2012). A pragmatic randomized controlled trial of computerized CBT (SPARX) for symptoms of depression among adolescents excluded from mainstream education. *Behavioural and cognitive psychotherapy, 40*(05), 529–541.

Dandeneau, S. D., & Baldwin, M. W. (2004). The inhibition of socially rejecting information among people with high versus low self-esteem: The role of attentional bias and the effects of bias reduction training. *Journal of Social and Clinical Psychology, 23*(4), 584–603.

Gardner, J. E. (1991). Can the Mario Bros. help? Nintendo games as an adjunct in psychotherapy with children. *Psychotherapy, 28*(4), 667–670.

Gee, J. P. (2003). *What video games have to teach us about learning and literacy.* Basingstoke: Palgrave/Macmillan.

Gentile, D. A., Lynch, P. J., Linder, J. R., & Walsh, D. A. (2004). The effects of violent video game habits on adolescent hostility, aggressive behaviors and school performance. *Journal of Adolescence, 27*(1), 5–22.

Gentile, D. A., & Walsh, D. A. (2002). A normative study of family media habits. *Journal of Applied Developmental Psychology, 23*(2), 157–178.

Griffiths, M. (1997). Video games and clinical practice: Issues, uses and treatments. *British Journal of Clinical Psychology, 36*(4), 639–641.

HopeLab. (2006). Re-Mission TM Outcomes study: A research trial of a video game shows improvement in health-related outcomes for young people with cancer [online]. [Accessed June 14, 2015] Available at https://secure.cigna.com/form/formmail/hopelab/re-mission_story.pdf.

Hyland, M., Kenyon, C. A., Allen, R., & Howarth, P. (1993). Diary keeping in asthma: Comparison of written and electronic methods. *British Medical Journal, 306*(6876), 487–489.

Lenhart, A., Kahne, J., Middaugh, E., Macgill, A. R., Evans, C., & Vitak, J. (2008). Teens, video games, and civics. Pew Internet & American Life Project. Retrieved from http://www.pewinternet.org/Reports/2008/.

Li, J., Theng, Y.-L., & Foo, S. (2014). Game-based digital interventions for depression therapy: A systematic review and meta-analysis. *Cyberpsychology, Behavior, and Social Networking, 17*(8), 519–527.

Matthews, M., Coyle, D., & Anthony, K. (2006). Personal investigator. *Therapy Today: The Magazine for Counselling and Psychotherapy Professionals, 17*(7), 30–33.

Matthews, M., Doherty, G., Sharry, J., & Fitzpatrick, C. (2008). Mobile phone mood charting for adolescents. *British Journal of Guidance and Counselling, 36*(2), 113–129.

McFarlane, A., Sparrowhawk, A., & Heald, Y. (2002). *Report on educational use of games: Teachers evaluating educational multimedia report.* St Ives, Cambridgeshire: TEEM.

Merry, S. N., Stasiak, K., Shepherd, M. et al. (2012). The effectiveness of SPARX, a computerised self help intervention for adolescents seeking help for depression: Randomised controlled non-inferiority trial. *BMJ, 344*, 1756–1833.

Oakley, C. (1994). SMACK: A computer driven game for at-risk teens. *Computers in Human Services, 11*(1), 97–99.

Parkin, A. (2000). Computers in clinical practice: Applying experience from child psychiatry. *British Medical Journal, 321*(7261), 615–618.

Pope, A. T., & Paisson, O. S. (2001). *Helping video games 'rewire our minds'.* Playing by the Rules Conference, Chicago, IL, Oct. 26–27.

Pratchett, R. (2005). *Gamers in the UK: Digital play, digital lifestyles (White Paper).* London: BBC.

Resnick, H., & Sherer, M. (1994). Computer games in the human services – A review. *Computers in Human Services, 11*(1), 17–29.

Schoenmakers, T.M., de Bruin, M., Lux, I. F. M. et al. (2010). Clinical effectiveness of attentional bias modification training in abstinent alcoholic patients. *Drug and Alcohol Dependence, 109*(1), 30–36.

Chapter 14

WEB-BASED CLINICAL ASSESSMENT

Reid E. Klion

INTRODUCTION

In an oft-told story, access to the Internet grew exponentially through the 1990s and into the twenty-first century. Originally developed as a means of communication amongst academics, the Internet has come to have a very broad influence in revolutionizing virtually every aspect of our lives ranging from banking and commerce to travel and dating.

In similar fashion, easy access to the Internet is also reshaping how we are able to provide mental health services and, more specifically, deliver clinical assessments. However, as is often the case when something new and potentially revolutionary emerges in our lives, the growth of web-based clinical assessment has been met with a mixture of both idealization and fear.

The overall theme of this chapter is that while web-based assessment brings with it significant benefits as well as some specific increased risks, the fact that an assessment is being delivered over the Internet does not alter many of the basic clinical and ethical considerations that apply when any form of clinical assessment is used. That is, web-based assessment is simply a means to an end – not an end in and of itself – and must be rooted within the principles of sound clinical work.

HISTORICAL CONSIDERATIONS

Using computer-based applications to assist in the delivery, scoring and interpretation of assessments goes back well over 40 years (Butcher et al., 2004). These early computer applications were largely employed for test scoring and report generation and Meehl's (1954) classic work on the benefits of actuarial (or statistical) scale profile interpretation was predicated upon the use of automated test scoring systems. Through the ensuing decades, computers were often used to deliver and score clinical assessments, such as the MMPI, in large institutional settings such as United States Veterans Administration hospitals. In parallel fashion, the United States armed forces started using a computer-based testing system to assign recruits into military jobs in the 1960s (Wiskoff, 1997).

However, the application of computerized assessment methods was of limited interest to most mental health practitioners other than for those who used it for automated MMPI report generation. The situation started to change, though, in the middle 1990s with the advent of widespread access to the Internet. Assessments that only could have been delivered in paper-pencil format (or in rarer situations with a mainframe computer or a diskette-based system running on a personal computer) were now widely accessible and often on demand. Furthermore, not only could a vast array of mental health assessments readily be found online (by both clinicians and clients), a web-based assessment could now be created by virtually anyone with a modicum of familiarity with web-based development tools.

The benefits of web-based assessment delivery are substantial because it allows a test to be administered on virtually any computer with Internet access anywhere in the world with the scored results available almost instantaneously. This way, a client can complete the assessment at a convenient time and place while sparing clinicians the burden of managing, distributing and hand-scoring paper and pencil assessments. Additionally, since certain populations (especially younger and higher socioeconomic status groups) often prefer Internet-based to paper-pencil assessments, some clients may be inclined to view clinicians negatively who do not use web-based technology in their practices (Berger, 2006). From the perspective of a test developer, updates and the correction of inadvertent errors can be easily managed. In a similar vein, since the assessment is scored centrally, ongoing data collection is facilitated. Centralized scoring also helps to control the unauthorized use of copyrighted printed testing materials by limiting the need to distribute scoring keys.

APPLICATION OF THE TECHNOLOGY IN RELATION TO THE THERAPEUTIC INTERVENTION

Web-based assessment can readily become part of effective clinical practice and it is easy to envision a broad range of application for these tools. For example, it might be appropriate for clients to be offered the opportunity to complete their initial intake forms and screening checklists prior to their first appointment as opposed to arriving an hour early to do so. (Since it is recognized that clients may have a variety of reactions to completing this process online – especially in the very early stages of treatment – it would seem reasonable that clients be given the choice and not required to do so.) Additionally, if an assessment is required during the course of treatment, the client can be asked to complete it in a web-based format if this is seen as appropriate by the clinician.

Web-based assessments are also particularly well-suited for use in situations where the input of multiple persons would be helpful in developing a fuller understanding of a client but when the informants may not be able to participate in person due logistical or other factors. This may be especially the case when treating children (where obtaining information from teachers can be crucial, for example) or clients who have chronic and severe mental illnesses (whose family members or group home workers can provide much insight into daily functioning and other issues that the client may not be able to provide him or herself during the session). Similarly, web-based assessment strategies can be particularly useful when repeated measures are required to gauge response to treatment. If done appropriately, this may provide a way for clinicians to have frequent updates about a client's condition without the need and cost of an office visit. Even when compared to a phone call, web-based updates may be preferable for clients, their informants, as well as clinicians because they can be completed and accessed when it is convenient for the parties involved.

ETHICAL CONSIDERATIONS

There has been considerable discussion in the literature about the specific ethical considerations which may arise when web-based assessments are used (e.g., Association of Test

Publishers, 2000; International Test Commission, 2005; Naglieri et al., 2004). However, the most important concept for clinicians to bear in mind when using web-based assessments is that the same ethical practice standards pertain as they do when carrying out more traditional clinical work. That being said, there are some specific issues that come to the fore when web-based assessments are used that may require special consideration.

APPROPRIATE PROFESSIONAL USE

Given the flexibility of web-based technologies, virtually anyone with a moderate degree of technical knowledge can create and post self-created "assessments" on the Internet. To this end, much concern has been raised about the proliferation of unvalidated, online "pop" psychological test (e.g., Naglieri et al., 2004), which can mislead the public as well as unwitting clinicians. As a first principle, if a clinician implements an assessment, he or she has an ethical obligation to fully understand both its benefits and limitations. Similarly, clinicians should only use assessments in the manner for which they are intended and supported by research. For example, an assessment of depressive symptomatology that is normed on adults will likely not be particularly valid for use in assessing preteens. To this end, unless an assessment is accompanied by validation data, its utility as a clinical instrument cannot be realistically judged. Clinicians may also need to engage in educative efforts if they believe a client has been provided with inaccurate or damaging information though a poorly validated assessment that he or she found independently online.

Also, while web-based assessments are often accompanied by a report based upon scoring algorithms created by the test author, it remains the clinician's responsibility to interpret the results and share them with the client within the context of a professional relationship (see Michaels, 2006, for a general discussion). Assessment, be it web-based or not, is a professional activity just as is any other exchange with a client. As a result, assessment must take place within context of a defined professional relationship (American Psychological Association, 1992; 1985). As a result, the use of a computer-generated report does not remove the need for professional judgment and integration of the results. Matarazzo (1990) makes a useful distinction between "testing" and "assessment." While a test may be administered in any number of ways, it remains the clinician's responsibility to carry out assessment by integrating all available clinical data about a client to address the underlying referral question or reason for testing. Berger (2006) touches upon a similar theme in arguing that the critical issue in

> computer-based testing is not so much the technology, empowering as it may be, but more the uses to which such developments are put to meet the needs of clients. . . . Further, whatever the powers of computers and the software that controls what they do, it assumed that the clinician remains central and necessary to the process of understanding what test data mean and how they are relevant to the needs of individuals. . . . (p. 66)

PSYCHOMETRIC EQUIVALENCY

Concerns have been expressed in the literature about reports of instances where differences have been found in the results generated by legacy paper and pencil and web-based versions of the same assessment. While clinicians should have an awareness of this (e.g., Barak & English, 2002: Buchanan, 2003), it is becoming less of an issue as test norms are increasingly being derived directly from the web-based version of an assessment and not based upon preexisting paper and pencil norms. Additionally, there is a large body of literature indicating that this is not a concern for many instruments, such as the MMPI (e.g., Finger and Ones, 1999), nor is it typically considered to be an issue when tests are used for pre-employment selection (other than for highly speeded up tests that are heavily dependent upon screen design ergonomics; see Bartram, 2006).

SUPERVISED TEST ADMINISTRATION

While there exist a large number of assessments that can be delivered in a web-based form for clients to complete at their convenience, this may not always be clinically advisable because there are times where a test should be administered in a supervised setting. (The critical factor here is whether the assessment is supervised, not how it is delivered.) One factor is that the content of some assessments must be protected from disclosure. Additionally, there may be clinical situations (e.g., involving the legal system) where it is critical to verify that it was the client him or herself who actually completed the assessment without assistance or coaching. However, if clinically appropriate, a client's completing a web-based assessment in the quiet and privacy of their home may very well be superior to asking her to complete a paper-pencil assessment on a clipboard in the crowded waiting room of a busy community mental health center. As such, it is critical that the clinician be aware of the context and nature of the assessment situation and be fully responsible for managing it.

SECURITY AND INFORMATION PRIVACY

Another factor that often arises is that of security and privacy. Most clinicians cannot

be expected to have a deep understanding of the technical issues associated with web-based systems. As a result, they should only work with trusted providers of these services. However, basic considerations include ensuring that clinical and financial data are only transmitted with SSL encryption and that clinicians fully review their provider's privacy policy prior to using it. In the United States, awareness of HIPAA issues is also critical and most countries have equivalent legislation that must be taken into account, such as the Data Protection Act in the UK. An important issue to bear in mind, though, is that most Internet security breaches are due to end-user behavior (e.g., carelessness with passwords, failing to logoff systems), not technical malfeasance due to factors like hacking or interception of Internet transmissions.

RESPECTING INTELLECTUAL PROPERTY

Another important issue to recall is that unless an assessment is in the public domain, it is copyright protected. As a result, a clinician cannot legally create a web-based version of an assessment unless specific permission is granted by the copyright holder. In a similar vein, simply finding an assessment on a website does not mean that the website owner has the right to post the assessment unless copyright notices are prominently placed or the provider is a well-known test publisher. For security reasons as well, it is often best that clinicians rely upon reputably sourced web-based assessments.

CONTEXTUALIZING ETHICAL CONCERNS

While a number of ethical issues may arise when web-based assessment models are considered, they are rarely unique. Rather, the principles of sound clinical assessment practice should always remain at the forefront regardless of the assessment modality to be used. The Internet provides a means of delivering an assessment, nothing more, nothing less. As a result, the same professional considerations apply – regardless of how an assessment happens to be administered.

CLINICAL SCENARIO

Robert is an eight-year-old male referred for concerns about inattention at school, noncompliance at home and borderline failing grades. Robert's family had not sought help for these issues in the past. He was evaluated the previous year by the school psychologist with results indicating average intellectual abilities with no specific strengths or weakness but academic achievement slightly below expectation. Other than seasonal allergies, Robert had no specific health problems.

Robert's parents were divorced when he was three. He lived with his mother (who was not remarried) and visited alternate weekends and during summer vacations with his father who remarried two years ago and lived in a nearby town. His father had a child with his current wife approximately a year ago.

Both his mother and step-mother reported a fair degree of distress in managing Robert's behavior with father reporting a lesser degree of concern.

The clinician had a number of initial diagnostic hypotheses after first meeting with Robert and his mother which included Attention Deficit Hyperactivity Disorder, Oppositional Defiant Disorder, and Parent-Child Relational Problem. She was also concerned that Robert's mother might be overwhelmed in her role as a single parent.

The clinician wanted to get a sense of the child's behavior at home, school, community and at his father's home. After explaining this to Robert's mother in person and his father

by phone, she asked that Robert's mother, father, stepmother, teacher and afterschool child care provider complete a behavioral disorder inventory that assessed a broad range of child psychopathology and was linked to DSM-IV-R diagnoses. She also asked that all three of Robert's parental caregivers complete a parenting stress inventory. Given her concerns about father's potential lack of involvement with Robert, she requested a face-to-face meeting with him and asked that he complete the assessments in her office during the visit while the other involved adults completed web-based versions of the same assessments at their convenience

Based upon clinical interview, review of assessment data and a brief call to the teacher, the clinician felt that Robert met diagnostic criteria for Attention Deficit Disorder, Predominantly Inattentive Type. Additionally, review of the parenting inventories indicated that both Robert's mother and stepmother (though not his father) showed a moderate degree of stress in fulfilling their parental roles.

The clinician referred Robert to his pediatrician for a medication evaluation and proposed a brief course of behavioral parenting training for his mother, father and stepmother. She also shared with Robert's father the distress experienced by both Robert's mother and his current wife due to child management issues.

The clinician also made Robert's pediatrician aware of the use of web-based assessment tools; the physician subsequently used them to guide her titration of Robert's psychostimulant medication regimen by asking his parents and teacher to complete a behavior rating form on a weekly and then biweekly basis until his behavior stabilized.

Robert's caregivers responded favorably to parenting training with father becoming more involved and both his mother and stepmother indicating a lesser degree of stress after completing eight weeks of parenting training.

CONCLUSION

We are only now beginning to see how web-based assessment can have a revolutionary impact upon the provision of mental health services. To this point, the Internet largely has been used as a test delivery mechanism for pre-existing paper-and-pencil assessments. While this does bring value, these web-based testing systems have often been used as little more than electronic "page turners."

Looking to the future, tests will be developed specifically for Internet-based delivery. Not only will this render moot discussions about the method variance due to paper-and-pencil vs. online test delivery, it will take full advantage of Internet technology. For example, we are now starting to see the emergence of web-based adaptive test delivery whereby the sets of questions posed to a client are adapted based upon responses to prior questions. For example, if an earlier set of screening questions have ruled out the presence of psychotic symptoms, the client will no longer be asked about the symptoms related to this. Further, web-based technology can now be used to deliver assessments that could only be delivered by a desktop computer application such as those involving reaction time, intricate branched diagnostic interviews, or complex interactive neuropsychological tests. Finally, the use of web-based assessment also permits the use of audio and video content in assessment, a potentially promising yet largely untapped approach.

In a more mundane yet equally valuable step, web-based assessments can be integrated into electronic medical records. By moving assessments beyond use as stand-alone tools, web-based technologies can facilitate the integration of psychological testing data into the electronic medical record where it can be made differentially available to clinicians based upon their needs. For example, if a web-based tool were used for ongoing monitoring of depressive symptomatology, the mental health clinician could be provided with a detailed report of each client's reported symptoms while providers involved in other aspects of the patient's medical care might only be presented with a high-level overview. Similar, automatic warnings could be generated if specific critical items were endorsed or overall symptomatology reached a predetermined critical level.

In summary, we are at the edge of a revolution when it comes to web-based assessment. The surest path to this goal will involve creating a vision that is based upon a deep understanding of the technological benefits of web-based technology, well-grounded in the principles of sound clinical practice.

REFERENCES

American Psychological Association. (1985). *Standards for educational and psychological testing.* Washington, DC: American Psychological Association.

American Psychological Association. (1992). *Ethical principles of psychologists and code of conduct.* Washington, DC: American Psychological Association.

Association of Test Publishers. (2000). *Guidelines for computer-based testing.* Washington, DC: Association of Test Publishers.

Barak. A., & English, N. (2002). Prospects and limitations of psychological testing on the Internet. *Journal of Technology in Human Services, 19*(2/3), 65–89.

Bartram, D. (2006). Testing on the Internet: Issues, challenges and opportunities in the field of occupational assessment. In D. Bartram & R. Hambleton (Eds.), *Computer-based testing and the internet: Issues and advances.* Chichester: John Wiley and Sons.

Berger, M. (2006). Computer assisted clinical assessment. *Child and Adolescent Mental Health, 11*(2), 64–75.

Buchanan, T. (2003). Internet-based questionnaire assessment: Appropriate use in clinical contexts. *Cognitive Behaviour Therapy, 32*(3), 100–109.

Butcher, J. N., Perry, J., & Hahn, J. (2004). Computers in clinical assessment: Historical developments, present status and future challenges. *Journal of Clinical Psychology, 60*(3), 331–345.

Finger, M. S., & Ones, D. S. (1999). Psychometric equivalence of the computer and booklet forms of the MMPI: A meta-analysis. *Psychological Assessment, 11*(1), 58–66.

International Test Commission. (2005). *International guidelines on computer-based and internet delivered testing* [online]. [Accessed November 27, 2009]. Available from: www.intestcom.org/itc_projects.htm.

Matarazzo, J. D. (1990). Psychological assessment versus psychology testing: Validation from Binet to the school, clinic and courtroom. *American Psychologist, 45*(9), 999–1017.

Meehl, P. E. (1954). *Clinical versus statistical prediction: A theoretical analysis and a review of the evidence.* Minneapolis, MN: University of Minnesota Press.

Michaels, M. H. (2006). Ethical considerations in writing psychological assessment reports. *Journal of Clinical Psychology, 62*(1), 47–58.

Naglieri, J., Drasgow, F., Schmitt, M., Handler, L., Prifitera, A., Margolis, A., & Velasquez, R. (2004). Psychological testing on the Internet: New problems, old issues. *American Psychologist, 59*(3), 150–162.

Wiskoff, M. (1997). R&D laboratory management perspective. In W. A. Sands, B. K. Waters, & J. R. McBride (Eds.), *Computer adaptive testing: From inquiry to operation.* Washington, DC: American Psychological Association.

Chapter 15

THE ROLE OF BEHAVIORAL TELEHEALTH IN MENTAL HEALTH

Thomas J. Kim

INTRODUCTION

Technology is transforming healthcare in extraordinary ways, whether or not providers participate (Fieschi, 2002; Barak, 1999; Bauer, 2002; Swanson, 1999; Tang & Helmeste, 2000). This highlights the prudence of provider engagement to ensure a meaningful transformation. Key to considering technology in healthcare is to first appreciate the challenge and then consider the technology. Too often, the technologically "possible" captivates and risks failing to achieve genuine benefit.

This chapter will examine technology's role in clinical behavioral healthcare (i.e., behavioral telehealth), a challenge of limited resources and rising need. This examination will consider historic efforts, analyze the current landscape and offer opinions based on clinical and program development experience. The intent is to reframe a frequently stalled discussion towards sustainable progress. To illustrate the value of behavioral telehealth, the following case example is offered as a precursor to this chapter.

This case example is an amalgam of incarcerated Gulf Coast juveniles seen via telehealth both before and after the landfall of Hurricanes Katrina and Rita. Significant post-disaster provider shortages present an opportunity to realize telehealth services impossible by traditional means that in effect drives telehealth maturation. This case material seeks to illustrate the power of telehealth within juvenile correctional care that currently exists as multiple siloed efforts challenged by interfacility collaboration.

Youth X is a 15-year-old female with a history of mood disturbance, inappropriate behaviors, drug dependence and self-harm (i.e., cutting). Escalating difficulties led to incarceration with a court date six months from detention center arrival.

The youth presented for evaluation to a telepsychiatric detention center clinic. This clinic was built following the loss of an onsite psychiatrist who commuted 45 minutes each way with a history of arrival delays and last minute cancellations. Without an onsite provider, youths are transported with two correctional officers to the nearest clinic one hour away and five weeks from the date of request. With the telepsychiatry clinic, a counselor escorts the youth to a treatment room in five minutes and within one week of detention center arrival. The telepsychiatrist is notable for moving from the Gulf Coast before hurricane landfall while successfully maintaining a clinical telehealth practice despite two moves around the country.

Upon presentation, the youth regarded the teleconferencing equipment with both curiosity and caution. Engaging the youth resulted in her cursing the provider and walking out of the treatment room. As a result of telehealth efficiencies, encounter refusals are rescheduled in one week. For five months, the youth would present weekly only to curse and walk out. Despite this lack of engagement, weekly encounter requests continued based on the observation that the youth would refuse in person. At five months, the youth presented for encounter and sat down without a word. Maintaining eye contact and with the practitioner nonverbally encouraging her to say something, the youth finally declared, "Will you please help me?" Treatment then began in earnest. Following adjudication in court, the youth was sentenced to another correctional facility where the telepsychiatrist also provided clinical services. This resulted in an efficient transfer of service with immediate access to detention center collateral information and treatment recommendations. Service transfer is traditionally a fractured process of incomplete communication and need for redundant effort, activity and cost (e.g., labs and medication plan) now avoided due to telehealth efficiencies. Youth X was ultimately released to home. Discharge planning included the identification of provider follow up and provision of a 30-day take home medication supply. The Office of Juvenile Justice (OJJ) contacted the telepsychiatrist four weeks after the youth's release. The youth was unable to secure an appointment until two months after release and was about to run out of medications. Given the availability of teleconferencing equipment at OJJ (installed for administrative purposes), the youth was seen at OJJ almost immediately for assessment and renewal of her medication regimen.

BACKGROUND

Terminology

To begin, there is an issue with terminology (Sood et al., 2007). The prefixes tele-, e- and i- precede an already expansive medical lexicon describing telehealth activity. With such a diversity of descriptors, there is little wonder that shared understanding is elusive. Multiple descriptors also reflect the historically insulated nature of telehealth (Manhal-Baugus, 2001). Given this, consider the following:

Telehealth

The Health Resources and Services Administration (HRSA), Office for the Advancement of Telehealth defines "telehealth" as: "The use of electronic information and telecommunications technologies to support long-distance **clinical health care**, patient and professional health related **education**, public health and health **administration**" [emphasis added] (HRSA, 2009, p. 1). "Telehealth" is favored given its inclusiveness of all potential activities. While an individual may focus on one activity, programs are best served to include all three for reasons to be explored further.

Synchronicity

Synchronicity refers to the nature of telehealth engagements. If participants interact in real time, the engagement is "synchronous." While easiest to imagine in terms of clinical activity (e.g., synchronous behavioral healthcare versus asynchronous radiology services), synchronicity impacts design, operation, and support.

TECHNOLOGY

Video Teleconferencing (VTC)

Telecommunications has evolved considerably since the age of the telegraph; perhaps the first applied electronic telehealth technology. Subsequent synchronous innovations include the telephone, cellular/mobile phone, instant messaging and video-teleconferencing (VTC) (via videophone, computer (PC) or dedicated appliance). VTC solutions deliver multi-modal transmissions (audio and video) and offer a distinct value: approximating the face-to-face (FTF) encounter. The focus of this chapter will be limited to VTC solutions. The wide array of VTC solutions prompts further emphasis on dedicated appliances (Polycom, 2009; Tandberg, 2009).

This is not to say that other VTC solutions are unviable (Kaplan, 1997; May et al., 1999, 2000, 2001; Menon et al., 2001). Dedicated VTC appliances, however, invite consideration of acceptance and utilization. Dedicated appliances offer:

- FTF verisimilitude with image fidelity and size
- familiar interface for remote providers
- familiar patient experience with television displays
- higher prices among VTC solutions

Videophones offer a widely deployable, inexpensive VTC alternative though small screens convey a suboptimal viewing experience. This lack of verisimilitude is believed to limit widespread videophone adoption. PC solutions offer a comparable experience to dedicated appliances and are touted as more affordable. Cost savings, however, is a misplaced argument for PC VTC. Those familiar with PC malfunctions can appreciate the expense of PC maintenance and costlier risk of alienating users. User experience and solution stability, then, represents useful benchmarks when considering the appropriate VTC solution to deploy. Appropriateness, in turn, emerges as a helpful construct when engaging those evaluating VTC solutions (Tachakra et al., 1996).

CONNECTIVITY

During the 1990s, considerable attention was devoted to "low bandwidth" VTC (Baigent et al., 1997; Zarate et al., 1997; Wheeler, 1998; Haslam and McLaren, 2000; Matsuura et al., 2000; Bishop et al., 2002). This level of service typically required tolerance of suboptimal transmissions. Consequently, attire, lighting and even wall color demanded optimization with varying success. Despite these limitations, low bandwidth solutions supported considerable activity (Allen & Wheeler, 1998). Multiple programs emerged, but few survived beyond initial funding. Several factors contributed to this limited sustainability including the considerable expense of low bandwidth connectivity.

Fortunately, broadband connectivity has since yielded larger, more affordable offerings with a growing footprint of availability (Yoshino et al., 2001). Bandwidth and cost, however, are only two factors impacting connectivity (OECD, 2009a). The US, for example, is lagging behind other industrialized nations in broadband subscriptions (OECD, 2009b). This slowing of broadband penetration reflects the complicated issue of "last mile" connectivity. And while this "last mile" remains to be crossed, the US telecommunications infrastructure is positioned for a new generation of telehealth activity reflecting growth elsewhere in the world.

Acting on this opportunity requires a degree of heroism, as available evidence is scant and includes programs with dated connectivity solutions. Negative anecdotal experiences also persist despite being drawn from low bandwidth initiatives. An appreciation of how environment is outpacing evidence can be found at any Internet Service Provider (ISP). ISP offerings older than one year reveal that additional bandwidth is now available for less money. More bandwidth creates more opportunity and frames a renewed dialogue about the future of telehealth.

The implication of improved connectivity is not to simply endorse high bandwidth solutions, particularly given "last mile" challenges. It is rather to appreciate connectivity as a shared resource. Connectivity should inform telehealth development rather than the reverse (Yellowlees, 1997). The reverse occurs when connectivity is purchased exclusively for telehealth activity despite existing resources or additional needs. As healthcare workflow migrates to the Internet (e.g., Internet Protocol (IP) telephony, electronic health record (EHR) solutions, or electronic claims processing), an appropriate connectivity strategy is essential to sustainable growth (Sorensen et al., 2008).

TELEHEALTH MODEL

Model Design

Approach

An appropriately designed telehealth model is vital to success, but there is no readymade template (Dusserre et al., 1995). If a proposed model is flawed or misapplied, success is threatened in even the most receptive environment (e.g., prisons) (Myers et al., 2006). Having established a three-fold purpose, identified core technologies and encouraged a litmus test of appropriateness, the next step involves how materials and personnel come together. Conceptually, telehealth should support rather than replace traditional services (Qureshi & Kvedar, 2003). This speaks to the challenge of developing services and sensitivity required for implementation (Darkins, 2001).

Model design takes into account the challenge of maldistributed personnel and unmet service need. Responding with telehealth reveals some prevalent though unproductive preconceptions. For some, telehealth represents distant engagements to isolated communities. Geography, however, isn't the only

service barrier though support is typically reserved for remote areas. Whether six hundred miles or six blocks, "access" rather than "distance" should define an underserved community.

Care fragmentation is another noted concern (Nohr, 2000), but not one specific to telehealth. Consider Australian practitioners who found diagnostic clarity, but limited treatment benefit, from a collaborative behavioral telehealth initiative (Clarke, 1997). A potential explanation might be care fragmentation. The lack of perceived benefit might also reflect underutilization of the technology. Model revision could include stakeholders capable of satisfying unmet needs. In this revision, telehealth promotes a more cohesive model rather than an isolated solution separate from traditional resources (Gelber, 2001).

Seeking a finer point with model design highlights a number of publications offering insight. Collectively, they reveal shared elements of model success despite the heterogeneity of constructs. The reader is encouraged to explore the following:

- seven core principles (Yellowlees, 1997)
- readiness model (Jennett et al., 2005)
- appreciating remote site needs (Mitchell et al., 2001)
- identify the inappropriate (Jones, 2001)
- value of shared resources (Brown, 1995)
- whole system thinking (Kalim et al., 2006)
- workforce dilemma approach (Faulkener et al., 1998)
- value of adaptability (Kavanagh & Hawker, 2001)
- four-part pilot development (Gelber, 1998)
- integrated global networks (Shannon et al., 2002)
- theory of innovation diffusion (Grigsby et al., 2002; Rogers, 1995)
- human development metaphor (Yellowlees, 2001)

A 1964 RAND memorandum deserves special mention given its continued relevance with distant communications (Baran, 1964). Intended to advise the military on wartime survivability of command and control centers, communication network architecture is classified into three archetypes:

- centralized (single coordinating node)
- decentralized (several coordinating nodes)
- distributed (equally weighted nodes)

These archetypes serve equally well in describing telehealth sustainability. Centralized models adopt the wheel and spoke configuration often found in pilots and suggest a single champion driving activity. This model has limited sustainability when the champion is unavailable. Decentralized models are found in adolescent-aged programs with multiple champions and demonstrate higher levels of utilization. Decentralized programs are better able to withstand change given the adaptability of multiple coordinating nodes. Distributed models, therefore, describe mature programs with autonomous encounters across the network. Change within any node has little effect on a distributed program's sustainability.

HUMAN FACTORS

Efforts in Norway determined that non-technical factors (e.g., personality) notably affect telehealth success (Aas, 2001a). Such a conclusion suggests that some factors impacting telehealth may also impact FTF encounters. This is not to say that telehealth is identical to FTF encounters, but that certain factors apply universally. In fact, organizational workflow is affected by telehealth (Aas, 2001b; Aas, 2002a; Ball et al., 1995). Adjustments in expectations, responsibilities, and coordination present a host of human factors

to overcome prior to widespread acceptance and utilization (Hailey, 2001; Aas, 2002b; Whitten & Rowe-Adjibogoun, 2002; Bulik, 2008).

VTC communication is one such factor requiring support and training (Liu et al., 2007; McLaren & Ball, 1997). It is opined that while VTC communication is a unique skill, it is not unlike FTF communication adjustments (e.g., emergency encounter versus educational presentation). Moreover, as VTC transmission has improved, positive telehealth communication ratings suggest a close approximation to FTF communication (Miller, 2001). Therefore, the cultivation of VTC communicative skill should remain a broader professional competency rather than a technology specific undertaking.

Another notable human factor issue is the cultural defense towards preserving the therapeutic relationship (May et al., 2001; Marcin et al., 2004). While evidence exists that this understandable concern may be unwarranted (Ghosh et al., 1997), some resistance to telehealth is generally assured. An effective response to cultural defenders can be found with full disclosure. Telehealth seeks not to displace existing relationships, but support environments where relationships are wanting or absent. Demonstrating transparency with intent and approach can effectively engage proponent and critic alike.

Another notable human factor issue is the cultural defense towards preserving the therapeutic relationship (May et al., 2001; Marcin et al., 2004). While evidence exists that this understandable concern may be unwarranted (Ghosh et al., 1997), some resistance to telehealth is generally assured. An effective response to cultural defenders can be found with full disclosure. Telehealth seeks not to displace existing relationships, but support environments where relationships are wanting or absent. Demonstrating transparency with intent and approach can effectively engage proponent and critic alike.

MODEL IMPLEMENTATION

As circumstances vary, a universal implementation strategy does not exist. There are, however, considerations of which to be mindful.

Integration

The celebration with launching a telehealth program is often fleeting as utilization is likely to progress slowly (Liebhaber & Grossman, 2006). Utilization is a key measure of sustainability and, therefore, requires thoughtful attention (Buist et al., 2000; Yellowlees, 2001). Active promotion and a reliable referral mechanism are two means of encouraging utilization (Cloutier et al., 2008). Whatever the means, it is clear that the "build it and they will come" approach is suboptimal (Doolittle, 2001). A better approach might be "integrate it and they will come." Establish a plan for how a proposed telehealth model supports existing workflow towards enhancing behavioral health care delivery (Greenberg et al., 2006). Revisiting the above mentioned design citations, an integrated telehealth strategy encourages ongoing stakeholder input towards supporting widespread propagation (Yellowlees, 1997; Grigsby et al., 2002).

Model Support

Appropriate telehealth models are not without challenges such as support for encounter completion. This includes an effective electronic health records (EHR) documentation strategy. The number of available EHR solutions continues to grow though many may not survive long term (Makris et al., 1998; Kaufman & Hyler, 2005). The predicted culling is based on the challenge of interoperability (i.e., information transfer between health systems). Solutions fated for demise are often "home grown" and designed for unique workflow needs. Some commercial solutions adopt a similar approach and create limited utility beyond the solution and its subscribers. Though logical for market share, this approach silos information and runs counter to the conceptual benefits of EHR. When evaluating an EHR solutions, inquiry into how data is shared is as important as what data is captured. This would include the capture and sharing of utilization data among telehealth stakeholders (Wootton et al., 2002).

Operational Support

Successful telehealth programs require personnel with the necessary technology skills. This highlights two sources of expertise with Information Systems/Information Technology (IS/IT) and Telehealth. While related, the two camps are seemingly oppositional with the former ensuring network integrity and the latter encouraging network plasticity. Fortunately, the two are not exclusive as balanced inclusion of IS/IT and Telehealth input can prevent avoidable setbacks.

Telehealth operational challenges are still likely to occur. As a general rule, common sense suffices. Miller offers an interesting forensic challenge regarding the inclusion of remote individuals during legal proceedings (Miller et al., 2005). The limits with viewing perspective raises a concern for "witness coaching" off camera. A potential solution might be to place a mirror behind the remote participant thereby providing the local site with a clear view of the remote environment.

Personnel Support

The issue of training and personnel support cannot be emphasized enough (Picot, 2000). Though telehealth is presented as integrating into existing protocols, it helps to prepare for how telehealth will impact personnel. The literature is a good place to gain situational awareness (Health Devices, 1999), but conclusions are often dated or lack generalizability. Professional organizations (Online Therapy Institute, 2010; American Telemedicine Association, 2009; American Association for Technology in Psychiatry, 2009; International Society for Mental Health Online, 2009) offer more timely insight and expertise though specific recommendations (i.e., standards and guidelines) remain a work in progress in some instances (Loane & Wootton, 2002). Formal curricular resources (NARBHA, 2009) also exist and will likely grow in both quality and number. Ultimately, a brief orientation is sufficient prior to launching a telehealth program (Aas, 2002c). Adaptable and responsive longitudinal support, however, is far more critical (Buist et al., 2000).

If appropriately designed, implemented, and supported, telehealth participants will stop thinking about the technology, utilization will rise and the service delivery challenge will abate.

TELEHEALTH CHALLENGES

At present, the principal challenges to widespread telehealth use are neither clinical nor technological. The remaining hurdles are legal, regulatory and financial in nature (Klien & Manning, 1995; Sanders & Bashsur, 1995; Nickelson, 1996; Cohen & Straw, 1996; Stanberry, 1998; Schmitz, 1999; ManhalBaugus, 2001; Silverman, 2003).

These challenges indicate a still burgeoning field within an environment that predates telehealth innovations. Whether optimistic or apprehensive about telehealth, formal guidance is needed to both encourage appropriate growth and prevent misfortune. Unfortunately, the call for a more hospitable telehealth environment remains unanswered (Wootton, 1998). Prior to exploring these challenges, it bears mentioning that legislation is not itself a barrier to telehealth. Australia

appears to have reversed this conventional belief and suggests how lawmakers can be a telehealth propagator rather than an inhibitor (O'Shannessy, 2000). Telehealth propagation is also evident within the US. Moving forward, there remains need for continued engagement between health care, technology and government stakeholders committed to improving health care service delivery through telehealth (Silverman, 2003; Siwicki, 1997).

Those seeking a deeper understanding of how these challenges impact a particular jurisdiction can find additional information from the American Telemedicine Association, the Telemedicine Information Exchange, and the Center for Telehealth and e-Health Law (American Telemedicine Association, 2009; Telemedicine Information Exchange, 2009a; Center for Telehealth and E-Health Law, 2009). Broadly, principal challenges include the following.

Licensure

Licencing or accrediting bodies are essential to maintaining a safe workforce. The challenge lies with regulations negatively impacting workforce adequacy relative to service need. Border regions between Georgia and Florida, for example, reveal patients with high need and available providers on the wrong side. As the challenge of service delivery is blind to borders, the question is whether telehealth should enjoy a comparable lack of discrimination.

Currently, there is progress in the form of special purpose licensure within a few areas (Telemedicine Information Exchange, 2009b). Elsewhere, an unrestricted license is required for both the originating and receiving site. Brief consideration reveals the cost prohibition of securing multiple unrestricted licenses. In the US, the Federation of State Medical Boards is a welcome stakeholder with an interest in exploring national telehealth licensure (Federation of State Medical

Boards, 2009). Resolution, however, will be difficult for many reasons including safety concerns highlighted by the 2005 Ryan Haight case (see ryanscause.org, 2009 for details). Though the incident involved e-prescribing, the ensuing legislation underscores the need for a therapeutic relationship prior to treatment. As many areas continue to struggle with provider shortages, telehealth licensure reform holds promise towards ensuring relationships while maintaining citizenry protection.

Licensure reform has also raised concern among providers. Some perceive telehealth as threatening to local practices. As mentioned, telehealth seeks not to replace traditional services, but support areas with unmet need. In locations with adequate provider availability, many patients choose FTF options. One means of assuring local provider interests is requiring partnership with local resources as necessary for telehealth licensure rather than unstipulated direct access to the patient. There is also potential for local provider telehealth service exportation emphasizing the value of an appropriately designed model. Inappropriately restricting telehealth service access at the state or regional level is submitted as counterproductive to resolving service need and supporting provider interests. Licensure reform remains fundamental.

Malpractice

While licensure highlights the challenge of interregional telehealth, intraregional activity is equally challenged. Onerous regulations play some part in discouraging adoption, but another notable barrier is the threat of litigation. At present, there is a lack of legal precedent and uncertainty about how a telehealth malpractice suit would be pursued.

Rather than bog down debating jurisdiction and culpability, it is reassuring to note that providers of professional insurance are now offering coverage for telehealth providers. Another notable exemplar milestone in the US, also encouraging for those elsewhere, is that behavioral telehealth provider enjoyed malpractice coverage under the statutes covering provider liability in their care of vulnerable patient populations. The inclusion of telehealth providers is both appropriate and very encouraging.

Reimbursement

Within the US, securing telehealth reimbursement has met varying levels of success (Center for Telemedicine Law, 2003). Reimbursement remains a substantial barrier to scalable telehealth growth (Smolensky, 2003).

A potentially constructive approach may be to consider why payers are reluctant to reimburse for telehealth (Nesbitt et al., 2000; Whitten & Buis, 2007). As telehealth offers service potential in environments that previously went without, payers are not alone in having concern about additional system costs with a model lacking proof of benefit (Curell et al., 2008). Proving that telehealth merits reimbursement is best served by reframing the anticipated impact beyond the encounter to broader metrics of resource utilization, quality of life effects, relationship to legal proceedings, and other downstream costs (Jennett et al., 2003). These societal costs are all too familiar to legislators and others in the public sector, addressing behavioral health care needs. Therefore, the demonstration of telehealth benefit in support of reimbursement aligns perfectly with the behavioral health care legislative agenda.

TELEHEALTH EVALUATION

During the 1990s, telehealth conclusions were far from glowing despite the surge of interest and inquiry (McLaren et al., 1996; Rosen, 1997; Liu Sheng et al., 1998; Werner

& Anderson, 1998; Rohland et al., 2000; Mielonen et al., 2003; Webster et al., 2008). These limited findings were possibly inevitable given the novelty of VTC, limited functionality and high costs of poorly approximated FTF encounters. Consequently, a cooling of interest and lack of sustainability explains the decline of telehealth publication output (Moser et al., 2004). Fortunately, advances in, and acclimation to, VTC have resolved many of these limitations. This along with persisting access to care challenges sets the stage for a renewed surge of telehealth activity and evaluation.

A review of the telehealth literature reveals generally positive findings though generalizable conclusions are rare and the necessary support for telehealth has stalled (Hailey, 2001; Neckelson, 1996; Currell et al., 2008; Baer et al., 1997; Hersh et al., 2006; Singh et al., 2002; Whitten et al., 2002; 2007). One approach to increasing rigor has been the standardized comparison of VTC to FTF encounters (Baer et al., 1995; Baigent et al., 1997; Montani et al., 1997; Ruskin et al., 1998; Nelson et al., 2003; Alessi, 2000; Brodley et al., 2000; Elford et al., 2000; Matsuura et al., 2000; Yoshino et al., 2001; Jones et al., 2001; Bishop et al., 2002; McLaren et al., 2002; Simpson et al., 2003; Greenwood et al., 2004; Ruskin et al., 2004; Cuevas et al., 2006; Urness et al., 2006; O'Reilly et al., 2007; Shore et al., 2007a; Singh et al., 2007; Spalding et al., 2008). These assessments employ validated instruments (e.g., structured interviews) and offer notable conclusions. While these findings are of interest, it is opined that this strategy is flawed in two ways.

The first issue relates to the scrutiny that telehealth solutions are subjected to. Undue technology expectations (e.g., frame rates, packet loss, dropped transmissions) are a by-product of low bandwidth VTC solutions inciting worry about missed nuance. Maintaining this concern given current capabilities distracts from more productive lines of inquiry. Put another way, excessive scrutiny of VTC has been compared by colleagues to requiring provider vision and hearing exams prior to FTF encounters. As high bandwidth availability increases, concern about transmission fidelity will subside and attention will refocus on demonstrating the substantive value of telehealth.

A second concern with VTC versus FTF comparisons has to do with context. Considering whether a telehealth solution is viable compared to a FTF alternative presumes that the FTF alternative is available. All things being equal, most people would choose FTF encounters. As FTF options become increasingly scarce, time consuming or otherwise prohibitive, particularly with vulnerable populations, a more useful approach may be to compare telehealth to available alternatives. Given real-world choices, providers and clients alike may favor telehealth (Starling, 2003; Bischoff et al., 2004; Mekhjian et al., 1999). Unless FTF options dramatically improve, the preference for telehealth will continue to grow.

Calling for more rigor in the evaluation of telehealth is far from new (Hailey et al., 1999). One explanation for the pace and quality of published data relates to the maturity of reporting programs (Krupinski et al., 2002). Young programs lack the impact to demonstrate clinical efficacy and are left with qualitative inquiries into acceptance and satisfaction. Therefore, a staged evaluation strategy based on model maturity (i.e., maturing towards a distributed model) is both reasonable and recommended (Shaw, 2002). With maturity, agreement on metrics and pooling of interoperable data will yield the necessary rigor supporting the evidence-based practice of telehealth.

FUTURE DIRECTIONS

Utilization is a key to realizing telehealth

benefits. Telehealth treatment adherence is one such utilization metric that demonstrates comparable rates to FTF treatments (Ruskin et al., 2004). Attendance is another with rates reported as higher than FTF encounters, suggesting superior efficiency in service delivery (Zaylor, 1999). The influence of telehealth on practice behaviors, however, has revealed conflicting results (Grady & Melcer, 2005; Gruen et al., 2006; Modai et al., 2006). A potential explanation may be the early and unpredictable effects of telehealth within service naive environments. Increases in hospitalization rates attributed to telehealth, for example, result in rising short-term costs, but also potentially improved surveillance, better treatment response, and eventual reduction in hospitalization rates. Additional metrics that clarify practice habits in support of telehealth include time to follow up and efficiencies in encounter duration (Zaylor, 1999; Grady & Melcer, 2005). Ultimately, the manner and effect that telehealth has on these and other metrics holds enormous promise that may prove integral to future health care reform.

The economics of telehealth will also remain a fundamental and active area of inquiry adding to the current body of supporting evidence (Trott & Blignaut, 1998; Dossetor et al., 1999; Mielonen et al., 2000; Elford et al., 2001; Simpson et al., 2001a and b; Grady, 2002; Hyler & Gangure, 2003; Young & Ireson, 2003; Ruskin et al., 2004; Harley, 2006; Modai et al., 2006; Shore et al., 2007b). As suggested earlier, a thoughtful economic evaluation strategy is vital. A few notable considerations include maintaining the patient perspective (Simpson et al., 2001b), ensuring real-world comparisons (Dossetor et al., 1999) and appreciating a rapidly changing marketplace (Werner & Anderson, 1998).

A final research direction to note is the demonstration of improved clinical outcome (Ruskin et al., 2004; Grady & Melcer, 2005). Though available data remains limited, it is predicted that telehealth's impact on clinical outcome is assured as maturing programs continue to address widespread service needs.

BEHAVIORAL TELEHEALTH CARE

It may be apparent that there has been limited emphasis on behavioral health care in favor of a broader exploration of telehealth. This is intentional and reflects a core recommendation that telehealth initiatives should cast a wide net. Whether in terms of organizational investment or stakeholder recruitment, the underlying technology facilitates encounters regardless of content or purpose. Seeking equitable inclusion of any interested parties ensures appropriateness, encourages adoption, and enables long-term sustainability. It should be noted that behavioral health care practitioners enjoy the enviable position of engaging in telehealth without the need for additional remote enhancements (e.g., scope attachments). As such, behavioral telehealth has and will continue to be a sustaining presence within telehealth.

CONCLUSION

Behavioral health care stakeholders occupy a unique position in assuming leadership and advocacy roles towards demonstrating the virtue of telehealth across disciplines and purposes. Such a demonstration will be complicated, but the rising burden of mental illness and ensuing call for meaningful health care reform may offer sufficient leverage towards mitigating service delivery challenges through telehealth.

REFERENCES

Aas, I. H. (2001a). Telemedical work and co-operation. *Journal of Telemedicine and*

Telecare, 7(4), 212–218.

Aas, I. H. (2001b). A qualitative study of the organizational consequences of telemedicine. *Journal of Telemedicine and Telecare*, 7(1), 18–26.

Aas, I. H. (2002a). Changes in the job situation due to telemedicine. *Journal of Telemedicine and Telecare*, 8(1), 41–47.

Aas, I. H. (2002b). Telemedicine and changes in the distribution of tasks between levels of care. *Journal of Telemedicine and Telecare*, 8(Suppl 2), 1–2.

Aas, I. H. (2002c). Learning in organizations working with telemedicine. *Journal of Telemedicine and Telecare*, 8(2), 107–111.

Alessi, N. (2000). Child and adolescent telepsychiatry: Reliability studies needed. *Cyberpsychology and Behavior*, 3(6), 1009–1015.

Allen, A., & Wheeler, T. (1998). Telepsychiatry background and activity survey. The development of telepsychiatry. *Telemedicine Today*, 6(2), 34–37.

American Association for Technology in Psychiatry. (2009). *Homepage* [online]. [Accessed November 25, 2009]. Available from: http://www.techpsych.net.

American Telemedicine Association. (2009). *Homepage* [online]. [Accessed November 25, 2009]. Available from: http://www.atmeda.org.

Baer, L., Cukor, P., Jenike, M. A., Leahy, L., O'Laughlen, J., & Coyle, J. T. (1995). Pilot studies of telemedicine for patients with obsessive-compulsive disorder. *American Journal of Psychiatry*, 152(9), 1383–1385.

Baer, L., Elford, D. R., & Cukor, P. (1997). Telepsychiatry at forty: What have we learned? *Harvard Review of Psychiatry*, 5(1), 7–17.

Baigent, M. F., Lloyd, C. J., Kavanagh, S. J., Ben-Tovim, D. I., Yellowlees, P. M., Kalucy, R. S., & Bond, M. J. (1997). Telepsychiatry: 'Tele' yes, but what about the 'psychiatry'? *Journal of Telemedicine and Telecare*, 3(Suppl 1), 3–5.

Ball, C. J., McLaren, P. M., Summerfield, A.

B., Lipsedge, M. S., & Watson, J. P. (1995). A comparison of communication modes in adult psychiatry. *Journal of Telemedicine and Telecare*, 1(1), 22–26.

Barak, A. (1999). Psychological applications on the Internet: A discipline on the threshold of a new millenium. *Applied and Preventive Psychology*, 8(4), 231–46.

Baran, P. (1964). *On distributed communications: I. Introduction to distributed communication networks*. Santa Monica, CA: The Rand Corporation.

Bauer, K. A. (2002). Using the Internet to empower patients and to develop partnerships with clinicians. *World Hospital Health Services*, 38(2), 2–10.

Bischoff, R. J., Hollist, C. S., Smith, C. W., & Flack, P. (2004). Addressing the mental health needs of the rural underserved: Findings from a multiple case study of a behavioral telehealth project. *Contemporary Family Therapy*, 26(2), 179–198.

Bishop, J. E., O'Reilly, R. L. Maddox, K., & Hutchinson, L. (2002). Client satisfaction in a feasibility study comparing face-to-face interviews with telepsychiatry. *Journal of Telemedicine and Telecare*, 8(4), 217–21.

Brodey, B. B., Claypoole, K. H., Motto, J., Arias, R. G., & Goss, R. (2000). Satisfaction of forensic psychiatric patients with remote telepsychiatric evaluation. *Psychiatric Services*, 51(10), 1305–1307.

Brown, F. W. (1995). A survey of telepsychiatry in the USA. *Journal of Telemedicine and Telecare*, 1(1), 19–21.

Buist, A., Coman, G., Silvas A., & Burrows, G. (2000). An evaluation of the telepsychiatry programme in Victoria, Australia. *Journal of Telemedicine and Telecare*, 6(4), 216–221.

Bulik, R. J. (2008). Human factors in primary care telemedicine encounters. *Journal of Telemedicine and Telecare*, 14(4), 169–172.

Center for Telehealth and E-Health Law. (2009). *Homepage* [online]. [Accessed

November 25, 2009]. Available from: http://www.ctel.org.

Center for Telemedicine Law. (2003). *Telemedicine reimbursement report.* Center for Telemedicine Law: Washington, D.C.

Clarke, P. H. (1997). A referrer and patient evaluation of a telepsychiatry consultation-liaison service in South Australia. *Journal of Telemedicine and Telecare, 3*(Suppl 1), 12–14.

Cloutier, P., Cappelli, M., Glennie, J. E., & Keresztes C. (2008). Mental health services for children and youth: A survey of physicians' knowledge, attitudes and use of telehealth services. *Journal of Telemedicine and Telecare, 14*(2), 98–101.

Cohen, J. L., & Strawn, E. L. (1996). Telemedicine in the '90s. *Journal of the Florida Medical Association, 83*(9), 631–633.

Cuevas, C. D., Arredondo, M. T., Cabrera, M. F., Sulzenbacher, H., & Meise, U. (2006). Randomized clinical trial of telepsychiatry through videoconference versus face-to-face conventional psychiatric treatment. *Telemedicine Journal and EHealth, 12*(3), 341–350.

Currell, R., Urquhart, C., Wainwright, P., & Lewis, R. (2008). Telemedicine versus face to face patient care: Effects on professional practice and health outcomes. *The Cochrane database of systemic reviews.* Issue 2. Chichester: Wiley. Updated quarterly.

Darkins, A. (2001). Program management of telemental health care services. *Journal of Geriatric Psychiatry and Neurology, 14*(2), 80–87.

Doolittle, G. C. (2001). Telemedicine in Kansas: The successes and the challenges. *Journal of Telemedicine and Telecare, 7*(Suppl 2), 43–46.

Dossetor, D. R., Nunn, K. P., Fairley, M., & Eggleton D. (1999). A child and adolescent psychiatric outreach service for rural New South Wales: A telemedicine pilot study. *Journal of Paediatrics and Child Health, 35*(6), 525–529.

Dusserre, P., Allaert, F. A., & Dusserre, L. (1995). The emergence of international telemedicine: No ready-made solutions exist. *Medinfo, 8*(Pt 2), 1475–1478.

Elford, R., White, H., Bowering, R., Ghandi, A., Maddiggan, B., St John, K., House, M., Harnett, J., West, R., & Battcock, A (2000). A randomized, controlled trial of child psychiatric assessments conducted using videoconferencing. *Journal of Telemedicine and Telecare, 6*(2), 73–82.

Elford, D. R., White, H., St John, K., Maddigan, B., Ghandi, M., & Bowering, R. (2001). A prospective satisfaction study and cost analysis of a pilot child telepsychiatry service in Newfoundland. *Journal of Telemedicine and Telecare, 7*(2), 73–81.

Faulkner, L. R., Scully, J. H., & Shore, J. H. (1998). A strategic approach to the psychiatric workforce dilemma. *Psychiatric Services, 49*(4), 493–497.

Federation of State Medical Boards. (2009). *Advocacy, key issues and goals* [online]. [Accessed November 25, 2009]. Available from: http://www.fsmb.org/grpol_key issues.html.

Fieschi, M. (2002). Information technology is changing the way society sees health care delivery. International *Journal of Medical Informatics, 66*(3), 85–93.

Gelber, H. (1998). The experience of the Royal Children's Hospital Mental Health Service videoconferencing project. *Journal of Telemedicine and Telecare, 4*(Suppl 1), 71–73.

Gelber, H. (2001). The experience in Victoria with telepsychiatry for the child and adolescent mental health service. *Journal of Telemedicine and Telecare, 7*(Suppl 2), 32–34.

Ghosh, G. J., McLaren, P. M., & Watson, J. P. (1997). Evaluating the alliance in video-link teletherapy. *Journal of Telemedicine and Telecare, 3*(Suppl 1), 33–35.

Grady, B. J. (2002). A comparative cost analysis of an integrated military telemental health-care service. *Telemedicine Journal and E-Health, 8*(3), 293–300.

Grady, B. J., & Melcer, T. (2005). A retrospective evaluation of telemental healthcare services for remote military populations. *Telemedicine Journal and E-Health*, *11*(5), 551–558.

Greenberg, N., Boydell, K. M., & Volpe, T. (2006). Pediatric telepsychiatry in Ontario: Caregiver and service provider perspectives. *The Journal of Behavioral Health Services and Research*, *33*(1), 105–111.

Greenwood, J., Chamberlain, C., & Parker, G. (2004). Evaluation of a rural telepsychiatry service. *Australasian Psychiatry*, *12*(3), 268–272.

Grigsby, J., Rigby, M., Hiemstra, A., House, M., Olsson, S., & Whitten P. (2002). Telemedicine/telehealth: An international perspective. The diffusion of telemedicine. *Telemedicine Journal and e-Health*, *8*(1), 79–94.

Gruen, R. L., Bailie, R., Wang, Z., Heard, S., & O'Rourke, I. (2006). Specialist outreach to isolated and disadvantaged communities: A population-based study. *Lancet*, *368*(9530), 130–138.

Hailey, D. (2001). Some successes and limitations with telehealth in Canada. *Journal of Telemedicine and Telecare*, *7*(Suppl 2), 73–75.

Hailey, D., Jacobs, P., Simpson, J., & Doze, S. (1999). An assessment framework for telemedicine applications. *Journal of Telemedicine and Telecare*, *5*(3), 162–170.

Harley, J. (2006). Economic evaluation of a tertiary telepsychiatry service to an island. *Journal of Telemedicine and Telecare*, *12*(7), 354–357.

Haslam, R., & McLaren, P. (2000). Interactive television for an urban adult mental health service: The Guy's Psychiatric Intensive Care Unit Telepsychiatry Project. *Journal of Telemedicine and Telecare*, *6*(Suppl 1), S50–2.

Health Devices. (1999). Telemedicine: An overview. *Health Devices*, *28*(3), 88–103.

Hersh, W. R., Hickam, D. H., Severance, S. M., Dana T. L., Pyle Krages K., &

Helfand, M. (2006). Diagnosis, access and outcomes: Update of a systematic review of telemedicine services. *Journal of Telemedicine and Telecare*, *12*(Suppl 2), S3–31.

HRSA. (2009) Telehealth [online]. [Accessed January 11, 2010]. Available from: http://www.hrsa.gov/telehealth/.

Hyler, S. E., & Gangure, D. P. (2003). A review of the costs of telepsychiatry. *Psychiatric Services*, *54*(7), 976–980.

International Society for Mental Health Online. (2009). *Homepage* [online]. Available from: http://www.ismho.org.

Jennett, P. A., Affleck, H. L., Hailey, D., Ohinmaa, A., Anderson, C., Thomas, R., Young, B., Lorenzetti, D., & Scott, R. E. (2003). The socio-economic impact of telehealth: A systematic review. *Journal of Telemedicine and Telecare*, *9*(6), 311–320.

Jennett, P. A., Gagnon, M. P., & Brandstadt, H. K. (2005). Preparing for success: Readiness models for rural telehealth. *Journal of Postgraduate Medicine*, *51*(4), 279–85.

Jones, B. N. (2001). Telepsychiatry and geriatric care. *Current Psychiatry Reports*, *3*(1), 29–36.

Jones, B. N., Johnston, D., Reboussin, B., & McCall, W. V. (2001). Reliability of telepsychiatry assessments: Subjective versus observational ratings. *Journal of Geriatric Psychiatry Neurology*, *14*(2), 66–71.

Kalim, K., Carson, E., & Cramp, D. (2006). An illustration of whole systems thinking. *Health Services Management Research*, *19*(3), 174–185.

Kaplan, E. H. (1997). Telepsychotherapy. Psychotherapy by telephone, videotelephone and computer videoconferencing. *Journal of Psychotherapy Practice and Research*, *6*(3), 227–237.

Kaufman, K. R., & Hyler, S. E. (2005). Problems with the electronic medical record in clinical psychiatry: A hidden cost. *Journal of Psychiatric Practice*, *11*(3), 200–204.

Kavanagh, S., & Hawker, F. (2001). The fall and rise of the South Australian telepsychiatry network. *Journal of Telemedicine and*

Telecare, 7(Suppl 2), 41–43.

Klein, S. R., & Manning, W. L. (1995). Telemedicine and the law. *Healthcare Information Management,* 9(3), 35–40.

Krupinski, E., Nypaver, M., Poropatich, R., Ellis, D., Safwat, R., & Sapci, H. (2002). Telemedicine/telehealth: An international perspective. Clinical applications in telemedicine/telehealth. *Telemedicine Journal and E-Health,* 8(1), 13–34.

Liebhaber, A. B., & Grossman, J. M. (2006). *Physicians slow to adopt patient e-mail. Data Bulletin No. 32.* Washington DC: Center for Studying Health System Change.

Liu Sheng, O. R., Jen-Hwa Hu, P., Chau, P. Y. K., Hjelm, N. M., Yan Tam, K., Wei, C. P., & Tse, J. (1998). A survey of physicians' acceptance of telemedicine. *Journal of Telemedicine and Telecare,* 4(Suppl 1), 100–102.

Liu, X., Sawada, Y., Takizawa, T., Sato, H., Sato, M., Sakamoto, H., Utsugi, T., Sato, K., Sumino, H., Okamura, S., & Sakamaki, T. (2007). Doctor-patient communication: A comparison between telemedicine consultation and face-to-face consultation. *Internal Medicine,* 46(5), 227–232.

Loane, M., & Wootton, R. (2002). A review of guidelines and standards for telemedicine. *Journal of Telemedicine and Telecare,* 8(2), 63–71.

Makris, L., Kopsacheilis, E. V., & Strintzis, M. G. (1998). Hippocrates: An integrated platform for telemedicine applications. *Medical Informatics,* 23(4), 265–276.

Manhal-Baugus, M. (2001). E-therapy: Practical, ethical and legal issues. *Cyberpsychology and Behaviour,* 4(5), 551–63.

Marcin, J. P., Schepps, D. E., Page, K. A., Struve, S. N., Nagrampa, E., & Dimand, R. J. (2004). Using telemedicine to provide pediatric subspecialty care to children with special health care needs in an underserved rural community. *Pediatrics,* 113(1, pt 1), 1–6.

Matsuura, S., Hosaka, T., Yukiyama, T., Ogushi, Y., Okada, Y., Haruki, Y., & Nakamura, M. (2000). Application of telepsychiatry: A preliminary study. *Psychiatry and Clinical Neurosciences,* 54(1), 55–58.

May, C. R., Ellis, N. T., Atkinson, T., Gask, L., Mair, F., & Smith, C. (1999). Psychiatry by videophone: A trial service in north west England. *Studies in Health Technology and Informatics,* 68,207–210.

May, C., Gask, L., Ellis, N., Atkinson, T., Mair, F., Smith, C., Pidd, S., & Esmail A. (2000). Telepsychiatry evaluation in the north-west of England: Preliminary results of a qualitative study. *Journal of Telemedicine and Telecare,* 6(Suppl 1), s20–22.

May, C. R., Gask, L., Atkinson, T., Ellis, N., Mair, F., & Esmail, A. (2001). Resisting and promoting new technologies in clinical practice: The case of telepsychiatry. *Social Science and Medicine,* 52(12), 1889–1901.

McLaren, P. M., Laws, V. J., Ferreira, A. C., O'Flynn, D., Lipsedge, M., & Watson, J. P. (1996). Telepsychiatry: Outpatient psychiatry by videolink. *Journal of Telemedicine and Telecare,* 2(Suppl 1), 59–62.

McLaren, P., Ahlbom, J., Riley, A., Mohammedali, A., & Denis, M. (2002). The North Lewisham telepsychiatry project: Beyond the pilot phase. *Journal of Telemedicine and Telecare,* 8(Suppl 2), 98–100.

McLaren, P. M., & Ball, C. J. (1997). Interpersonal communications and telemedicine: Hypotheses and methods. *Journal of Telemedicine and Telecare,* 3(Suppl 1), 5–7.

Mekhjian, H., Warisse Turner, J., Gailiun, M., & McCain, T. A. (1999). Patient satisfaction with telemedicine in a prison environment. *Journal of Telemedicine and Telecare,* 5(1), 55–61.

Menon, A. S., Kondapavalru, P., Krishna, P., Chrismer, J. B., Raskin, A., Hebel, J. R., & Ruskin, P. E. (2001). Evaluation of a portable low cost videophone system in the assessment of depressive symptoms and cognitive function in elderly medically ill veterans. *Journal of Nervous and*

Mental Disease, 189(6), 399–401.

Mielonen, M. L., Ohinmaa, A., Moring, J., & Isohanni, M. (2000). Psychiatric inpatient care planning via telemedicine. *Journal of Telemedicine and Telecare, 6*(3), 152–157.

Mielonen, M. L., Väisänen, L., Moring, J., Ohinmaa, A., & Isohanni, M. (2003). Implementation of a telepsychiatric network in northern Finland. *Current Problems in Dermatology, 32,* 132–140.

Miller, E. A. (2001). Telemedicine and doctor-patient communication: An analytical survey of the literature. *Journal of Telemedicine and Telecare, 7*(1), 1–17.

Miller, T. W., Burton, D. C., Hill, K., Luftman, G., Veltkemp, L. J., & Swope, M. (2005). Telepsychiatry: Critical dimensions for forensic services. *Journal of the American Academy of Psychiatry and the Lazo, 33*(4), 539–546.

Mitchell, J. G., Robinson, P. J., McEvoy M., & Gates, J. (2001). Telemedicine for the delivery of professional development for health, education and welfare professionals in two remote mining towns. *Journal of Telemedicine and Telecare, 7*(3), 174–180.

Modai, I., Jabarin, M., Kurs, R., Barak, P., Hanan, I., & Kitain, L. (2006). Cost effectiveness, safety and satisfaction with video telepsychiatry versus face-to-face care in ambulatory settings. *Telemedicine Journal and E-Health, 12*(5), 515–520.

Montani, C., Billaud, N., Tyrrell, J., Fluchaire, I., Malterre, C., Lauvernay, N., Couturier, P., & Franco, A. (1997). Psychological impact of a remote psychometric consultation with hospitalized elderly people. *Journal of Telemedicine and Telecare, 3*(3), 140–145.

Moser, P. L., Hauffe, H., Lorenz, I. H., Hager, M., Tiefenthaler, W., Lorenz, H. M., Mikuz, G., Soegner, P., & Kolbitsch, C. (2004). Publication output in telemedicine during the period January 1964 to July 2003. *Journal of Telemedicine and Telecare, 10*(2), 72–77.

Myers, K., Valentine, J., Morganthaler, R., & Melzer, S. (2006). Telepsychiatry with incarcerated youth. *Journal of Adolescent Health, 38*(6), 643–648.

NARBHA. (2009). *Telepsychiatry seminars* [online]. [Accessed November 25, 2009]. Available from: http://www.rbha.net/index_seminar.htm.

Nelson, E. L., Barnard, M., & S. Cain, (2003). Treating childhood depression over videoconferencing. *Telemedicine Journal and E-Health, 9*(1), 49–55.

Nesbitt, T. S., Hilty, D. M., Kuenneth, C. A., & Siefkin A. (2000). Development of a telemedicine program: A review of 1,000 videoconferencing consultations. *Western Journal of Medicine, 173*(3), 169–174.

Nickelson, D. (1996). Behavioral telehealth: Emerging practice, research and policy opportunities. *Behavioral Sciences and the Lazo, 14*(4), 443–457.

Nohr, L. E. (2000). Telemedicine and patients' rights. *Journal of Telemedicine and Telecare, 6*(Suppl 1), S173–174.

OECD. (2009a). *OECD Broadband portal* [online]. [Accessed November 25, 2009]. Available from: http://www.oecd.org/sti/ict/broadband.

OECD. (2009b). *Broadband subscribers* [online]. [Accessed November 25, 2009]. Available from: http://www.oecd.org/data oecd/21/35/39574709.xls.

Online Therapy Institute. (2010). *Homepage* [online]. [Accessed January 15, 2010]. Available from: www.onlinetherapyinsti tute .com/.

O'Reilly, R., Bishop, J., Maddox, K., Hutchinson, L., Fisman, M., & Takhar, J. (2007). Is telepsychiatry equivalent to face-to-face psychiatry? Results from a randomized controlled equivalence trial. *Psychiatric Services, 58*(6), 836–843.

O'Shannessy, L. (2000). Using the law to enhance provision of telemedicine. *Journal of Telemedicine and Telecare, 6*(Suppl 1), S59–62.

Picot, J. (2000). Meeting the need for educational standards in the practice of telemedicine and telehealth. *Journal of Telemedicine and Telecare, 6*(Suppl 2), s59–62.

Polycom. (2009). *Polycom* [online]. [Accessed November 24, 2009]. Available from: http://www.polycom.com.

Qureshi, A. A., & Kvedar, J. C. (2003). Telemedicine experience in North America. *Current Problems in Dermatology, 32,* 226–232.

Rogers, E. M. (1995). *Diffusion of innovations.* New York: Simon and Schuster.

Rohland, B. M., Saleh, S. S., Rohrer, J. E., & Romitti, P. A. (2000). Acceptability of telepsychiatry to a rural population. *Psychiatric Services, 51*(5), 672–674.

Rosen, E. (1997). Current uses of desktop telemedicine. *Telemedicine Today, 5*(2), 18–19.

Ruskin, P. E., Reed, S., Kumar, R., Kling, M. A., Siegel, E., Rosen, M., & Hauser, P. (1998). Reliability and acceptability of psychiatric diagnosis via telecommunication and audiovisual technology. *Psychiatric Services, 49*(8), 1086–1088.

Ruskin, P. E., Silver-Aylaian, M., Kling, M. A., Reed, S. A., Bradham, D. D., Hebel, J. R., Barrett, D., Knowles, F., & Hauser, P. (2004). Treatment outcomes in depression: Comparison of remote treatment through telepsychiatry to in-person treatment. *American Journal of Psychiatry, 161*(8), 1471–1476.

ryanscause.org. (2009). The Ryan Haight bill (the Internet pharmacy consumer protection act) *ryanscause.org* [online]. [Accessed November 25, 2009]. Available from: http://www.ryanscause.org/ryan-haightbill.html.

Sanders, J. H., & Bashshur, R. L. (1995). Challenges to the implementation of telemedicine. *Telemedicine Journal, 1*(2), 115–123.

Schmitz, H. H. (1999). Telemedicine and the role of the health information manager. *Topics in Health Information Management, 19*(3), 52–58.

Shannon, G., Nesbitt, T., Bakalar, R., Kratochwill, E., Kvedar, J., & Vargas, L. (2002). Telemedicine/telehealth: An international perspective. Organizational models of telemedicine and regional telemedicine networks. *Telemedicine Journal and eHealth, 8*(1), 61–70.

Shaw, N. T. (2002). 'CHEATS': A generic information communication technology (ICT) evaluation framework. *Computers in Biology and Medicine, 32*(3), 209–220.

Shore, J. H., Savin, D., Orton, H., Beals, J., & Manson, S. M. (2007a). Diagnostic reliability of telepsychiatry in American Indian veterans. *American Journal of Psychiatry, 164*(1), 115–118.

Shore, J. H., Brooks, E., Savin, D. M., Manson, S. M., & Libby, A. M. (2007b). An economic evaluation of telehealth data collection with rural populations. *Psychiatric Services, 58*(6), 830–835.

Silverman, R. D. (2003). Current legal and ethical concerns in telemedicine and emedicine. *Journal of Telemedicine and Telecare, 9*(Suppl 1), s67–69.

Simpson, J., Doze, S., Urness, D., Hailey D., & Jacobs P. (2001a). Evaluation of a routine telepsychiatry service. *Journal of Telemedicine and Telecare, 7*(2), 90–98.

Simpson, J., Doze, S., Urness, D., Hailey, D., & Jacobs, P. (2001b). Telepsychiatry as a routine service–The perspective of the patient. *Journal of Telemedicine and Telecare, 7*(3), 155–160.

Simpson, S., Knox, J., Mitchell, D., Ferguson, J., Brebner, J., & Brebner, E. (2003). A multidisciplinary approach to the treatment of eating disorders via videoconferencing in north-east Scotland. *Journal of Telemedicine and Telecare, 9*(Suppl 1), s37–8.

Singh, G., O'Donoghue, J., & Soon, C. K. (2002). Telemedicine: Issues and implications. *Technology and Health Care, 10*(1), 1–10.

Singh, S. P., Arya, D., & Peters, T. (2007). Accuracy of telepsychiatric assessment of new routine outpatient referrals. *BMC*

Psychiatry, 7(1), 55.

Siwicki, B. (1997). Telemedicine. Legal issues could slow growth. *Health Data Management,* 5(4), 107–110.

Smolensky, K. R. (2003). Telemedicine reimbursement: Raising the iron triangle to a new plateau. *Health Matrix: Journal of Law-Medicine,* 13(2), 371–413.

Sood, S., Mbarika, V., Jugoo, S., Dookhy, R., Doarn, C. R., Prakash, N., & Merrell, R.C. (2007). What is telemedicine? A collection of 104 peer-reviewed perspectives and theoretical underpinnings. *Telemedicine and e-Health,* 13(5), 573–90.

Sorensen, T., Rivett, U., & Fortuin, J. (2008). A review of ICT systems for HIV/AIDS and anti-retroviral treatment management in South Africa. *Journal of Telemedicine and Telecare,* 14(1), 37–41.

Spaulding, R. J., Davis, K., & Patterson, J. (2008). A comparison of telehealth and face-to-face presentation for school professionals supporting students with chronic illness. *Journal of Telemedicine and Telecare,* 14(4), 211–214.

Stanberry, B. (1998). The legal and ethical aspects of telemedicine. *Journal of Telemedicine and Telecare,* 4(Suppl 1), 95–97.

Starling, J. (2003). Child and adolescent telepsychiatry in New South Wales: Moving beyond clinical consultation. *Australasian Psychiatry,* 11(Suppl), s117–121.

Swanson, B. (1999). Information technology and underserved communities. *Journal of Telemedicine and Telecare,* 5(Suppl 2), s3–10.

Tachakra, S., Mullett, S. T., Freij, R., & Sivakuma, A. (1996). Confidentiality and ethics in telemedicine. *Journal of Telemedicine and Telecare,* 2(Suppl 1), 68–71.

Tandberg. (2009). *Tandberg* [online]. [Accessed November 24, 2009]. Available from: http://www.tandberg.com.

Tang, S., & Helmeste D. (2000). Digital psychiatry. *Psychiatry and Clinical Neurosciences,* 54(1), 1–10.

Telemedicine Information Exchange. (2009a). *Homepage* [online]. [Accessed November 25, 2009]. Available from: http://tie.tele med.org.

Telemedicine Information Exchange. (2009b). *Law and policy in telemedicine* [online]. [Accessed November 25, 2009]. Available from:http://tie.telemed.org/legal/state_ data. asp?type=licensure.

Trott, P., & Blignault, I. (1998). Cost evaluation of a telepsychiatry service in Northern Queensland. *Journal of Telemedicine and Telecare,* 4(Suppl 1), 66–68.

Urness, D., Wass, M., Gordon, A., Tian E., & Bulger T. (2006). Client acceptability and quality of life – Telepsychiatry compared to in-person consultation. *Journal of Telemedicine and Telecare,* 12(5), 251–254.

Webster, K., Fraser, S., Mair, F., & Ferguson J. (2008). Provision of telehealth to the Scottish Police College. *Journal of Telemedicine and Telecare,* 14(3), 160–162.

Werner, A., & Anderson, L. E. (1998). Rural telepsychiatry is economically unsupportable: The Concorde crashes in a cornfield. *Psychiatric Services,* 49(10), 1287–1290.

Wheeler, T. (1998). Thoughts from telemental health practitioners. *Telemedicine Today,* 6(2), 38–40.

Whitten, P., & Buis, L. (2007). Private payer reimbursement for telemedicine services in the United States. *Telemedicine and e-Health,* 13(1), 15–24.

Whitten, P., & Rowe-Adjibogoun, J. (2002). Success and failure in a Michigan telepsychiatry programme. *Journal of Telemedicine and Telecare,* 8(Suppl 3), s75–77.

Whitten, P. S., Mair, F. S., Haycox, A., May, C. R., Williams, T. L., & Hellmich, S. (2002). Systematic review of cost effectiveness studies of telemedicine interventions. *BMJ,* 324(7351), 1434–1437.

Whitten, P., Johannessen, L. K., Soerensen, T., Gammonand, D., & Mackert, M. (2007). A systematic review of research methodology in telemedicine studies. *Journal of Telemedicine and Telecare,* 13(5), 230–235.

Wootton, R. (1998). Telemedicine in the National Health Service. *Journal of the Royal Society of Medicine, 91*(12), 614–621.

Wootton, R., Smith, A. C., Gormley, S., & Patterson, J. (2002). Logistical aspects of large telemedicine networks. 2: Measurement of network activity. *Journal of Telemedicine and Telecare, 8*(Suppl 3), 81–82.

Yellowlees, P. (1997). Successful development of telemedicine systems – Seven core principles. *Journal of Telemedicine and Telecare, 3*(4), 215–223.

Yellowlees, P. (2001). An analysis of why telehealth systems in Australia have not always succeeded. *Journal of Telemedicine and Telecare, 7*(Suppl 2), 29–31.

Yoshino, A., Shigemura, J., Kobayashi, Y., Nomura, S., Shishikura, K., Den, R., Wakisaka, H., Kamata, S., & Ashida, H. (2001). Telepsychiatry: Assessment of tele-video psychiatric interview reliability with present- and next-generation internet infrastructures. *Acta Psychiatrica Scandinavica, 104*(3), 223–226.

Young, T. L., & Ireson, C. (2003). Effectiveness of school-based telehealth care in urban and rural elementary schools. *Pediatrics, 112*(5), 1088–1094.

Zarate, C. A., Weinstock, L., Cukor, P., Morabito, C., Leahy, L., Burns, C., & Baer, L. (1997). Applicability of telemedicine for assessing patients with schizophrenia: Acceptance and reliability. *Journal of Clinical Psychiatry, 58*(1), 22–5.

Zaylor, C. (1999). Clinical outcomes in telepsychiatry. *Journal of Telemedicine and Telecare, 5*(Suppl 1), S59–60.

Chapter 16

THE USE OF VIRTUAL REALITY FOR PEER SUPPORT

Leon Tan

INTRODUCTION

Given that a host of developments in Internet technologies and cultures since the turn of the century have produced numerous widely accessible and highly immersive virtual reality environments or 3D virtual worlds such as Second Life, Entropia Universe and Small Worlds, it seems useful to consider how such virtual worlds may, like their offline counterparts, function to deliver therapeutic benefits beyond professionally run programs. In-vivo exposure therapy (IVET) is considered a standard treatment of choice for phobias with wide empirical support (Garcia-Palacios et al., 2007). As the Latin origin of the term suggests (*in-vivo* – within the living), such therapy involves exposure to actual aversive situations in the so-called "real" world. Thus IVET for the fear of flying involves exposure to actual experiences of flying, and IVET for arachnophobia involves exposure to actual spiders. Since at least the 1990s, however, virtual reality (VR) environments have been successfully deployed by mental health professionals in treating a variety of phobias as well as posttraumatic stress disorder. VR Exposure Therapy (VRET) involves exposure to virtual and not actual aversive situations. As Cote and Bouchard (2005) observe, a large

number of outcome studies now support the efficacy of VRET, and "most of them converge towards the conclusion that VRE[T] is as effective as in-vivo exposure" (p. 217). In a controlled clinical trial (n=83), Rothbaum et al. (2006) demonstrated VRET and IVET to be equally effective in treating fear of flying, "suggesting that experiences in the virtual world can change experiences in the real world" (p. 80). Furthermore, "the gains observed in treatment were maintained at 6- and 12-months" (p. 87), indicating that transformative virtual experiences carrying over into the "real" world may be sustained over time.

VRET is typically deployed in offline and/or "gated" VR environments, with elaborate technologies (e.g., computer driven head-mounted displays running 3D simulations) under the control of mental health professionals. The offerings of *Virtually Better* (http://www.virtuallybetter.com/), a leading provider of VRET, are thus located within physical clinics and administered by psychotherapists. Yet as Garcia-Palacios et al. (2007) observe, "most people who suffer phobias (around 60%–80%) never seek treatment" (p. 722), meaning that the benefits of VRET may be restricted to a minority of sufferers with the fortune or inclination to access professional clinic based services.

The goal of this chapter is to portray the mental health affordances of 3D virtual worlds for populations of individuals engaging socially as peers. This will be accomplished by way of a portrait of an adult woman overcoming agoraphobia through the social use of Second Life (SL), reported recently by Tracy Smith (2008) for CBS News on the *Early Show*. A case is chosen from popular culture in order to emphasize the wide accessibility of online virtual world based therapeutic affordances. In contrast to relatively scarce clinical virtual environments reliant on interventions by trained mental health professionals (such as psychiatrists, psychotherapists, and psychologists), the mental health affordances of online virtual worlds derive from interactions in supportive peer-based communities.

Quantifying the spread of mental illness and the associated impacts on individual quality of life and community health is never a simple task. Nevertheless,

> Data developed by the massive Global Burden of Disease study conducted by the World Health Organization, the World Bank and Harvard University, reveal that mental illness, including suicide, accounts for over 15% of the burden of disease in established market economies, such as the United States. This is more than the disease burden caused by all cancers. . . . (NIMH [video recording], 2001).

If this portrait of the global severity and cost of mental illness is anything to go by, it would seem that mental illness poses a significant and ongoing problem in contemporary societies. Given the seemingly intractable problem of mental illness worldwide and the large numbers of individuals not seeking out professional treatment for various mental illnesses, widely accessible peer-driven opportunities for improving mental health deserve greater attention.

AFFORDANCES OF 3D VIRTUAL WORLDS

For those unfamiliar with the term, "affordances" are sets of opportunities and risks particular environments supply or provide (Gibson, 1977). As a virtual social environment, SL provides individuals with a set of opportunities and risks to express identities and interact socially. The expression of identities and the production of social relations are vital dimensions of human existence and indeed of therapeutic and transformative experiences of self. In actual environments, expressing an identity and forming social relations take place largely through conversations involving both linguistic and nonlinguistic means. In the absence of physical bodies in SL, the expression of identity depends largely on the creation and deployment of a 3D avatar (see www.secondlife.com). A high level of visual customization is possible for an avatar, from facial features through to clothing and accessories. As for the production of social relations in SL, this involves the use of an avatar to participate in conversations. It thus relies on SL as an expressive repertoire and social ecology. That is to say, social relations in SL depend on the communicative means SL affords, as well as on SL as a population of peers with whom individuals may interact.

The SL user interface may be viewed by visiting www.secondlife.com; it will be useful to take a look to understand how an individual deploys a virtual life within an online 3D community. In the SL user interface, an avatar is located in the center of the screen looking outwards. SL's expressive means in the form of communication and navigation toolbars are located at the bottom of the screen. The communication toolbar provides options for engaging in conversations with other SL inhabitants using synchronous text and/or voice chat as well as bodily gestures (users can shrug, laugh, show boredom, bow, and point, amongst other things). Text clouds follow users throughout the SL world displaying context-relevant information such as the names of surrounding peers and interactive possibilities of various in-world objects. The navigation toolbar allows for movement of an avatar (typically walking or flying) through the 3D spaces of the SL grid. By and large, content and experiences within SL are user-generated, meaning that the spaces, architectures, avatars, and social events one is likely to encounter in-world are limited in variety only by the imagination and the basic rules for behavior known as "community standards." Users are also able to share various media and to perform specialized actions such as building rooms and houses. Together, all these various components can be considered SL's expressive repertoire through which individual users express identities and develop social relationships through conversations.

Mental health affordances can be considered opportunities and risks provided by a social environment to affect the mental health of individuals. In a recent article (Tan, 2008), I demonstrated how blogging (or writing socially) in the online community MySpace could function as a cathartic vehicle as well as to assist an individual in discovering and developing a "voice" in a social milieu. As an online community, SL also offers users opportunities for cathartic expression (tension reduction through affective expressions involving text, voice, and gestures), as well as opportunities to express and transform identities in social interactions. There are in fact a wide range of general and mental health groups and communities within SL offering specialized social contexts not only for cathartic tension reduction but also for social support and psychoeducation. The Heron Sanctuary, for example, is a group for disabled people gathering for mutual support and social interaction. Support groups also exist for autism, cancer, AIDS/HIV, agoraphobia, and so on. Finding one's way to these groups in SL is also relatively easy on account of portal organizations such as the Health Support Coalition and Health Info Island. SL thus offers users a range of opportunities to improve mental health. In the specific case of phobias, SL as a user-generated community allows for exposure situations through which individuals may confront and learn to cope with problematic associations between particular situations and anxious affects, as we will see in the case illustration.

CASE ILLUSTRATION

CBS News recently covered the case of an individual utilizing SL therapeutically to overcome agoraphobia. According to Tracy Smith (2008), Patricia Quig suffered from agoraphobia from an early age; a condition for which medication and psychotherapy offered limited help in her instance.

Agoraphobia is a condition where a sufferer experiences an increase in anxiety in social situations, which, left unchecked may develop into panic attacks. Another way of putting this is to say that agoraphobia involves the production of associations between social situations and anxiety. Anxiety and panic triggers for Quig included "too much people, too much noise, too much stimulation" leaving her feeling "too exposed" to the point where she became more or less house-bound and incapable of maintaining regular employment. Quig, however, discovered SL a little before her 40th birthday and became an active SL user through her avatar "Baji." For Quig, there is little doubt that virtual living in SL enabled her to gain traction in her battle with agoraphobia. As she herself says, "You can go and be with a group of people and discover that it's not the worst thing in the world . . . and that you don't feel strange doing it and enjoy it. And once you've learned that it's an enjoyable experience, you're not scared of it anymore" (Smith [video recording], 2008).

A vital aspect of Quig's recovery can be explained in terms of IVET and VRET. In the application of exposure therapy, sufferers are equipped by a psychotherapist with coping components such as relaxation training and cognitive reappraisal of imagined outcomes and then gradually exposed to (actual or virtual) conditions associated with a phobia and its anxious affects. Through repeated encounters coupled with the practice of coping skills, an individual experiences a new possibility – that of being in a "phobic" situation without being overwhelmed by anxiety. If we conceive of this new possibility as a new identity (differing from that of say an "agoraphobic"), we can say that the rehearsal of this new identity over time produces new associations between social situations and affective states. The portrayal of Quig's recovery by CBS shows precisely such a transformative process. As Smith observes,

> In Second Life, your alter ego, called an "avatar," can be and do anything. Quig's avatar, Baji, started doing things in second life she wouldn't consider doing in real life. "Facing her fears over and over again in Second Life freed Quig from her real-life phobias" (Smith [video recording], 2008).

Clearly, the therapeutic possibilities of invivo and virtual exposure are not confined to offline clinical contexts involving mental health professionals, but may also emerge for individuals interacting socially within a supportive network of peers in virtual worlds such as SL. Quig, it seems, found a way of expanding and transforming a self-limiting identity as the unemployed agoraphobic "Patty" to experiment with a virtually articulated new identity "Baji."

"Naïve realism" is a term that refers to conventional wisdoms sharply separating virtual experiences on the one hand and "real"-life experiences on the other. In naïve realism, real is conflated with actual. According to this view, social reality is confined to the actuality of material worlds; in the case of social relations, in the paradigmatic face-to-face encounter. The various experiences afforded by the Internet are, by contrast, deprived of reality and validity, fantastic (in the psychoanalytic sense of fantasy), and insignificant (because immaterial). To counter any naïve realist skepticism as to the "real life" effects of such virtual identity transformations, it is important to examine the mixed reality dimension of this case. By mixed reality, I mean the mixing of virtual and actual life worlds through the integration of Internet technologies and experiences into the fabric of everyday reality. The virtual must not be naively dismissed as less real or even unreal, but instead be understood as "real without being actual, ideal without being abstract" (Proust, in Deleuze, 1988, p. 96). Mixed reality provides a framework recognizing the reality of virtuality, allowing us to think virtuals and actuals as consequential and real dimensions of contemporary life.

The CBS news video clearly shows Quig walking through the aisles of an actual supermarket, when six months prior to her interview for CBS she was unable to shop in a grocery store. Furthermore, Quig was also able to travel to New York to participate in a face-to-face encounter with the CBS journalist before a massive American viewership. In discussing how the experience of overcoming her fears of social situations in SL has carried over into her actual daily life, Quig is very specific, saying, "I'm not *just* Patty anymore, I'm Baji . . . I just feel like a different person."

The actual effects of Quig's virtual social experiences testify to the therapeutic potential of 3D virtual worlds for individuals to rework habitual associations between effects, ideas, and actual life circumstances. By actualizing the virtual identity developed in SL, Quig effectively transforms her real life. Should she continue along this trajectory of expressing "Baji" and not just "Patty" in actual everyday situations, it is likely that Baji will eclipse Patty as a habitual identity.

DISCUSSION

If as the philosopher Deleuze (1991) argues, "We are habits, nothing but habits – the habit of saying 'I'" (p. x), it becomes possible to think of the mental health of an individual in terms of socially adaptive habits of saying "I" and of mental illness in terms of socially maladaptive habits of saying "I." The habitual saying of "I" is, of course, another way of discussing identity. In the case of Patricia Quig, we can consider "Patty" as a socially maladaptive habit of saying "I" on the one hand and "Baji" as an adaptive one allowing Quig to break out of self-imposed constraints in virtual and actual life on the other. Whilst Quig's case demonstrates the mental health opportunities of virtual worlds for situational phobias, it must be emphasized that SL's mental health affordances are not just limited to those suffering from agoraphobia, but instead may be deployed by any individual whose mental health is compromised by the existence of problematic habits of saying "I" and limiting self-images.

At the crux of the matter is the identity experimentation set into motion by an engagement in a massively social virtual environment such as SL. Where individuals are caught up in socially maladaptive habits of saying "I," transformations are made possible by an exploration of different habits of saying "I" (different identities or selves). In the illustration above, Quig need not stop at the first socially viable identity or self-image. Like other users of social 3D worlds, she is able to experiment with a multiplicity of possibilities for identity,

self-image and social relations and to reintegrate these experimentations back into the fabric of actual social reality.

The capacity to experiment with different identities and self-images in social interactions is not unique to 3D virtual worlds. Non-3D online communities such as MySpace and Facebook also provide such opportunities. SL, however, differs from non-3D virtual environments in the nature or style of identity expression. Unlike the photographs or videos depicting actual faces and bodies in MySpace-type communities, 3D avatars tend to bear less visual relation to actual appearances. This difference lends to a heightened sense of anonymity, accentuating and amplifying what Suler (2004) calls the online disinhibition effect – the tendency of individuals to behave in less inhibited ways in virtual spaces. Such disinhibition can be of tremendous therapeutic value if deployed in supportive contexts, leading to increased imaginative play and risk taking and thus the destabilizing of habitual associations and forming of new habits of saying "I". Where disinhibition inspires experimentation, SL–as an expressive repertoire–provides the means to express different self-images through the construction and evolution of 3D avatars, as well as the means to explore different social situations and dynamics through conversations and activities with other SL inhabitants.

Opportunities for transformative expressions of identity depend, of course, on the massively social dimension of online virtual worlds, not least because such expressions always take place in the context of social interactions, primarily conversations. In social reality, it is never enough for an individual to simply express an identity. As the work of Goffman (1967) demonstrates, participants in conversations must ratify each other in order to enter into a state of talk. That is to say, the expression of identity requires the validation/ acceptance of those addressed. Peers are thus important components contributing to the mental health affordances of virtual worlds. In the first place, supportive peers provide contexts for conversations within which individuals may experiment with new expressions of identity and thus form new habits of saying "I." Second, peers may assist in the development of socially adaptive identities through the repetitive validation of identity expressions, thus consolidating an individual's new habits of saying "I." Finally, peers interacting regularly tend to produce communities (such as the many specialized support groups in SL) within which new habits of saying "I" may be reinforced at a community level. Such peer-based communities may afford individuals a sense of belonging as well as a consensually derived social reality, thus supporting an individual's integration of virtual identity transformations back into actual life.

Thus far this chapter has focused on the mental health *opportunities* of peer-based 3D virtual worlds such as SL. Virtual worlds and the experiences they make possible also come with risks, as Turkle (1995) observes,

> People can get lost in virtual worlds. Some are tempted to think of life in cyberspace as insignificant, as escape or meaningless diversion. It is not. Our experiences there are serious play. We belittle them at our risk. We must understand the dynamics of virtual experience both to foresee who might be in danger and to put these experiences to best use. Without a deep understanding of the many selves we express in the virtual we cannot use our experiences there to enrich the real. If we cultivate our awareness of what stands behind our screen personae, we are more likely to succeed in using virtual experience for personal transformation. (pp. 268–269)

Turkle points out that it is possible to get lost in the elaboration of multiple identities online. It is also possible to overemphasize virtual living over actual experiences, or valorize actuality over virtuality as real. Whilst principles governing the provision of online mental health services by professionals have already been endorsed (ISMHO & PSI, 2000; Anthony & Goss, 2009; Nagel & Anthony, 2009), no such guidelines exist concerning engaging in peer-based social interactions in popular 3D virtual worlds for mental health benefit. Protection from risk in this case is best achieved by taking Internet virtuality and its experiences seriously, as well as by developing and promoting useful understandings of virtual life experiences and their affective relationships with actual life.

CONCLUSION

In conclusion, this chapter has explored how widely accessible virtual social worlds such as SL afford both opportunities and risks for individual mental health within the context of peer-based social interactions and ongoing relationships. Whilst virtual, transformative experiences of identity and self in SL relationships nevertheless have the power to affect actual lives, as the case of Patricia Quig demonstrates. This is because virtual experiences are no less real than in-vivo ones; IVET and VRET work because they both involve exposure within the living so-to-speak. The possibilities for peer-based use of virtual worlds for mental health are not limited to the conditions typically treated by VRET (namely phobias), but in fact apply to any situation where the development and social rehearsal of new and more socially adaptive habits of saying "I" may therapeutically displace maladaptive ones. Whilst a great deal of research has already gone into validating the professional use of VRE for the treatment of phobias and PTSD, relatively little has been done on the professional treatment of other conditions such as depression or generalized anxiety in virtual environments and even less on peer-based models of mental health development, within both 3D and non-3D online virtual worlds. Future research might thus investigate these neglected areas. Whilst this chapter proposes mixed reality as a more accurate and sophisticated reality framework, constraints of space have not allowed for a full elaboration, nor for a comprehensive critique of naïve realism (responsible for the kind of perspectives and attitudes belittling virtuality that Turkle cautions against). Future research might thus address the ontological status of virtuality and the relations of virtuals to actuals, as a great deal of confusion still exists both within academic and mass populations concerning the reality and value of online social experiences.

REFERENCES

Anthony, K., & Goss, S. (2009). *Guidelines for online counselling and psychotherapy including guidelines for online supervision* (3rd ed.). Lutterworth: BACP.

Cote, S., & Bouchard, S. (2005). Documenting the efficacy of virtual reality exposure with psychophysiological and information processing measures. *Applied Psychophysiology and Biofeedback, 30*(3), 217–232.

Deleuze, G. (1991). *Empiricism and subjectivity.* New York: Columbia University Press.

Deleuze, G. (1988). *Bergsonism.* New York: Zone Books.

Garcia-Palacios, A., Botella, C., Hoffman, H., & Fabregat, B. A. (2007). Comparing acceptance and refusal rates of virtual reality exposure vs. in vivo exposure by patients with specific phobias. *Cyberpsychology and Behavior, 10*(5), 722–724.

Gibson, J. J. (1977). The theory of affordances. In R. Shaw & J. Bransford (Eds.), *Perceiving, acting and knowing: Toward an ecological psychology.* Hillsdale, NJ: Erlbaum.

Goffman, E. (1967). *Interaction ritual: Essays on face-to-face behavior.* New York: Anchor Books.

International Society for Mental Health Online and Psychiatric Society for Informatics. (2000). *The suggested principles for the online provision of mental health services* [online]. [Accessed July 14, 2008]. Available from: http://www.ismho.org/ builder //?p=page&id=2 14.

Nagel, D. M., & Anthony, K. (2009). Ethical framework for the use of technology in mental health. *Online Therapy Institute* [online]. [Accessed December 4, 2009]. Available from: http://www.onlinetherapy institute.com/id43.html.

NIMH. (2001). *The impact of mental illness on society: A fact sheet* [online]. [Accessed February 3, 2006]. Available from: http:// www.masterdocs.com/fact_sheet_ files/ pdf/mental_illness.pdf.

Rothbaum, B. O., Anderson, P., Zimand, E., Hodges, L. F., Lang, D., & Wilson, J. (2006). Virtual reality exposure therapy and standard (in vivo) exposure therapy in the treatment of fear of flying. *Behavior Therapy, 37*(1), 80–90.

Smith, T. (2008). Real-life fears faced in an online world: Having alter-egos in 'Second Life' helps people cope. *CBS News The Early Show* [online]. [Accessed July 14, 2008]. Available from: http:// www. cbsnews.com/stories/2008/01/29/early-show/contributors/tracysmith/main 3763968.shtml.

Suler, J. (2004). The online disinhibition effect. *The Psychology of Cyberspace* [online]. [Accessed July 14, 2008]. Available from: http://www-usr.rider.edu~suler/psycyber /disinhibit.html.

Tan, L. (2008). Psychotherapy 2.0: MySpace blogging as self-therapy. *American Journal of Psychotherapy, 62*(2), 143–163.

Turkle, S. (1995). *Life on the screen: Identity in the age of the Internet.* New York: Simon and Schuster.

Chapter 17

THE USE OF PODCASTING IN MENTAL HEALTH

Marcos A. Quinones

INTRODUCTION

Podcasting, as it exists today, began to take hold in 2005, when Apple Computers included a directory of podcasts in its iTunes software. They saw big potential in a technology that could broadcast audio and video content over the Internet and be stored on computers and portable digital devices like iPods. The term podcast comes from the merging of iPod + Broadcast (Wikipedia, 2008). It is often thought of as a radio or television program that is reduced to a computer file. A podcast is a file that is created using a digital camcorder, computer and editing software. Creating podcasts is relatively easy and inexpensive and has therefore inspired thousands of professionals, including mental health professionals, to seek out the potential in using this technology to move their industry forward. In this chapter, I will discuss the use of podcasts in improving mental and physical health for clients, best practices in creating and keeping a podcast successful, ethical considerations and the role of podcasting in the future of mental health.

APPLICATION

I have been podcasting since 2005, when I first came across a podcast called Yogamazing.

Chaz, the author or podcaster, published a 10-minute yoga class each week that focused on a different part of the body. I recognized that this would be good as a psycho-educational addition to my practice. I decided to undertake this project and chose Self-Help as the theme. Similar to Chaz's Yogamazing podcast, I chose to focus on one problem, disorder, behavior, or idea in each podcast. Since then, I have created over 80 podcasts, which have been downloaded and viewed over half a million times by clients in countries as far as India, Thailand, Australia, China, Africa, Argentina, Iraq, and many others at http://www.thejoveinstitute.org/podcast.html.

The success of this project has been attributed to the ease of use in hearing the message. From the emails that I receive from clients that use my podcast to help themselves, the overwhelming benefit they take from it stems from learning a basic theory that they can then apply for themselves. Many of my podcast clients do not have access to professional mental health resources in their region or do not have the means to acquire the limited psychological resources that exist.

Others, in regions with sufficient professional help available, are hesitant or reluctant to attend therapy. Individuals have indicated that seeing the podcast showed them there might be a way out of their problems and that solutions could exist. Therefore, clients are eager to learn methods of helping themselves overcome depression, anxiety and other disorders and their causal self-defeating behaviors like social isolation, addictions and self-injury.

Podcast technology is global and can easily be misinterpreted. Not only do clients from different races, languages, cultures and religious backgrounds view the podcasts, but also clients with varying degrees of mental and physical functioning. Therefore it is very important to keep with an empirically proven theory when planning the fundamental underpinning of the podcast. I chose to keep with Cognitive Behavioral and Rational Emotive Behavioral Theories, which work exceptionally well as self-help adjuncts to cultural and religious beliefs (Selmi et al., 1990).

Some of the benefits that clients have reported are as follows:

Psychoeducation on the Theory

Clients report ease of use and understanding of the theory; the practicality of theory; the benefits of semantics on their culture, language and religious belief; the benefit of theory to people of different ages; and the sheer number of self-help techniques available to them.

Fictional Case Examples to Reinforce Theory and Self-help Techniques

Clients like the use of fictional case examples, as they say that it makes it seem like I'm not speaking about a theory, but about real people and how they use the exercises to help themselves.

Cognitive Exercises

Clients report benefits of changing the way that they think using self-talk exercises, homework assignments, worksheets, journals and lists.

Behavioral Exercises

Clients mention the benefits of relaxation training and breathing exercises, meditation and awareness and behavioral exercises to control addictions.

Emotive Exercises

Clients benefit from visualization exercises, labeling emotions and emotion logs.

Personable Nature of the Podcast

Clients point out the benefits of seeing me and being able to relate and feel the empathy and compassion coming through the visual medium. They consider valuable the fact that someone puts this kind of effort into solving their particular problem. They report the value of hearing the podcasts in their language at their intellectual level and benefits from the interactive technology that allow them to email comments, opinions and questions related to specific podcasts.

Professional Uses

Teachers have commented that they use my podcasts to present to their students. Website owners use my podcasts targeted at their client audiences (geriatric, children, etc.). Job groups and team leaders use my podcasts to help with common labor and environmental issues. An Iraq aid workers' team leader uses podcasts to help with addictions and secondary trauma. Private practice therapists use my podcasts to orient the client to therapy or the theory itself.

This is just a short list of the therapeutic benefits of this technology that clients, mental health professionals, nonmental health professionals and I have reported over the years. There are many more benefits, uses, and stories from clients that I will never hear, as well as around a million users who have used these podcasts and chosen to keep anonymous.

BEST PRACTICES

Podcasting offers a unique opportunity for someone with a message to reach hundreds of thousands of people. The technology allows for the proliferation of the podcast based on its merits and usually not on expensive advertising. Similar to dogmatic religions where it is an all or nothing belief of the theory, a mental health client can agree or disagree with the message and choose to subscribe to the podcast or not. This is what will determine whether the podcast is successful.

If the client subscribes to the podcast, then every time the podcaster uploads a new segment (podcast), the client's computer automatically receives it. Podcasts are usually free and the more people subscribe to the podcast, the more popular it becomes. Hosting companies and websites that draw millions of users advertise podcasts that are doing well by having a steady increase in the number of subscribers. These websites thrive on successful podcasts to draw users to their sites and subsequent advertising revenue. There are many creative ways for a podcaster to increase subscription numbers, but the bottom line is the message. This is important for mental health professionals who want others to benefit from their theories, because the message has to appeal to a wide range of individuals so that it will proliferate throughout the Internet and subsequently be advertised by these portal websites. In other words, subscribers = proliferation = success.

This success also works in reverse. Individuals can unsubscribe at any time. If the message does not have merit, or the podcaster does not upload new podcasts regularly, then subscription falls and the podcast becomes less desirable to the websites and individuals.

Therefore, it is important that before a podcaster decides to start podcasting, he or she defines a goal and determines how the podcast technology is going to help him or her to reach his or her goal. Each podcaster has his or her individual goal, but podcast technology is universal and in order to be successful using it, the podcaster needs to consider content and technology. It is similar to starting up a radio station that will potentially broadcast to millions of listeners – it will take a lot of work, dedication and money. Assuming the podcaster has a good work ethic, time to dedicate to creating a weekly or bi-weekly podcast, and enough money to fund the project, what is going to be needed? The following outlines the basics of identifying content and technological needs for the project.

Content

- Podcast Program Theme
- List of Podcast Titles for the First 10 Podcasts
- Target Audience
- Length
- Frequency
- Medium (audio only or audio/visual)
- Location

Technology

- Computer
- Digital Video Camcorder
- External Microphone
- Lighting
- Editing Software
- Internet Connection
- Hosting Facility
- Email Address

CONTENT

The Podcast Program Theme is the fundamental basis of the podcast. It is derived from the podcaster's goal and will be used by websites that promote podcasts to categorize and list it appropriately. The theme could be self-help, psychology lectures, mind-body, research study results, happiness, relationships, etc. A common mistake when setting the theme is not considering the longevity of the project as, for the most part, this theme cannot be changed. If a podcaster wishes to change the theme, a new podcast program will have to be created and previous subscribers will be lost. Along with the theme, the podcaster needs to develop a catchy definition of the podcast that listing directories will use to draw subscribers.

Creating a list of the first 10 podcasts and a definition of each is a good exercise. It gives the podcaster an idea of the work needed to come up with ideas for podcasts, a framework for initiating the project and a starting point to practice as the other logistical details come together. More than 10 may not be needed because if the project takes off, the podcaster should receive emails from clients on suggested titles for future podcasts.

Target audience should be determined when setting the goal of the podcast. The content, message, delivery, time, frequency and medium are all factors to consider depending on the targeted client demographics. For example, if the target audience is children, then specific technical arrangements will have to be considered to keep their attention.

The longer the length of time of the podcast, the larger the size of the file, and the larger the size of the file, the longer it's going to take for it to download to a computer. In this age of speed, clients tend to be impatient and will not wait minutes for a file to download. Therefore, it is important to keep podcasts to less than 15 minutes in length. Some websites have file size restrictions, which will help to limit talkative podcasters.

When beginning a new podcast, it is important to get the word out as often as possible. New podcasters may need to publish a new podcast every week or bimonthly in order to draw subscribers. When the frequency drops below one a month, subscribers lose interest and unsubscribe.

Podcasts can be audio only or audiovisual.

The podcast file is much smaller when it is audio only, but there are also limitations, such as competition. There are many more audio-only podcasts than audiovisual podcasts. Also, in mental health, I have found that it makes a difference for the client to see whom they are hearing. I have received requests for audio only and have created them for those users, but continue to do audiovisual podcasting for the vast majority of my subscribers.

Location is the least important of the logistical considerations but nevertheless important. I have received feedback that noise obstructs and distracts clients from hearing the message. The message should be clear and unobstructed so that it can be understood and internalized. Some of the distractions are noise from cars, people talking, air conditioners and other devices, color of room or office, art, size of the podcaster in relation to the room, clothing and grooming.

TECHNOLOGY

Making a decision on which computer to use early on will alleviate headaches in the future. It will be important to choose a computer with enough memory to store the large files that camcorders create before editing. Anything less than 100GB will become obsolete before you get properly started.

Choose a digital camcorder that is compatible with the computer that you chose above and an external microphone that is compatible to the camcorder.

I have found lighting and noise to be the main obstacles to expressing a clear message to my clients. Although sometimes professional lighting is not necessary, if you have the means, investing in professional lighting could be worthwhile.

I decided to use IMovie HD for editing my videos because of ease of use. There are many other editing software suites available in the market that are more flexible and can offer more than IMovie, but the "ramp-up" time (the time it will take you to learn the software and start using it) is longer.

A high-speed Internet connection is necessary because of the large size of the file that will be uploaded to the hosting facility.

A hosting facility is the place on the Internet that will host the podcast. Hosting facilities usually provide you with a website and limited storage capabilities. Depending on the frequency of your podcasts, it will be important to choose a hosting facility that will scale with you. Most hosting facilities allow you to purchase more space and bandwidth as your subscribers grow, but make sure of this in the beginning. The reason you need a hosting facility is because the podcast listing website will only list your podcast, it will not store it. When a new subscriber chooses to download your podcast, the website will direct them to a place where your podcast file is stored and the client downloads it from there. The process of downloading a file takes up bandwidth. Think of bandwidth as traffic on a road – the hosting facility owns this road and will allow a limited amount of your traffic and will charge you more as your traffic increases.

When your clients come across a problem it will be important for them to reach you. An email address for the podcast is important for feedback, comments, suggestions, recommendations and problem solving. Stay away from offering your phone number in any of the descriptions of the podcast; it will be impossible to return all of the messages you receive.

FILMING, EDITING AND HOSTING

I have found it useful to write down what I will say in the podcast and run through it a couple of times. Then, I put the sheets down and have a conversation with the camera. I have tried several ways to approach this and most of the feedback I have received supports a conversational approach. Film and edit the podcast using the instructions supplied by the camcorder and computer editing software, respectively. When you are done editing the podcast, the software should supply a file with the extension .mp3, .m4a, .mp4, .m4v, or .mov etc. This is the final file that will be uploaded to the hosting facility.

At this point, the podcaster is ready for others to start looking at his or her work. The podcaster needs to create an .rss file (which according to Wikipedia is called a "feed," "web feed," or "channel" and includes full or summarized text, plus metadata such as publishing dates and authorship) and submit it. The instructions for creating the file are very clear and there is plenty of online support from other podcasters should you have any questions.

TRACKING

You will want to know how many people are subscribing to your podcasts and there are several companies that do this. I chose Feedburner.com which provides an easy interface to track subscribers and hits to your website and podcasts. It is free and the information you get from the tracking software is invaluable.

FEEDBACK AND ADJUSTING

Finally and most importantly, be open to feedback. Ask your friends and family to go through the steps of finding your podcast and downloading and viewing it. If they have problems with it, most likely others will, too. Also, be open to feedback from people you don't know. There are people in different cultures who listen to your message and may have constructive criticism. If you don't take it personally, then you may have an easier time to make adjustments in subsequent pod-casts. Being able to listen to others criticize your hard work and make sense of it is a skill that will go well beyond podcasting and will help you develop as a seasoned podcaster.

ETHICAL CONSIDERATIONS

When considering ethical and moral ques-tions, the first thing a podcaster needs is common sense. The Internet has grown to be a global highway of information essentially be-cause of the morality and basic common sense of the people who publish information. Of course, there is plenty of misinformation pub-lished on the Internet, sometimes with tragic outcomes, but for the vast majority of web users, the Internet is a safe and useful place for publishing and searching for information.

Also, as mentioned above, the podcast technology serves as a gateway in weeding out messages that are not likely to serve others. The key to being a successful podcaster is subscriptions and subscribers are not going to subscribe for information that is not rele-vant, lacks evidence, or is false. The podcasts that are most successful present a clear mes-sage for clients to accept or reject.

Being a Licensed Social Worker in New York, I researched ethical and legal regulations that could be relevant within my professional organization and state law. What I found rel-evant was the importance of competence and of confidentiality (NASW, 2002). It was easy to stay within the boundaries of competence because of my podcast theme. At the begin-ning I had chosen to use as the underpin-nings of my podcasts a published theory that is empirically proven: Cognitive Behavioral and Rational Emotive Behavioral Theories (Chambless et al., 1998). Second, I chose never to discuss real cases online, instead using fictional case examples that were previ-ously imagined and presented the material to the audience by making the disclaimer that

the case example is fictional and names are made up.

Again, common sense comes to mind when I consider competence and confidenti-ality. Researching your professional organiza-tion's ethics and region's legal regulations is also important.

Disclaimers are also a good idea to protect the podcaster and the client. I make it clear in my podcasts that this is a self-help tool and is not meant to replace formal individual psy-chotherapy with a professional. I also men-tion that this is not meant to help people who are currently suicidal and that if someone is currently suicidal, he or she should immedi-ately seek emergency help.

CONCLUSION

Based on my experience, podcasts are an effective intervention in providing self-help techniques to clients, including individual cli-ents, mental health professionals, nonmental health professionals, and others. Any profes-sional who follows best practices in planning, implementing, and maintaining a podcasting project, considering at the same time the ap-plicable ethical and legal regulations, will be able to successfully reach and help a great number of people. The mental health profes-sion needs risk takers with common sense and integrity, willing to experiment with new technology to offer help to people and regions with limited mental health services. This pod-cast technology and others will continue to evolve and provide tools for these risk takers to test the limits of the technology. In the past, technology has been limited by memory space and bandwidth, but as more efficient hardware becomes available, memory and bandwidth will become cheaper. We are al-ready seeing this with the success of YouTube and Apple TV. YouTube has created data cen-ters and technology to host millions of large video files and making the bandwidth available for users to publish and view as many of these videos as they like free of charge and other companies are following suit.

In the next few years, it will be very likely for a school teacher, a housewife, or a hospital patient to turn on a TV and choose from over a million podcasts to bring joy, understanding, and alleviate a bit of stress about the world we live in.

REFERENCES

Chambless, D. L., Baker, M. J., Baucom, D. H., Beutler, L. E., Calhoun, K., & CritsChristoph, P. (1998). Update on empirically validated therapies, II. *The Clinical Psychologist, 51*(1), 3–16. Wikipedia. (2008). Podcast [online]. [Accessed August 14, 2009]. Available from: http://en.wiki pedia.org/w/index.php?title=Podcast &oldid=222708839.

National Association of Social Workers. (1999). *Code of ethics.* Washington, DC: NASW Press.

Selmi, P. M., Klein, M. H., Greist, J. H., Sorrell, S. P., & Erdman, H. P. (1990). Computer-administered cognitive-behavioral therapy for depression. *American Journal of Psychiatry, 147*(1), 51–56.

Chapter 18

THE USE OF ONLINE PSYCHOLOGICAL TESTING FOR SELF-HELP

Mark Dombeck

INTRODUCTION

This chapter concerns online psychological testing as it applies to self help efforts. The aims of this chapter are to review how online testing in its various forms supports mental health self-help efforts; to discuss problems and concerns associated with online testing and self-help practices; and to offer informed speculation concerning the ways in which online psychological testing and self-help technologies will likely develop in the future.

PSYCHOLOGICAL TESTING CONCEPTS REVIEWED

Psychological tests can be used for many purposes, one of them being to support psychological self-help efforts. Psychological tests provide a way for people to make tangible what are otherwise intangible psychological attributes, like mood. The act of self-monitoring raises awareness and tends to suppress the unconscious emission of undesirable behaviors. Repeated measurement over time enables people to track the progress of their change efforts over time, or understand how they compare to peers.

ONLINE PSYCHOLOGICAL TESTING

The Internet and the visual interface to that worldwide computer network known as the World Wide Web are arguably the most important technological and cultural developments of recent times. The web can be thought of as a digital publishing platform which can be used to present content, such as psychological tests, to consumers. The key word here is "digital." Because content published on the web is digital, it can be easily projected across vast (or local) distances, duplicated, stored, retrieved and manipulated via algorithm. These characteristics make it possible to effectively transcend many of the reproduction, scoring and scaling problems inherent to printed tests and offer dramatically new possibilities for psychological testing and for self-help and therapeutic efforts more broadly.

CURRENT AVAILABILITY OF ONLINE TESTS

The low costs associated with publishing content on the web has led to a rapid expansion of available online psychological tests, many of which have potential to be used for self-help purposes. Unfortunately, a good deal of these tests are of dubious quality. Popular testing websites, such as tickle.com and queendom.com, are advertiser supported and thus motivated to produce psychological tests for entertainment purposes so as to generate web traffic necessary to attract advertisers. Many of the tests appearing on such sites have little practical utility as capable measurements.

Though there are some quality and organizational problems with today's available online psychological tests, there is reason to expect that the situation will improve over time. As the web becomes ever more integrated into society, commercial publishers will create reliable and valid online versions of popular clinical measures and will integrate them into online self-help programs so that consumer choice of tests for self-help use is responsibly guided. Also, we can expect to see novel testing and self-help platforms built to exploit the rapidly evolving possibilities of the networked environment.

CURRENT SELF-HELP ONLINE TESTING EXAMPLES

Several current online self-help programs bear brief mention here as they illustrate how testing can function in the context of an online self-help program.

Qwitter.tobaccofreeflorida.com, an online smoking cessation tool, uses Twitter to help people track their efforts to quit smoking. Participants follow "iquit" and then use Twitter's response functions to record when they smoke and to keep an ongoing journal of their experience.

Psychtracker.com offers a freely available online behavioral recording tool suitable for use by people who are looking to keep track of various behaviors, moods, and symptoms as part of a therapy program or self-help effort. Users may create a free individualized account and then log in daily to make simple Likert ratings on relevant subjects such as suicidality, mood and interest in activities. As part of setup, users select only those subjects that are relevant for themselves to track. At any time, system users may view graphical representations of their progress over time and print out copies of their results so as to share with their therapist or self-help partners.

Myselfhelp.com offers a series of targeted online self-help workbooks based on cognitive behavioral principles. Regular measurement of targeted symptoms such as depressed mood is an integral part of each Myselfhelp. com program. In their Defeating Depression program, for instance, participants take and retake an online version of the Zung Depression Rating Scale and may view a graphical representation of their Zung scores over time as they make progress through the program. People using Myselfhelp.com programs can authorize their therapist to view their data.

Fearfighter.com (see also Chapter 12 in this volume) is another self-help implementation of online cognitive behavioral therapy. It is currently only available in the United Kingdom and only by a subscribing doctor's prescription. Fearfighter participants step through a series of steps designed to teach and implement CBT therapy principles (such as exposure therapy) proven to be helpful for treating anxiety problems. The program authors note that the system has been empirically studied and shown to be as efficacious as working with an actual CBT therapist. As regular symptom measurement is integral to all CBT, Fearfighter participants complete periodic online anxiety and adjustment questionnaires and review their progress over time via online graphs of their test scores.

DOWNSIDES OF ONLINE TESTING AND SELF-HELP

Though there are many benefits associated with online testing and self-help programs, there are numerous downsides as well. All of the psychometric caveats that apply to traditional testing practices also apply to online testing. A variety of security and privacy issues related in part to testing platform reliance on rapidly evolving and often bug-ridden web technologies create additional causes for concern.

Reliability and Validity Concerns

Reliability and validity are essential components of any useful psychological test. If either of these qualities are questionable for a given test, that test ceases to be useful as a measurement device and may deserve to be downgraded to a mere means of entertainment at best. Because of the advertisement-driven economics of web publishing, many currently available online psychological tests are there primarily to attract web traffic and advertising dollars. Other tests have been designed to be biased so as to lead consumers to come to particular marketing-driven conclusions (such as that they may have a problem that could benefit from a specific pharmaceutical aid). At least with regard to free-standing tests that have not been preselected for inclusion in a formal self-help program, there is no simple way for lay people to distinguish tests that are valid and reliable from those with alternative agendas. *Clinicians looking to recommend online tests for client's self-help use should take care to make sure that they are recommending properly validated tests.*

Even if obviously dubious online tests are eliminated from consideration, reliability, and validity concerns may linger. Establishing the reliability and validity of a test is a time consuming and expensive and thus infrequent process. Many tests which appear online are translations of tests which were developed and validated offline. It is not entirely clear that the reliability and validity of such tests will have survived this translation process intact. Any online version of a psychological test which has only been evaluated in its original print form (which describes most tests available today) should be considered somewhat suspect until a revalidation has taken place. *Interpretations made based on data taken from suspect tests should be qualified, at least, so as to acknowledge the issue if they are made at all.*

Data Interpretation Concerns

A virtue of online tests is that they can be self-scoring and can provide automated feedback as to what scores mean. For instance, a depression screening test can be programmed to make suggestions as to what different score ranges indicate with regard to the severity of a depression condition. A low score may suggest that depression is not a particular problem, while a very high score may suggest that immediate treatment would be a good idea.

Potential problems exist with regard to the accuracy and appropriateness of computerized interpretive feedback. Such feedback can only be made on the basis of numerical scores; it is not possible for the online testing system to take context or history into account, or to make adjustments for cultural variations in terms of how people will respond to questions. Consequently, there is an ever-present chance that test takers will receive inappropriate feedback, either minimizing the extent of existing problems, or, alternatively, making more of them than is warranted. Screening tests are generally designed to cast a wide net and may lead lay test takers to overly pathologize their experience. *Clinicians should take care to educate their clients as to how to best make sense of automated test interpretations and to the proper purpose of recommended tests. Screening tests should be distinguished from tests more appropriate for repetitive symptom tracking, for instance.*

Data Ownership and Privacy Concerns

Consumers utilizing testing and self-help services may assume that they own the data they produce, but this is by no means a safe assumption. Contemporary online testing and self-help services are generally provided by private, for-profit companies that may assert partial or complete ownership over data stored in their system. Further, testing data generated through the use of such services may not qualify for legal privacy protections afforded to medical records. Consequently, *clinicians should take care to carefully review the privacy and terms of use statements issued by testing services they plan to recommend.* These documents should make explicit who owns data generated by the use of the testing or self-help service, under what conditions that ownership may be asserted, and what the disposition of the data is in the event of a sale or similar transaction of the testing or self-help company.

Some uses for stored data a testing company may assign itself may be less palatable than others. For instance, a testing service that states it will use consumer-generated data in an anonymized fashion for purposes of quality control and benchmarking might be considered an acceptable use by most individuals. A service that plans to use the same data for direct marketing purposes may be something test-takers would rather avoid.

It is similarly important to know who is considered to be the actual client of testing and self-help services. Some testing services such as Fearfighter.com are sold to healthcare institutions that in turn provide them to health care consumers. In such a resale scenario, it can be confusing to know whether the client of the service (and thus the presumed owner of generated data) is the healthcare institution who paid for the service, or the healthcare consumer actually using the service. Exactly who owns generated data and to what degree each party may assert ownership over that data needs to be made clear in a process of informed consent prior to consumer's use of the service. To the extent that third parties are allowed to access testing data, the terms of service document should address this possibility and outline in detail under what circumstances third parties may see the data.

An obvious issue to explore and document concerns efforts testing services take to protect the privacy of testing system users. Psychological test data are personal and sensitive by nature. It could be embarrassing or even damaging to a system user's career or employment prospects should such data inappropriately find its way into a public arena. The potential for such damage to occur is greatly lessened when the testing service has taken care to properly design their service so as to anonymize and secure stored data. Programmatic encryption of passwords as well as actual data are possible, but the most effective method of all is to keep personally identifiable information wholly separated from all recorded test data. This is easy for most free services to accomplish since they never need to collect identifying information in the first place. Services that require a credit card or other identifiable payment must take additional precautions. The methods by which testing services secure data will hopefully be documented and discoverable so that potential consumers and recommenders of such services can make informed decisions as to whether or not to participate.

A separate issue to consider has to do with data retention policies. It is important for consumers of a testing service (and clinicians recommending such services) to know how long and under what circumstances a given testing service will retain customer data. If a testing service will delete an account after a period of disuse, a consumer of that service ought to know about that policy in advance. The only way to know this information is to carefully read the privacy and terms of service documents published by testing services.

The possibility of data portability is another area to explore carefully. It is possible for testing sites to allow users to export and download data stored within the service, but testing services may not be motivated to create such a download feature until multiple requests for it have been logged.

Even if the terms of service and privacy documents are all satisfactory, users of online testing services should be aware and comfortable with the fact that nothing on the Internet is ever truly stable and that data may be lost at any time. Catastrophic equipment failures, unfortunate software problems, malicious hackers and simple bankruptcy may force a testing service offline at any time. Testing service users should consider themselves to be on the bleeding edge of a new and emerging technology and should ensure that they are comfortable with the idea that they may lose all of their stored data without notice.

Security and Availability Concerns

It is *extremely* difficult to secure online services from all possibility of compromise. Web software is often created rapidly so as to gain competitive advantage and as such it can contain bugs and poorly written code that leave it vulnerable to attack by malicious hackers. More than just the testing application itself may be insecure; all layers of software from the server operating system on up through the web server, database and scripting language used will generally contain bugs and vulnerabilities. Internet service provider companies, (of which online testing providers are a subset) defense against such vulnerabilities is to make sure that server software is updated regularly with applicable security patches, to make sure scheduled security audits are performed, to properly apply firewalls and similar network boundary, encryption and monitoring measures and to expend resources fixing vulnerable code when it is found. While most companies make best efforts

to do these things, inevitably, some vulnerability remains.

If the need to fend off attackers was not enough, Internet Service Providers must contend with the vagaries of hardware and network failures and other events that can temporarily disable a service. Companies can partially mitigate such failures by hosting their application with a high-end service provider that makes available 24/7 network engineering support and monitoring, server spare parts, redundant high-speed connections to the Internet, physical security measures and backup services, but even when this is the case, temporary periods of downtime will probably still occur.

Measures taken by testing companies to identify and correct unwanted software vulnerabilities and mitigate damage from hardware and network failures may be documented somewhere on their respective websites. It is a good idea for concerned clinicians to research this information (or call to obtain it if it is not otherwise posted) so as to take it into account when deciding on which service to recommend or use.

In light of the inevitable security and availability issues that will exist, people using online testing or self-help services should be made aware of, and hopefully become comfortable with, the idea that data may be compromised or become temporarily unavailable. This comes down to an informed consent issue. The potential for compromise or failure is, of course, easier to stomach when little or no personally identifying information is attached to stored data.

FUTURE DIRECTIONS FOR ONLINE TESTING AND SELF-HELP

Online testing and self-help will undoubtedly continue to rapidly evolve both as network technologies evolve and as psychologists become more knowledgeable about how to put these technologies to work. I close this chapter with a few speculations as to the probable shape some of these future developments will take.

The trend towards designing web resources for consumption on mobile devices such as the cell phone and ebook as well as for traditional web browsers will undoubtedly continue. Online testing applications that incorporate behavioral recording (such as counting the number of cigarettes smoked, or types of foods consumed across the day) will benefit most greatly from this trend, as the use of such networked mobile devices will enable practical end-to-end digitization of vital *in situ* data.

Applications will be built up around online testing technologies so as to harness their potential as technologies of description and change. We are already seeing this in the form of self-help psychoeducational services such as Fear-fighter and Myselfhelp and in the form of various personality testing websites which, for a fee, will help you learn about yourself. As these applications mature and as more money becomes available to businesses offering these services, we will hopefully also see continuing efforts to empirically validate these services. The early example set by Fearfighter and Myselfhelp in this direction is encouraging.

It is still the case that relatively few clinicians have actively embraced online therapy at this moment in time, in part because of the strangeness and lack of body-language feedback current implementations of such services offer and also, in part, because professional associations and licensure boards have not always encouraged the practice.

What seems far more likely to happen, in my opinion, is for clinicians to incorporate online testing and self-help technologies into their face-to-face practice. For example, therapists might create homework assignments for their clients and enable them to keep an online journal and daily mood record through an online resource while still seeing clients face-to-face on a weekly basis. One can imagine future empirically validated therapies being shipped in manualized online workbook format, via an online application not unlike Myselfhelp that therapists could offer to their clients as a practical therapeutic resource. This sort of application would, of course, appeal most of all to behaviorally oriented clinicians treating highly specific and targeted disorders, as it would aid them in holding their clients to an organized and empirically validated track towards the resolution of their troubling issues.

FURTHER GENERAL READING ON PSYCHOLOGICAL TESTING

Cohen, J. (1960). A coefficient of agreement for nominal scales. *Educational and Psychological Measurement*, *20*(1), 37–46.

Cronbach, L. J. (1951). Coefficient alpha and the internal structure of tests. *Psychometrika*, *16*(3), 297–334.

Nunnally, J. C. (1978). *Psychometric theory* (2nd ed.). New York: McGraw-Hill.

WEBSITES

http://fearfighter.com/
http://qwitter.tobaccofreeflorida.com/
http://www.myselfhelp.com/
http://twitter.com/
http://www.psychtracker.com/
http://web.tickle.com/
http://queendom.com/

Chapter 19

TEXT-BASED CREDENTIALING IN MENTAL HEALTH

Daniel M. Paredes

INTRODUCTION

Continuing Education (CE credits) or Continuing Professional Development (CPD) is frequently included among the requirements for membership in professions. Continuing education requirements imposed by credentialing bodies often are met through text-based methods. The inclusion of such requirements, in addition to specialized training, assures that members of a particular profession are continuously offering high quality services (Daniels & Walter, 2002; Lundgren & Houseman, 2002). Requirements imposed upon working professionals are intended to assure that practitioners remain up-to-date on the latest trends in their respective field. In the case of the mental health professions such as counseling, this could include, for example, new epidemiologic data; new trends in theory and skills; and alerts to professional issues, such as updates to ethical codes, government policies, or third-party payment considerations (National Board for Certified Counselors, 2008). Taking into consideration the fact that, due to time constraints, many training programs prepare students in a generalist model, continuing education also plays an important role in facilitating the specialization of working professionals (Latham & Toye, 2006). Despite its ubiquity, there are some concerns with the relevance of compulsory continuing education, including that provided by text-based methods. In this chapter, the author will briefly provide an introduction to text-based continuing education, present a model other authors have developed for the classification of continuing education activities, discuss the ethical implications of the use of text-based continuing education and present recommendations for entities requiring participation in continuing education that can promote the appropriate use of text-based methods.

WHAT IS TEXT-BASED CONTINUING EDUCATION?

One could argue that continuing education activities have been a part of professional practice for millennia. Depending on one's view of continuing education, the guild model where master craftsmen trained and supervised apprentices could be seen as a continuing education process. Text-based continuing education methods and the implementation of systems for documenting continuing education are much more recent and have been associated with professionalization (Daniels & Walter, 2002). Defining text-based continuing education requires that continuing education as a whole first be defined.

Continuing education has been described as postgraduate participation in learning activities that are intended to provide up-to-date knowledge and skills pertinent to professional practice (Cividin & Ottoson, 1997; Daniels & Walter, 2002; Davis et al., 1999; Jameson et al., 2007; Lundgren & Houseman, 2002; Smith et al., 2006). Activities are generally didactic, experiential, or a combination of both. Defining which specific activities generally constitute continuing education is challenging as acceptable activities are defined by the bodies requiring continuing education for the maintenance of professional status and there is often little consistency with professions, across jurisdictions (Daniels & Walter, 2002; Latham & Toye, 2006). In the case of counseling in the United States, for example, it is not uncommon for policies to include continuing education credit for assuming a leadership position in a professional association (National Board for Certified Counselors, 2008; North Carolina Board of Licensed Professional Counselors, 2007). Other organizations may choose not to accept association leadership as a continuing education activity.

Text-based continuing education consists of professionals completing a reading selection, either in paper or electronic format and then demonstrating proficiency by obtaining a passing score on an assessment of learning (Davis et al., 1992). Recent attention has been directed to the use of computers and other technology as a means to delivering continuing education (Ellery et al., 2007; Krupinski et al., 2004; Smith et al., 2006). However, the fundamental process of text-based continuing education has been in place for decades. Correspondence courses and dedicated continuing education providers have been sending readings, sometimes accompanied by media such audio and videotapes since well before the Internet was invented. Didactic, text-based continuing education may be especially

helpful for providing information about practice issues rather than training in how to implement new information into practice (Aylward et al., 2003; Cividin & Ottoson, 1997; Davis et al., 1999; Vaughn et al., 2006). The selection of which topics to approach is largely at the discretion of the individual practitioner. In some cases, continuing education topics are prescribed by management at a professional's employer (Daniels & Walter, 2002; Latham & Toye, 2006). Ideally, however, the decision to participate in continuing education of any kind is preceded by a critical self-evaluation of what areas of professional knowledge and practice could be strengthened rather than a determination of what means is most expedient to meet recredentialing or agency requirements (Brown, 2002; Xiao, 2006).

Mental health/education professionals who have determined what topic they need to address and which continuing education method would be appropriate should consider that continuing education is known by several terms. Some terms (e.g., continuing medical education (CME), continuing nursing education (CNE)) are designed with certain professionals in mind. Nonetheless, they may be of value to professionals from other disciplines. For example, a text-based update on medications frequently used to treat attention-deficit/hyperactivity disorder would be helpful to many counselors as well as physicians or nurses. Other terms that are frequently used by scholars and continuing educational providers alike include professional development, continuing professional development, in-service training, and lifelong learning, among others. Professionals seeking to engage in text-based continuing education also would be well served by choosing the source of their education provider carefully. In an industry worth more than nine billion dollars, it is imperative that credible sources be identified (Vaughn et al., 2006). Some professional bodies, incidentally, have chosen to accredit certain continuing education providers. One example of how professional bodies have interceded to assure the quality of continuing education is the American Psychological Association's (2007) *Standards and Criteria for Approval of Sponsors of Continuing Education for Psychologists*.

ISSUES IN THE USE OF TEXT-BASED CONTINUING EDUCATION

A major criticism of continuing education activities is the apparent lack of a relationship to either practitioner behaviors or client outcomes (Aylward et al., 2003; Davis et al., 1999; Lundgren & Houseman, 2002; Smith et al., 2006). This criticism, however, warrants further study as there is some evidence that continuing education is helpful (Chakraborty et al., 2006; Davis et al., 1992; Smith et al., 2006; Xiao, 2006). Another criticism of continuing education activities is that they are susceptible to falsification. Continuing education credit at conferences and workshops, the most common type of continuing education, is given simply for attendance and not necessarily a demonstration of learning (Vaughn et al., 2006). As part of the general field of continuing education, text-based methods are not immune to such criticisms. Many text-based methods use post course tests to provide evidence of learning. It is unclear, however, what steps are taken to assure unethical participants are not simply choosing to participate in activities in which they already hold mastery. In other words, it is unclear what measures are in place to assure that an expert in a particular area is not fulfilling his or her continuing education requirements by participating in the easiest activity rather than one that promotes the development of new knowledge and skills.

Another criticism of didactic text-based learning methods, not solely those that are used in continuing education, is that they are an ineffective means of teaching skills (Davis et al., 1999; Livneh & Livneh, 1999; Jameson et al., 2007). In the counseling field, practica and internships are an integral part of training. The Unites States' Council for Accreditation of Counseling and Related Educational Programs' *2009 Standards* require training programs to provide supervised practica and internships with the expressed purpose of facilitating the translation of specialized knowledge into practice.

ETHICAL CONCERNS

The limitations and strengths of text-based continuing education mean that it can be used ethically – especially when included among other learning strategies. Ethical concerns arise, however, in situations where the practitioner, intentionally or unintentionally, does not engage in a breadth of activities ensuring their professional development. As noted earlier in the chapter, text-based continuing education is helpful for providing new and updated knowledge to practitioners (Davis et al., 1999; Smith et al., 2006). Undoubtedly, it is helpful for practitioners to be informed of new developments in theory and policy. In this respect, text-based continuing education should be a part of every practitioners' professional development plans. An optimal design of continuing education would include requirements based upon a system of classifying activities more precisely and understanding how practitioners planned to implement new knowledge and skills into practice. In the remainder of the chapter, a way that credentialing bodies could increase the relevance of continuing education is presented.

CLASSIFYING CONTINUING EDUCATION ACTIVITIES

Frameworks explaining continuing education and the continuing education process have been developed that are helpful in discussing text-based methods. One of these, the Application Process Framework (APF), explains the process by which continuing education activities are implemented in practice (Cividin & Ottoson, 1997; Ottoson, 1995, 1997). The APF is useful because it helps address one of the principal criticisms of continuing education – that participation has limited bearing on changes in practitioner behavior or patient/client/student outcomes. The other classification system discussed in the chapter, developed by Daiches, Verduyn, and Mercer (2006), provides a structure for classifying continuing education activities may be classified. The classification of content will be critical to discussion how text-based continuing education methods can be included in credentialing/membership organizations' requirements.

APPLICATION PROCESS FRAMEWORK (APF)

The APF is designed from the standpoint of what practitioners need to implement knowledge and skills developed through continuing education (Cividin & Ottoson, 1997). As such, the framework addresses barriers to implementation and may or may not address all of the limitations identified by researchers exploring the relationship between practitioner participation in continuing education and client outcomes. The framework is based on the premise that application considerations and training programs are in a continuous feedback loop. The influence of training on application is understood to be mediated by predisposing, enabling, and reinforcing factors (Aylward et al., 2003; Cividin & Ottoson, 1997; Davis et al., 1992). A characteristic that distinguishes predisposing factors is that they pertain to the individual practitioner rather than their work setting. Predisposing factors such as intrinsic interest in a particular continuing education topic have been identified

as the most influential in predicting application of learning. Enabling and reinforcing factors refer to steps a practitioner's employer provides in support of the application of knowledge and skills gleaned from continuing education activities.

An example of the feedback loop between application and training programs in the context of text-based continuing education is practitioners' identification of a spike in the incidence of self-injurious behaviors among teenagers in the United States. An increased amount of research was focused on the topic and materials for those who self-injure, as well as those providing support were developed (National Center for Trauma-Informed Care, 2008; Trepal & Wester, 2007). A predisposing factor might be the selection of the activity by a counselor working in a secondary school who constantly seeks to understand trends he or she sees in the student population. An example of an enabling factor would be the school administration's support for a comprehensive school counseling program. Reinforcing factors – those that support the individual practitioner – could be exemplified by other school staff with which the counselor can debrief periodically.

Requiring practitioner reflection upon how a text-based continuing education activity is being applied could encourage greater intentionality in identifying follow-up strategies. Practitioner use of the APF could also close the gap between the intended goals of continuing education and improved client outcomes. In addition to examining how text-based education is being applied upon completion, greater specificity in classifying content can facilitate the ethical use of this type of continuing education.

DACHIES, VERDUYN AND MERCER FRAMEWORK

Dachies and colleagues (2006) suggest classifying continuing education activities according to general content area. This strategy allows for more precise selection by professionals creating their professional growth plans (a plan indicating what knowledge and skills could be improved). The plan development process could be based on a list of profession-related job behaviors, such as that created by Brown (2002) or those routinely used to underpin accreditation and credentialing schemes, such as those developed by the Council for Accreditation of Counseling and Related Educational Programs (2009) and the National Board for Certified Counselors (2008). Dachies et al. identified five general categories into which continuing education activities could be clustered: *practice-centered activities, issue-centered activities, population-centered activities, specialism-centered activities,* and *service-centered activities.*

Practice-centered activities focus on refining one's training within a particular kind of therapy modality. Such activities may be especially salient for early-career professionals who were trained from either a generalist model or an overly specific model and who have found an interest in another theoretical framework. Issue-centered activities might include those related to programmatic issues such as improving a school environment or community advocacy. Population-centered activities focus on specific subgroups, such as at-risk youth, immigrants, or methamphetamine users. Specialism-centered activities focus on what Dachies et al. refer to as interest network issues. Activities in this arena might include those related to the practice of counseling internationally – such as the American Counseling Association's International Interest Network. Service-centered activities focus on administrative and professional association aspects of the profession. Counseling examples of service-centered activities might include updates on third-party payer reimbursement processes or political advocacy issues.

Revisiting how text-based continuing education is classified and the process by which it is reviewed could improve the relationship between this particular kind of professional development and the services provided to clients. Increased intentionality in selecting continuing education activities that are related to practice and are a different content area than one typically attended to could prevent professionals from simply choosing the most convenient activities or those that merely confirm what the professional is already doing.

ASSURING TEXT-BASED CONTINUING EDUCATION IS USED ETHICALLY

Given the limitations of text-based continuing education, its widespread availability and the pressures placed upon practitioners to meet requirements, the onus falls on credentialing bodies to encourage breadth in continuing education participation. Fortunately, existing frameworks for the classification of education methods and content allow for the ready categorization of activities in a way that facilitates the development of comprehensive professional development plans. Credentialing bodies, which have already established parameters for mandatory continuing education, also have the power to establish parameters regarding the proportion of requirements that are met by text-based or experiential methods as well as parameters regarding content (Davis et al., 1999; Vaughn et al., 2006; Xiao, 2006). Given the lack of research supporting the identification of an optimal proportion of text-based versus experiential methods, each credentialing body should make its own determination. Issues such as time commitment, for both the practitioner and the reviewing agency, costs and accessibility should be considered when establishing proportional requirements.

CONCLUSION

Continuing education is widely regarded as an important means to assure the public that practitioners are maintaining their knowledge and skills. Prior research suggests that, as it is currently used, continuing education may not be helpful as a strategy to assure competence. One particular kind of continuing education, text-based, may be helpful as a means to provide up-to-date knowledge. It may, however, be an ineffective means to assure that new skills are learned or that existing skills are refined. Therefore, text-based methods should be used in moderation as a strategy to assure professional competence through continuing education. Additional research is necessary to determine the ideal cost/benefit ratio with respect to requirements for continuing education modality and content. Nonetheless, given the doubtful utility of current strategies, revision of current schemes is warranted.

REFERENCES

American Psychological Association. (2007). *Standards and criteria for approval of sponsors of continuing education for psychologists.* Washington, D C: American Psychological Association.

Aylward, S., Stolee, P., Keat, N., & Johncox, V. (2003). Effectiveness of continuing education in long-term care: A literature review. *Gerontologist, 43*(2), 259–271.

Brown, M. (2002). Best practices in professional development. In A. Thomas & J. Grimes (Eds.), *Best practices in school psychology* (4th ed.). Washington, DC: National Association of School Psychologists.

Chakraborty, N., Prasad Sinha, B. N., Nizamie, S. H., Sinha, V. K., Akhtar, S., Beck, J., & Binha, B. (2006). Effectiveness of continuing nursing education program in child psychiatry. *Journal of Child and Adolescent Psychiatric Nursing, 19*(1), 21–28.

Cividin, T. M., & Ottoson, J. M. (1997). Linking reasons for continuing professional education participation with postprogram application. *The Journal of Continuing Education in the Health Professions, 17*(1), 46–55.

Council for Accreditation of Counseling and Related Educational Programs. (2009). *2009 Standards.* Alexandria, VA: Council for Accreditation of Counseling and Related Educational Programs.

Daiches, A., Verduyn, C., & Mercer, A. (2006). Continuing professional development mid career. In L. Golding & I. Gray (Eds.), *Continuing professional development for clinical psychologists: A practical handbook.* Oxford: British Psychological Society/ Blackwell.

Daniels, A. S., & Walter, D. A. (2002). Current issues in continuing education for contemporary behavioral health practice. *Administration and Policy in Mental Health, 29*(4), 359–376.

Davis, D., O'Brien, M. A., Freemantle, N., Wolf, F. M., Maxmanian, P., & TaylorVaisey, A. (1999). Impact of formal continuing medical education. Do conferences, workshops, rounds and other traditional continuing education activities change physician behavior or health care outcomes? *Journal of the American Medical Association, 282*(9), 867–874.

Davis, D. A., Thomson, M. A., Oxman, A. D., & Haynes, R. B. (1992). Evidence for the effectiveness of CME: A review of 50 randomized controlled trials. *Journal of the American Medical Association, 268*(9), 1111–1117.

Ellery, J., McDermott, R. J., & Ellery, P. J. (2007). Computers as formal continuing education tool: Moving beyond intention. *American Journal of Health Behavior, 31*(3), 312–322.

Jameson, P., Stadter, M., & Poulton, J. (2007). Sustained and sustaining continuing education for therapists. *Psychotherapy: Theory, Research, Practice, Training, 44*(1), 110–114.

Krupinski, E. A., Lopez, M., Lyman, T., Barker, G., & Weinstein, R. S. (2004). Continuing education via telemedicine: Analysis of reasons for attending or not attending. *Telemedicine Journal and E-Health, 10*(3), 403–409.

Latham, A., & Toye, K. (2006). CPD and newly qualified clinical psychologists. In L. Golding & I. Brown (Eds.), *Continuing professional development for clinical psychologists: A practical handbook.* Oxford: British Psychological Society/Blackwell.

Livneh, C., & Livneh, H. (1999). Continuing professional education among educators: Predictors of participation in learning activities. *Adult Education Quarterly, 49*(2), 91–106.

Lundgren, B. S., & Houseman, C. A. (2002). Continuing competence in selected health care professions. *Journal of Allied Health Professions, 31*(4), 232–240.

National Board for Certified Counselors. (2008). *NBCC continuing education file.* Greensboro, NC: National Board for Certified Counselors.

National Center for Trauma-Informed Care. (2008). Self-inflicted violence: Understanding and treatment. *Trauma Matters* [online]. [Accessed November 27, 2009]. Available from: http://mentalhealth.samhsa.gov/nctic/newsletter_02-2008.asp.

North Carolina Board of Licensed Professional Counselors. (2007). *License renewal guidelines.* Garner, NC: North Carolina Board of Licensed Professional Counselors.

Ottoson, J. M. (1995). Use of a conceptual framework to explore multiple influences on the application of learning following a continuing education program. *Canadian Journal for the Study of Adult Education, 9*(2), 1–18.

Ottoson, J. M. (1997). After the applause: Exploring multiple influences on application following an adult education program. *Adult Education Quarterly, 47*(2), 92–107.

Smith, C. A., Gant, A., Cohen-Callow, A., Cornelius, L. J., Dia, D. A., Harrington, D., & Bliss, D. L. (2006). Staying current in a changing profession: Evaluating perceived change resulting from continuing professional education. *Journal of Social Work Education, 42*(3), 465–482.

Trepal, H. C., & Wester, K. L. (2007). Self-injurious behaviors, diagnoses and treatment methods: What mental health professionals are reporting. *Journal of Mental Health Counseling, 29*(4), 363–375.

Vaughn, H. T., Rogers, J. L., & Freeman, J. K. (2006). Does requiring continuing education units for professional licensing renewal assure quality patient care? *The Health Care Manager, 25*(1), 78–84.

Xiao, L. D. (2006). Nurse educators' perceived challenges in mandatory continuing nursing education. *International Nursing Review, 53*(3), 217–223.

Chapter 20

ONLINE RESEARCH METHODS FOR MENTAL HEALTH

Tristram Hooley and Vanessa Dodd

INTRODUCTION

Internet technologies have shaped both the way in which individual's live their lives and the practices of mental health counsellors and psychotherapists. Researchers are legitimately interested in both of these issues and may wish to construct research projects that investigate both the intersection between individual's mental health and the Internet and the affordances of the online and digital environments for supporting individuals' mental health quite apart from using the Internet as a medium for conducting research in itself. Online research methods in mental health are now well established and can provide us with numerous models to follow for future research.

The saturation of the Internet into our daily lives has created unique challenges for those working in mental health, counselling and psychotherapy. The Internet can shape an individual's mental health as well as how they access mental health information and support. For example, many research studies focus on the intersections between mental health and problematic Internet use as well as smartphone addiction (e.g., Yau, Potenza, & White, 2013).

Mental health help-seeking is increasingly done online. Research suggests that individuals who fear social stigma as a result of seeking counselling and who wish to remain anonymous are likely to prefer to access mental health support online (DeAndrea, 2015). The ability to access mental health support online offers opportunities to overcome issues of time and space that often present barriers to mental health help-seeking.

This chapter draws on the version published in the first edition of this book (Hooley et al., 2012) but has been substantially reworked to take account of the changes in online research methods and data collection tools in the intervening period. It will examine how research on mental health has addressed the online environment, as well as how it has made use of this environment to explore research questions associated with mental health and mental health support in both online and onsite contexts. The term "online" is used in this chapter to describe the full range of Internet-enabled technologies whether they are accessed from a desktop, tablet, phone or other device. The term "onsite" is used to refer to all face-to-face activities and interactions. Online and onsite activities are becoming increasingly intertwined as Internet enabled devices become more widespread and more peripatetic.

WHAT ARE ONLINE RESEARCH METHODS?

Online research methods are techniques that use the Internet to answer research questions. They cover a wide and growing number of techniques which can broadly be divided into those that allow researchers to examine naturally occurring online data through fieldwork, network analysis, web analytics and so on and those that utilise the Internet to collect new data, for example, through surveys, interviews, focus groups, and experiments. Such methods use a wide variety of technical tools to collect, analyse and report these data. This chapter will look at all of these approaches and will attempt to maintain a distinction between the methodology (the approach used to investigate a particular subject) and the technology (the tool used to do this).

Online research methods have been used to investigate mental health issues in a variety of populations (Bockting, Miner, Swinburne Romine, Hamilton, & Coleman, 2013; Yau, Potenza, & White, 2013). In addition, online research methods are used to evaluate online mental health support (Dowling & Rickwood; 2013; Ellis, Collin, Hurley, Davenport, Burns, & Hickie, 2013; Rodda & Lubman, 2013). The factors that influence a participant's willingness to undertake online counselling, such as IT and web literacy and the preference for anonymity or distance from counselling opportunities, are also likely to mean that such people are suited to participating in studies conducted online.

However, online research is not confined to investigating online activity. Madge et al. (2006) identified advantages offered by online research methods. They suggest that online research can overcome geography, facilitate connection with hard to reach groups (e.g., people who have limited mobility, are in prison or in hospital), the socially isolated (e.g., drug dealers/terminally ill) or those living in dangerous places (e.g., war zones). They also identify a range of logistical advantages to online methods like cost savings (travel, venue, data entry) and quicker timelines for data collection. These advantages apply regardless of whether the experience being investigated took place online. So, for example, researchers could investigate a therapeutic approach using a survey to measure levels of satisfaction. This survey could be disseminated through a variety of modes such as by post or face-to-face meetings. Despite the development of online research methods these approaches still have their place, but would be slower, potentially more expensive and more complex to administer than an online survey. So, even where the experience under investigation is something that takes place offline, online research methods may offer advantages.

When the phenomenon under investigation has taken place online, online research methods offer even more possibilities including the possibility to collect and analyse data created in online interactions. Online counselling interactions commonly leave a trail of data, as will an individual's Google searches for mental health topics, their posts on discussion boards, social media and so on. The preservation of social and professional interactions in permanent or semi-permanent forms is one of the biggest consequences of the increasing centrality of the Internet in society. Social researchers are only just beginning to explore the consequences of this, but they are likely to be profound.

While online research methods can be powerful, they are not always the most appropriate methodological tools. There are disadvantages with online research methods just as there are advantages. Both Illingworth (2001) and O'Connor and Madge (2001) found that new technologies present technical challenges to be negotiated by both researcher and participants. Furthermore, despite increasing levels of penetration of the Internet into the general population, a digital divide still exists between those with Internet access and those without. For example, when undertaking research on older age groups, the socially excluded or those outside a western context, using an online research method may impact on the validity of the sample. Furthermore, online research methods (at least when text based) mean that subjects are responding in environments distinct from the researcher's, without visual and auditory cues and where, as Hewson et al. (2003) note, the researcher cannot ultimately be sure of the participant's identity.

Concerns about the authenticity of online identities and online data can be raised as a criticism of online methods. This issue has evolved from being a straightforward concern as to whether participants are who they say they are to a recognition that individuals reveal their identities in different online spaces strategically revealing different facets of their personality in different places (Marwick & Boyd, 2010). For example, an individual may use one online platform (e.g., Facebook) for social interactions and another (e.g., Linkedin) for professional interactions. However, this does not mean that an online identity is less real or stable than an onsite identity (Bowker & Tuffin 2003; Valkenburg & Peter 2008). Just

as individuals will adopt different behaviours online, so they will also do this when interacting with each other or researchers onsite.

A related question is whether researchers are more able to judge the trustworthiness of participants in a face-to-face environment. Hewson et al. (2003) argue that when onsite a researcher is able to pick up on a variety of visual and social clues to judge the trustworthiness of the response. However, research around online identity suggests that different but equivalent clues exist to signify authenticity, identity and trustworthiness (Toma & Hancock, 2009; Mislove, Viswanath, Gummadi, & Druschel, 2010; Shin & Kim, 2010). It is also worth noting that many of these disadvantages can also be the case in other methods. For example, identity can also be difficult to verify in postal questionnaires or even face-to-face.

DATA COLLECTION METHODS

There are a range of online data collection methods that may be appropriate for particular research questions. The following section identifies the range of data collection methods available to researchers in mental health. Figure 20.1 provides a visual representation

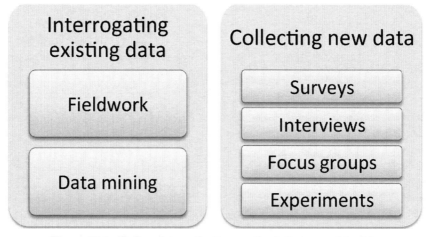

Figure 20.1. Online data collection methods for mental health.

of the main online data collection methods currently used in the field of mental health research. Researchers may choose to use one method or a combination of methods to answer their research question.

Interrogating Existing Data

The Internet has become a ubiquitous aspect of our lives. The implications of this, both positive (e.g., convenience, availability of information and ease of demographic participation) and negative (e.g., narcissism, the growth of unregulated information, and potential for online bullying), have all been remarked upon and offer subjects for researchers to investigate. However, the Internet offers an additional important change for social researchers: namely that in all of these interactions individuals are leaving trails of data which have potential value for researchers. In addition to widespread "digital footprints" of content creation and communication by users of social media, the Internet also collects large swathes of "unconscious" or passive data. Trackers and cookies placed onto computers via first- and third-party sites have the ability to collect and store information about an individual's web usage including the websites they visit and the web searches they make. Increasingly researchers are learning to access and analyse this kind of "naturally occurring" Internet data.

Fieldwork

The interrogation of online data can be viewed as a kind of fieldwork or ethnography (Kozinets, 1998, 2006; Langer & Beckman, 2005). Such methods draw on conventional face-to-face fieldwork and resituate it within the online environment (see Hine, 2000; Miller, & Slater, 2001). Fieldwork is likely to involve exploration of various online subcultural contexts. Researchers could, for example, participate in email lists, observe discussions

in specialist forums or professional/social networking sites (e.g., www.onlinetherapysocialnetwork.com), engage in video exchanges via You Tube, examine the written record afforded by chat or email therapy exchanges with counselling clients, or observe user behavior in online gaming environments or sites intended to address problem gambling (e.g., http://www.GamblingTherapy.org, cf. Anthony, 2005).

Online fieldwork is often, but not always, qualitative, and can be participatory rather than merely observational. However, these are not absolute rules. Where online fieldwork is largely observational, for example viewing a discussion board but not engaging directly in it, it blurs into our next category of data collection (data mining).

Data Mining

New technologies offer a range of opportunities for researchers to interrogate online data in new ways (Hooley et al., 2012). A range of tools have been developed that allow researchers to collect, visualise and analyse online data. This opens up the possibility of analysing what is essentially user-generated qualitative data (e.g., social media posts) on a quantitative scale to examine a variety of research questions. For example a researcher interested in the use of the word "depression" on a social networking site like Twitter could map and analyse what other words the term co-occurs with, who is using the term, where it is being used and how the different actors interact and connect. Chung and Pennebaker (2012) discuss this kind of analysis, arguing that linguistic analysis of large scale datasets mined from social media can provide insights into the psychology and culture of communities.

Secondly, the Internet offers opportunities for individuals to connect datasets together, for example connecting the names of users of an online discussion board to telephone directory data and a geographical application like Google Maps. For the purposes of mental health research, this could include the linking of several clinical and administrative datasets to other datasets. The ability to link and analyse date in this way opens up the possibility of answering new kinds of research questions which highlight intersections between online and onsite experience. In addition, the growth of embedded digital systems in everything from coffee makers to cars opens up new possibilities to monitor individuals' actual behaviour. Developers have already sought to use this function to support people in behaviour change for both physical and mental health purposes through behavioural intervention technologies (BITs). A relatively new BIT is the creation of interventions delivered as apps through mobile devices. BITs are purposeful interventions designed to support individuals with their health or mental health. This might include the provision of reminders (e.g., for taking medication) or information and advice. It might also include various forms of gamification and incentives to support behavior change (e.g., providing rewards for taking a certain amount of exercise in a day).

The potential for mining naturally occurring data in research is, however, not without limitations and critics cite several type of bias rife within these data such as measurement error, selection bias, misclassification and ethical issues pertaining to consent (Ioannidis, 2013).

There are four main sources of data that can be mined by researchers: (1) research data; (2) administrative data; (3) user-generated data; and (4) intervention interactions.

- **Research data**. While in the past, gaining access to other researchers' data was often complicated, increasingly the presumption is that data should be made available online so that other researchers can check it, replicate it, and build on it. As a result, many researchers deposit

their data in online archives like the UK Data Archive (http://www.data-archive. ac.uk/). This means that there is a growing resource of research data which researchers can use for secondary data analysis projects.

- **Administrative and clinical data**. Individual's interactions with mental health services are usually well documented. This results in the accumulations of large amounts of administrative and clinical records that are increasingly stored digitally and which may even be available online in anonymised and aggregated forms. Such data present a potential resource for researchers if legal and ethical issues can be appropriately addressed (Epstein, 2010). Jensen, Jensen, and Brunak (2012) argue that this digital administrative and clinical data should be used in research and to inform policy related to mental health while Lalayants et al. (2012) highlight its capacity to support evidence-based practice. In addition, the linking and pooling of administrative and clinical data from different health systems is being explored (Hoagwood et al., 2015). This will allow researchers to investigate mental health issues as individuals move through multiple systems. Several limitations exist with this type of data source including missing data, the use of crude indicators, and a lack of data accuracy due to logistical restraints (Lalayants et al., 2012).

- **User-generated data**. The Internet has linked individuals in a range of new forms of communication and content sharing. These social technologies generate online datasets that researchers can explore to understand both users online behaviour and wider issues related to the kinds of context shared on these sites. Many users provide detailed information about their mental health on social media (Park et al., 2012). Some social media platforms have publically available protocols and tools that allow researchers to interrogate their data through application programming interfaces (API). In addition, some social media platforms offer powerful search features through which researchers can retrieve publicly available data. Examples of this kind of research include: Moreno et al. (2011) who investigated disclosure of depression by college students on Facebook; Park et al. (2012) who collected baseline data on depression via an online survey and also asked permission to collect data on their use of Twitter. The researchers were able to explore the different types of tweets – those with and without depressive symptoms posted; and Shepherd et al. (2015) used the native search feature on Twitter to explore users' experiences with their mental health disorders as well as their experiences with mental health delivery and their healthcare professionals. Researchers must be aware of ethical issues of informed consent and privacy surrounding this type of data mining activity especially where the individual's involved can be identified. One way to overcome this is by obtaining consent before mining the data, but this is challenging in studies involving large numbers of participants (Park et al., 2012).

• **Intervention interactions**. The evolution of modern BITs changed the way in which mental health technology-based interventions can interact with targeted individuals. The diffusion of mobile phone technologies has made these technologies cost effective, scalable, and easily accessible (Ben-Zeev et al., 2015) resulting in the creation of mobile health ('mhealth') apps. Mhealth technologies store user interactions with the application, allow users to self-report, and even capture how the user interacts with the

phone itself. Ben-Zeev et al. (2015) discuss the implications of three mhealth applications to treat depression, improve anti-depressant medication adherence, and increase self-management of those with schizophrenia. The application designed to help treat depression also included the development of a data collection tool called a context sensing system which collect data on active user locations, activity, social context, and mood. In order to improve antidepressant medication adherence, a mobile application was connected to a digitally enabled pill bottle which actively collects data on medication use. Mhealth interventions represent an important new treatment approach, but also provide opportunities for researchers to evaluate their impact through the collection of data.

Collecting New Data Online

Online methods also offer opportunities for researchers to collect new data from target groups in an efficient and effective way.

Surveys

The use of online surveys and questionnaires has proliferated in recent years. Researchers familiar with conducting onsite surveys can carry those skills into the online environment. However, researchers need to contemplate the consequences of utilising online technologies to deliver a survey. There are many examples using online surveys for data collection in the mental health, counselling and psychotherapy field. Bockting et al. (2013) used an online survey to measure stigma, resilience and mental health of a U.S. transgender population; Rodda and Lubman (2014) examined the use and potential of an online counselling service for problem gambling in Australia; and Ellis et al. (2013) used online surveys to support the development of online mental services for young men.

Online surveys offer challenges regarding coverage of the population you are wishing to reach (Dillman, Smyth, & Christian, 2009). In addition, survey design should have an iterative pretesting process in order to gain insights prior to sending the survey to the sample. This process can be used to evaluate the reliability and usability of the instrument. Sampling and recruitment should be carefully considered when disseminating the survey. Probability sampling frames such as simple random sampling and stratified random sampling are the ideal but are often costly. Other sampling methods may be considered such as convenience sampling, quota sampling or snowball sampling. It may be valuable to identify gatekeepers for recruitment to groups and individuals as they may help provide access to respondents. Other recruitment methods may include the placement of paid or unpaid ads on various social media platforms and relevant discussion boards and forums among other websites.

Online Focus Groups and Interviews

Focus groups and interviews can be powerful tools to explore experiences, attitudes, and psychologies. These techniques are applied regularly in counselling and psychotherapy research (see, for example, Grafanaki, 1996; Read, 2001). Using text-based or video-based communication tools may enable researchers to overcome barriers of distance and access and to contact research participants that would otherwise be out of reach. However, they also pose some significant challenges. For example, in the online environment, some of the interpersonal tools used face-to-face to develop rapport are absent. Online researchers need to overcome these barriers and find new ways of establishing trust and rapport before beginning to gather data. It is useful to gain insights into the culture and

communication style of the environment being researched. There are a number of other techniques that researchers may consider when building rapport with their research subjects. For example:

- establishing web pages with photographs and brief biographical information;
- establishing relationships before the start of the interview or focus group by meeting, telephone or email exchanges;
- using any similarities or insider status that you have to encourage identification;
- sharing your own profile data and encouraging others to do so.

Online focus groups can be synchronous, when all participants are online simultaneously, or asynchronous when participants respond at their own convenience. Synchronous focus groups work best for individuals with competent keyboarding skills comfortable with instant messaging and "chat" systems (Fox et al., 2007). Asynchronous focus groups or interviews typically take place in a discussion board or forum environments or through the exchange of emails (Williams et al., 2012). Asynchronous methods can offer powerful insights for longitudinal work and can encourage reflective and thoughtful responses.

Experiments and Trials

Most mental health experiments and trials are conducted in face-to-face clinical settings. However, it is possible for researchers to conduct experiments and trials online. For example, in a controversial study conducted on Facebook, researchers investigated whether emotional states could be transferred by "emotional contagion" by manipulating users' news feed in order to control whether positive or negative emotional expressions were displayed (Kramer, Guillory, & Hancock, 2014).

As previously introduced, the area of mhealth offers a new type of online mental health intervention which can be evaluated through the use of trials. One fundamental challenge to applying randomised control trials (RCT) to mhealth technology is that the pace of technology often outpaces the length of the mhealth trial (Kumar et al., 2013) meaning that mhealth apps can be obsolete before the end of the trial period.

ETHICAL ISSUES

Undertaking research in the mental health field requires researchers to be aware of the ethical implications of their work. The principles of beneficence and nonmaleficence remain the cornerstones of research ethics. However, the potential to unwittingly do harm becomes greater when working with a research subject who cannot be seen and who the researcher has never met.

Hine (2005) argues that online research is "a special category in which the institutionalised understandings of the ethics of research must be reexamined" (p. 5). However, this runs the risk of viewing "online" as a single space or category when in fact it presents researchers with a multitude of environments. The researcher needs to analyse these spaces when considering the ethical implications of conducting research. For example, writing that appears in an online journal or newspaper may be seen as having a different status from that which appears on a person's Facebook profile.

Hooley et al. (2012) highlight privacy, informed consent, anonymity, confidentiality, compliance with the law and addressing participant vulnerability as key issues that researchers should attend to in relation to online ethics. However, the balance between private/public and identified/anonymous can be very difficult to tease out online as can clear definitions of who is vulnerable and what is legal. This is especially the case in relation to multijurisdictional situations where a researcher might be in one country and

culture, their participants in another or even in a range of countries, while the data may be being stored in the "cloud," whilst actually being housed in servers in a third country.

The challenges are illustrated by considering the ethics of a researcher who is drawing data from a BBC forum that deals with a contentious issue about public policy and mental health. Such a researcher might reasonably conclude that postings within this forum are public, available to quote and likely to be personally (if not politically) uncontentious. Many online researchers have attempted to determine the status of public online data and activity by considering them to be either (1) accessible to anyone with an Internet connection or (2) data/activity that is perceived to be public by participants (even though researchers are not the intended audience) (Rosenberg 2010). Whiteman (2010), and Langer and Beckman (2005), have taken this stance to justify data mining public discussion boards without members' knowledge. Grodzinsky and Tavani draw upon Nissenbaum's (2004) work to examine the specific privacy issues related to blogging and reach a similar conclusion that "authors of (nonpassword-protected) blogs have no reasonable expectation of their personal privacy being normatively protected" (Grodzinsky & Tavani, 2010: 45). Thelwall goes further, arguing that human subject standards do not apply to studies of publically available data because it is the publication, and not the person, which is being researched (Thelwall, 2010). This chapter has argued that data mining has the potential to answer many mental health-related questions; however, it is also possible to challenge this method on both methodological (it is difficult to be confident about the robustness of data mining) and ethical (why should the presumption of informed consent disappear just because you are conducting a large scale study) grounds (Ioannidis, 2013).

Researchers investigating mental health issues may legitimately feel concerned about the permissive assumptions of much of the ethical discussion outlined above. If we shift the focus of the forum being researched from public policy to individual's experience of psychotherapy or to a peer support forum for people experiencing eating disorders we might feel that data is more sensitive and that researchers should exercise care in analyzing and representing it. Shirky (2008) makes the point that most conversations on the Internet are available to all but are consciously written for a small group of like-minded people. Researchers need to consider the ethical implications of moving the conversations of these "small worlds" into a new and possibly larger, context. Yet, in this example, the technology and the rules governing the forums would be identical. The law gives researchers little guidance in this area and is, in many countries, highly permissive. Therefore, it is difficult to produce absolute guidelines leaving the decision about how to proceed ethically with the researcher (and an appropriate research ethics committee). The Association of Internet Researchers (AoIR) Ethics Working Committee (Markham, Buchanan, & AoIR, 2012) supports ethical pluralism and flexibility while offering six guiding principles: (1) the greater the vulnerability of the individual or group, the greater the obligation to protect the individual or group; (2) decision-making should be practical and applied to the specific context; (3) digital information at some point has involved human subjects and the principles guiding research on human subjects apply; (4) understanding the balance of the rights of the individual with the potential social benefits of the research; (5) ethical issues may occur at any time during the research and must be addressed as they arise; and (6) the ethical process in research is an explicit and deliberate process.

Consequently, it is possible to identify a number of researchers who have emphasised the importance of respecting participant privacy and control over data. Kozinets (2010)

suggest that researchers should disclose their presence and gain informed consent. Whiteman (2010) explores how her original ethical stance regarding the public nature of discussion boards was challenged when the privacy settings changed part way through her research. She also goes on to explain the mixed reaction she got from the discussion board users when she provided them with links to her research findings – with some of them sharing her view that the data were public and others considering her work to be voyeuristic. Rosenberg also found a lack of agreement regarding what constituted public space amongst users of Second Life. Driscoll and Gregg (2010) stressed how important it was for researchers to consider the specific contexts, practices and expectations of the online communities and spaces they are researching in order that they can reflect on, and justify, their ethical position.

Many of the ethical considerations discussed above are not particular to online research. The boundaries between categories are more blurred than in traditional research, but the same questions need to be asked of any research project, online or onsite. There is extensive literature on undertaking ethical research in counselling and psychotherapy (see, for example, Goss & Anthony, 2012; Hay, 2014; Proctor, 2014), but the following questions are a useful starting point.

- Is there potential to do harm?
- How can informed consent be sought and agreed with the participants?
- Can the participant withdraw from the research if they feel uncomfortable?
- Is deception a defensible research strategy? For example, can "lurking" as socialisation into the online culture of a group be an important prerequisite for research?
- What will happen to the data and how will the participants be informed/involved in this feedback process?

CONCLUSIONS

Online research offers powerful tools for undertaking research on mental health. It is particularly effective when investigating online experiences, but its use does not need to be confined to the online world.

This chapter has set out a framework for thinking about the way in which researchers collect data online. At the heart of this is the distinction that we make between interrogating existing data and collecting new data. As online research in mental health continues to grow, it is likely that the former is utilised more and that these two approaches continue to entwine. As Internet technologies become ever more embedded into our society, researchers in mental health will need to become increasingly proficient in the use of online methods. It is, of course, important that this use is careful, ethical and rooted in clear methodological thinking. However, it is also important that online methods continue to develop to take advantage of new technologies and understand new psychosocio-technical phenomena as they emerge.

REFERENCES

Anthony, K. (2005). Counselling problem gamblers online. *BACP Counselling and Psychotherapy Journal, 16*(6), 9–10.

Bockting, W. O., Miner, M. H., Swinburne Romine, R. E., Hamilton, A., & Coleman, E. (2013). Stigma, mental health, and resilience among an online sample of the U.S. transgender population. *American Journal of Public Health, 103*(5), 943–951.

Bowker, N., & Tuffin, K. (2003). Dicing with deception: People with disabilities' strategies for managing safety and identity online. *Journal of Computer-Mediated Communication, 8*(2).

Chung, C. K., & Pennebaker, J. W. (2012). Counting little words in big data: The psychology of communities, cultures, and history. In J. László, J. Forgas, & O. Vincze (Eds.), *Social cognition and communication.* New York: Psychology Press.

DeAndrea, D. C. (2015). Testing the proclaimed affordances of online support groups in a nationally representative sample of adults seeking mental health assistance. *Journal of Health Communication: International Perspectives, 20*(2), 147–156.

Dillman, D. A., Smyth, J. D., & Christian, L. M. (2009). *Internet, mail, and mixed-mode surveys: The tailored design method.* New York: John Wiley & Sons.

Dowling, M., & Rickwood, D. (2013). Online counseling and therapy for mental health problems: A systematic review of individual synchronous interventions using chat. *Journal of Technology in Human Services, 31*(1), 1–21.

Driscoll, C., & Gregg, M. (2010), My profile: The ethics of virtual ethnography. *Emotion, Space and Society, 3*(1), 15–20.

Ellis, L. A., Collin, P., Hurley, P. J., Davenport, T. A., Burns, J. A., & Hickie, I. B. (2013). Young men's attitudes and behaviour in relation to mental health and technology: Implications for the development of online mental health services. *BMC Psychiatry, 13*, 119.

Epstein, I. (2010). *Clinical data-mining: Integrating practice and research.* New York: Oxford University Press.

Goss, S. P. and Anthony, K. The evolution of guidlines for online counselling and psychotherapy – the development of clinical practice. In: B. Popoola and O. Adebowale (Ed.), *Online Guidance and Counselling: Towards effectively applying technology.* Hershey, PA: IGI Global

Grafanaki, S (1996). How research can change the researcher: The need for sensitivity, flexibility and ethical boundaries in conducting qualitative research in counselling/psychotherapy. *British*

Journal of Guidance and Counselling, 24(3), 329–338.

Grodzinsky, F. S., & Tavani, H. T. (2010). Applying the "contextual integrity" model of privacy to personal blogs in the blogosphere. *International Journal of Internet Research Ethics, 3*(1), 38–47.

Hay, J. (2014). Research ethics for counsellors, nurses and social workers. *Counselling and Psychotherapy Research, 14*(2), 162–163.

Hewson, C., Yule, P., Laurent, D., & Vogel, C. (2003). *Internet research methods.* London: Sage.

Hine, C. (2000). *Virtual ethnography.* London: Sage.

Hine, C. (Ed.) (2005). *Virtual methods: Issues in social research on the Internet.* Oxford: Berg.

Hoagwood, K. E., Essock, S., Morrissey, J., Libby, A., Donahue, S., Druss, B., Finnerty, M., Frisman, L., Narasimhan, M., Stein, B. D., Wisdom, J., & Zerzan, J. (2015). Use of pooled administrative data for mental health services research. *Administration and Policy in Mental Health and Mental Health Services Research*, pp. 1–2.

Hooley, T., Marriott, J., & Wellens, J. (2012). *What is online research? Using the Internet for social science research.* London: Bloomsbury.

Hooley, T., Wellens, J., Madge, C., & Goss, S. (2012). Online research methods in mental health. In K. Anthony, D. Merz Nagel, & S. Goss (Eds.), *The use of technology in mental health: Applications, ethics and practice* (2nd ed.). Springfield, IL: Charles C Thomas.

Illingworth, N. (2001). The Internet matters: Exploring the use of the internet as a research tool. *Sociological Research Online, 6*(2) [online]. [Accessed January 27, 2008]. Available from: http://www.socresonline.org.uk/6/2/illingworth.html.

Ioannidis, J. P. (2013). Informed consent, big data, and the oxymoron of research that is not research. *American Journal of Bioethics, 13*(4), 40–42.

Jensen, P. B., Jensen, L. J., & Brunak, S. (2012). Mining electronic health records: Towards better research applications and clinical care. *Nature Reviews Genetics, 13*, 395–405.

Kozinets, R. V. (1998). On netnography. Initial reflections on consumer investigations of cyberculture. In J. Alba & W. Hutchinson (Eds.), *Advances in consumer research.* Provo, UT: Association for Consumer Research.

Kozinets, R. V. (2006). Netnography 2.0. In R. W. Belk (Ed.), *Handbook of qualitative research methods in marketing.* Cheltenham: Edward Elgar.

Langer, R., & Beckman, S. (2005). Sensitive research topics: Netnography revisited. *Qualitative Market Research: An International Journal, 8*(2), 189–203.

Lalayants, M., Epstein, I., Auslander, G.K., Chi Ho Chan, W., Fouche, C., Giles, R., Joubert, L., Rosenne, H., & Vertigan, A. (2012). Clinical data-mining: Learning from practice in international settings. *International Social Work, 56*(6), 775–797.

Madge, C., O'Connor, H., Wellens, J., Hooley, T., & Shaw, R. (2006). Exploring online research methods in a virtual training environment [online]. [Accessed November 24, 2008]. Available from: http://www.geog.le.ac.uk/orm.

Markham, A., Buchanan, E., & the Association of Internet Researchers (AoIR) Committee. (2012). Ethical decision-making and Internet research: Recommendations from the AoIR Ethics Working Committee [online]. [Accessed February 21, 2009]. Available from: http://www.aoir.org/reports/ethics.pdf.

Markowetz, A., Blaszkiewicz, K., Montag, C., Switala, C., & Schlaepfer, T. E. (2014). Psycho-informatics: Big data shaping modern psychometrics. *Medical Hypotheses, 82*, 405–411.

Miller, D., & Slater, D. (2001). *The Internet: An ethnographic approach.* New York: Berg.

Moreno, M. A., Jelenchick, L. A., Egan, K. G., Cox, E., Young, H., Gannon, K. E., & Becker, T. (2011). Feeling bad on Facebook: Depression disclosures by college students on a social networking site. *Depression and Anxiety*, *28*, 447–455.

O'Connor, H., & Madge, C. (2001). Cybermothers: Online synchronous interviewing using conferencing software. Sociological Research Online, 5(4) [online]. [Accessed January 27, 2009]. Available from: http://www.socresonline.org.uk/5/4/o'connor.html.

Mislove, A., Viswanath, B., Gummadi, K. P., & Druschel, P. (2010). You are who you know: Inferring user profiles in online social networks. In Proceedings of the third ACM international conference on Web search and data mining, WSDM '10. New York: ACM, 251–260.

Nissenbaum, H. (2004). Privacy as contextual integrity. *Washington Law Review*, *79*(1), 119–157.

Park, M., Cha, C., & Cha, M. (2012). Depressive moods of users portrayed in Twitter. In Proceedings of the ACM SIGKDD Workshop on Health Informatics.

Read, S. (2001). A year in the life of a bereavement counselling and support service for people with learning disabilities. *Journal of Intellectual Disabilities*, *5*(1), 19–33.

Rodda, S., & Lubman, D. I. (2014). Characteristics of gamblers using a national online counselling service for problem gambling. *Journal of Gambling Studies*, *30*, 277–289.

Rosenberg, A. (2010), Virtual world research ethics and the private/public distinction. *International Journal of Internet Research Ethics*, *3*(1).

Shin, H. K., & Kim, K. K. (2010), Examining identity and organizational citizenship behaviour in computer-mediated communication. *Journal of Information Science*, *36*(1), 114–126.

Shirky, C. (2008). *Here comes everybody: The power of organizing without organizations*. London: Penguin.

Thelwall, M. (2010). Researching the Public Web. E Research Ethics. http://eresearch-ethics.org/position/researching-the-public-web/ [accessed 28 Feb 2012].

Toma, C., & Hancock, J. (2009). Catching liars: The linguistic signature of deception in online profiles. Paper presented at the annual meeting of the NCA 95th Annual Convention, Chicago Hilton and Towers, Chicago, IL, Nov 11, 2009. http://www.allacademic.com/meta/p367023_index.html [accessed 28 Feb 2012].

Valkenburg, P. M., & Peter, J. (2008). Adolescents' identity experiments on the Internet. *Communication Research*, *35*(2), 208–231.

Whiteman, N. (2010). Control and contingency: Maintaining ethical stances in research. *International Journal of Internet Research Ethics*, *3*(1), 6–22.

Williams, S. Clausen, M. G., Robertson, A. Peacock, S., & McPherson, K. (2012). Methodological reflections on the use of asynchronous online focus groups in health research. *International Journal of Qualitative Methods*, *11*(4), 368–383.

Yau, Y. H., Potenza, M. N., & White, M. A. (2013). Problematic internet use, mental health and impulse control in an online survey of adults. *Journal of Behavioral Addictions*, *2*(2), 72.

Chapter 21

EVALUATING THE ROLE OF ELECTRONIC AND WEB-BASED (E-CBT) CBT IN MENTAL HEALTH

Eva Kaltenthaler, Kate Cavanagh, and Paul McCrone

INTRODUCTION

As new electronic and web-based methods of delivering CBT (E-CBT), also known as computerised CBT (CCBT) are introduced, it is important to use appropriate methods for appraising their quality and suitability. This chapter explores issues to consider when evaluating web-based psychological therapies. Emphasis is placed on programmes for depression and anxiety as there has been a considerable amount of research in this area. Recent reviews have found computerised or web-based CBT to be effective and acceptable (Andrews et al., 2010; Foroushani et al., 2011; Griffiths et al., 2010; Grist & Cavanagh, 2013; Richards & Richardson, 2012). New modes of delivery, such as individualised e-mail therapy, have also been found to be effective in the treatment of depression (Vernmark et al., 2010). The chapter explores key issues to consider when evaluating trial reports of interventions and discusses aspects around software programmes as well as client and logistical issues. One of the primary reasons for the development of web-based and electronic packages to treat mental health disorders is to increase access to effective interventions. A second is to reduce the costs associated with therapist treatment and therefore cost

effectiveness issues are also considered. Finally these programmes allow flexibility in terms of standardisation and personalisation and have the potential to improve interactivity and consumer engagement (Lal et al., 2014). However, evidence is lacking. A recent scoping review identified 32 web-based intervention programs for depression, only 12 of which had published evidence of efficacy (Renton et al., 2014).

ISSUES RELATED TO TRIAL DESIGN

Issues to consider in the evaluation of E-CBT packages include those related specifically to trial design. These are illustrated in Table 21.1 below. Randomised controlled trials (RCTs) are often considered the best possible study design to answer questions of comparative efficacy. They are used routinely in trials of pharmacological treatments. In the established hierarchy of study design, RCTs with concealed (blinded) allocation are considered to be of highest quality as variables that may influence outcome independently of the intervention are distributed between groups. Researchers have reported difficulties with designing RCTs in the area of Internet-based CBT, such as recruiting patients and general practitioners to take part in studies (Hickie et al., 2010).

Power calculations are undertaken to calculate how large the trial needs to be in order to detect an effective intervention condition. Intention to treat is the preferred form of analysis as all clients initially randomised to take part in the trial are taken into account. Including only those who complete the trial may give a false impression of how effective a treatment was as everyone who dropped out could have deteriorated.

RCTs are expensive to conduct and RCT data is often unavailable with regards to specific research questions. It therefore becomes necessary to draw conclusions about evidence from studies using less vigorous research designs. RCTs were initially developed for investigating pharmacological treatments and are not entirely applicable to psychological treatments. For example, the use of double blinding, where both the client and clinician are unaware if treatment or a control is being administered, is rarely possible in trials of psychological therapies. Both clinician and client will have at least an idea of what type of therapy they are giving or receiving. However, there are still ways to reduce bias, such as blinded assessment, where the clinician interpreting the results is unaware of what treatment the client has had. Different types of evidence are obtained from different study designs. For example, an RCT would not be the best place to find information on treatment acceptability. For this type of information, it may be best to seek out observational studies or qualitative studies based on interviews or questionnaires.

The consolidated standards of reporting trials (CONSORT) statement was developed to improve the reporting of RCTs. Recently, an extension to these standards was added to focus on web-based and mobile health interventions, CONSORT-EHEALTH (Eysenbach & CONSORT-EHEALTH Group, 2011). These guidelines were developed to improve and standardise evaluation reports of web-based and mobile health interventions, specifically components of the intervention. The items included in the CONSORT-EHEALTH extension to CONSORT are shown in Table 21.2. These guidelines are partially based on work undertaken by Proudfoot et al. (2011) who established a framework of guidelines for Internet intervention research. They outline 12 key facets to consider when evaluating and reporting internet intervention studies including:

- Focus and target population
- Authorship details
- Mode of change
- Type and dose of intervention
- Ethical issues
- Professional support
- Other support
- Program interactivity
- Multimedia channel of delivery
- Degree of synchronicity
- Audience reach
- Program evaluation

Effectiveness and Efficacy

Effectiveness refers to the extent to which an intervention produces beneficial outcomes under ordinary day-to-day circumstances. This reflects "real-life" conditions. *Efficacy* refers to the extent to which an intervention can produce a beneficial outcome under ideal circumstances (Khan et al., 2003). For example, a randomised controlled trial where a strict protocol is adhered to and only certain types of clients are suitable for inclusion is an efficacy trial. An intervention may appear to work in an efficacy trial but be found to be ineffective in ordinary day-to-day situations. In efficacy trials, there is often careful monitoring throughout the trial, clients may be carefully selected and have frequent contact with study personnel. These conditions are not necessarily met in effectiveness trials. Trials of effectiveness often include a much broader spectrum of clients and more accurately reflect the type of client who may come forward for treatment in a routine care situation.

Client Group

It is important to consider the features of the client group participating in research trials and evaluation studies, as this may have implications for the generalisation of findings. Most research on software packages of psychological therapies has been done on client groups that consist mainly of women between the ages of 30–45, mostly Caucasian, and from higher education level and higher socioeconomic groups (Kaltenthaler et al., 2006). There is less evidence for the suitability or acceptability of such programmes for other groups.

Follow-up

Follow-up is a particularly important issue in trials of psychological therapies which traditionally have high drop-out rates (Kaltenthaler et al., 2008). The length of follow-up in the trial needs to be recorded as well as the percentage of participants who completed the program. For those who did not complete, information should be collected as to why. Was it because they felt worse, improved, or just didn't like the treatment? A recent meta-analysis (So et al., 2013) found no significant clinical effect at long-term follow-up for E-CBT and significantly higher drop-out rates for E-CBT than for controls.

Comparators

It is important to consider whether or not the comparators used in the trial reflect current and local practice. Some studies include no

Table 21.1
TRIAL CONSIDERATIONS

Effectiveness vs. Efficacy	*What type of trials:*
Study design	RCT is the "gold standard" but others provide useful data on some outcomes.
Client group	Was the client group in the trial representative of clients who will receive the intervention?
Allocation concealment	Was this undertaken by the research team during randomisation to ensure that there are no differences between the study groups in terms of prognosis or response to treatment?
Blinding	Was this undertaken, where appropriate, to ensure that there are no differences in treatment or care (apart from the intervention) and no differences in the interpretation of study outcomes?
Power calculation	Was the trial large enough to identify anticipated effects?
Intention to treat analysis	Were all randomised clients included in the final analysis?
Follow-up	Were numbers lost to follow up reported?
Description of non-completers	Were reasons for clients not completing treatment reported?
Comparators	Were these appropriate and do they reflect current practice?
Outcome measures	Were these clinically relevant outcome measures and were they well validated?

Table 21.2
CONSORT EHEALTH DESCRIPTIONS OF INTERVENTION

Subitem	Description	Importance
Names, credentials, and affiliations of the developers, sponsors and owners	If authors/evaluators are owners this needs to be declared as a conflict of interest.	Highly recommended
History/development process of application	The development and formative evaluations need to be described.	Highly recommended
Revisions and updating	Date and version numbers need to be mentioned, any changes and dynamic components (such as news feeds).	Highly recommended
Quality assurance methods	Information provided to ensure accuracy and quality of information provided.	Highly recommended
Ensure replicability	Provision of source code and/ or screenshots; flowcharts of algorithms used.	Highly recommended
Digital preservation	Provide URL of application and ensure intervention is archived. Consider demo pages.	Highly recommended
Access	Describe how application is accessed including setting, payment, membership of specific groups. Consider providing login details for reviewers/ readers to explore application.	Essential
Mode of delivery	Description of content, how it is tailored to individuals, how progress is tracked, feedback received and details of presentation.	Essential
Parameters of use	Describe intended use and optimal timing for use.	Highly recommended
Level of human involvement	Clarify level of human involvement from health professionals as well as technical assistance.	Highly recommended
Prompts/reminders	Clarify if there are prompts (letters, e-mails, phone calls, SMS) and frequency.	Essential
Co-interventions	State additional interventions if not stand-alone, including training sessions.	Essential

Adapted from Eysenbach 2011.

comparator group. Caution is needed when interpreting these trial results. Clients often get better on their own without treatment (although perhaps more slowly) and improvement may be a result of the natural course of the condition rather than as a result of the treatment. Trials that do include comparators may use a whole spectrum, but not all may be appropriate comparators reflecting current treatment. Appropriate comparators may include treat-ment as usual or therapist led CBT, while other options include bibliotherapy, other self-help interventions, group CBT, short course CBT or primary care counselling.

Outcome Measures

Outcome measures used should be clinically relevant and well validated. This makes it easier to compare results with other trials and/or software programmes. A whole spectrum of outcome measures has been used in trials of software packages, making comparisons between programmes difficult (Kaltenthaler et al., 2006). The most commonly used outcome measures for E-CBT of depression are the Beck Depression Inventory (Proudfoot et al., 2004; Newby et al., 2013), Core Outcomes in Routine Evaluation (CORE) (Cavanagh et al., 2009), Center for Epidemiological Studies Depression Scale (Clarke et al., 2002, 2005; Christensen et al., 2004) and PHQ-9 (Newby et al., 2013; Perini et al., 2009). In order to determine whether or not there has been an improvement, baseline scores of outcome measures are compared with post-treatment scores and ideally follow-up scores. Statistical tests are used to compare scores between groups. Indices of reliable and clinically significant change may be reported. Care must be taken to ensure appropriate methods are used and to determine changes that are clinically relevant.

SOFTWARE PROGRAMMES CONSIDERATIONS

Components of E-CBT Packages

Translation of the intervention, in this case cognitive behaviour therapy (CBT), into a software package is an essential first step for a successful E-CBT programme. The components of CBT that are recognised as integral to effective treatment must be included. In order to determine whether or not this is the case, there should be a description of what aspects of CBT are included in the package. Programmes must meet recognised standards of proof for psychotherapeutic interventions (Department of Health (DoH), 2001) but, to date, there has been little research as to what essential components of E-CBT might be. The UK's National Institute for Health and Care Excellence (NICE) has offered some guidance as to important features of E-CBT

programmes for depression (NICE, 2009 [surveillance review 2013], see Chapter 13). Packages aimed at different client groups will have emphasis on different techniques to meet the needs of the clients for which they were developed.

Specific approaches to client engagement and motivation, change techniques (such as identification, monitoring and evaluation of negative automatic thoughts and strategies such as sleep management, problem-solving, graded exposure, task breakdown and behavioural experiments) and methods of monitoring and feedback vary between programmes. Beating the Blues, for example, uses different types of media to present interactive CBT which includes work with negative automatic thoughts, core beliefs, unhelpful attributions and a variety of behavioural methods. FearFighter uses computerised graded exposure. Some programmes may use video clips of clients or clinicians. They may use touch screens or have boxes for typing in free text. It is important to have a clear understanding of what CBT components are included in a computerised programme and how they are delivered.

Keeping diaries or experience in between sessions, recording of other data and completing behavioural experiments are integral to the CBT approach and the generation of such "homework" exercises is equally incorporated in many software programmes. Homework may be an integral part of the process or an extra if required.

Delivery of Software Programs

When considering an E-CBT software programme, it is important to take the mode of delivery into account. Some programmes may require a stand-alone computer, some telephone access and some Internet access. They also vary in terms of the extent and complexity of interaction with the programme itself, from a single brief interaction

Table 21.3
PROGRAMME CONSIDERATIONS

E-CBT components	What components are included for client engagement, motivation, change techniques, monitoring and feedback?
Mode of delivery	Is a standalone computer, laptop, Internet or telephone needed?
Sessions	What is the number and frequency of sessions?
Homework	Is this integral or extra? Who reviews the homework and is it private or for the health care provider to see?
Therapist input	What type of therapist is needed and for what amount of time?
Provider acceptability	Is the health care provider willing to use this programme and convinced of its effectiveness? What training is required?

to a lengthy relationship. Moreover, the programme of treatment including a computer-assisted psychotherapy system might range from one where the client for themselves finds a single episode to interact with anonymously, to one where a client is referred to a complex programme offered over several weeks, including a mixture of multiple attendance at a computerised-therapy clinic, scheduled or on-demand phone calls and ongoing monitoring by primary care staff.

Therapist Input

E-CBT programmes may be designed as pure self-help (with no support), guided self-help (with some support from either a paraprofessional or practitioner) or to complement or augment more traditional therapeutic work. It is important to consider the type of worker needed to administer or support a software package as well as how much support time is needed. As with therapist-led psychological therapies, it may be that therapist training and experience will have an effect on client outcomes (Horvath & Luborsky, 1993). Another consideration is how support is provided: by telephone (scheduled or on-demand), by e-mail or other online methods or in person (each session or on request). Farrer et al. (2011) have explored the use of web CBT with and without telephone

tracking in an RCT, while Linder et al. (2014) have explored the use of therapist input via e-mail or telephone for patients with major depression receiving Internet CBT. It may also be important to consider the researched health care provider's attitude towards the treatment programme. Provider acceptability may be important for the successful implementation of a programme. If providers do not believe that the treatment package is appropriate, useful and value for money, this may impact on program uptake, retention, and outcomes.

Providers also need support and education and resources to incorporate the new programmes so that they are not overburdened.

CLIENT CONSIDERATIONS

In order to determine the boundaries of generalisability for a study (how many clients and what type of clients may use the programme), care must be given to how clients are recruited and screened and to how depression and/or anxiety are diagnosed. Self-referral routes may capture a different group of clients to health-care professional referral. Screening criteria may determine who is eligible for the study and who is suitable for use of the programme. Which, if any, diagnostic criteria are applied and how any diagnostic

Table 21.4
CLIENT CONSIDERATIONS

Method of diagnosis	Is the method for diagnosis appropriate? Who is responsible for this?
Screening	How is suitability and risk assessed?
Monitoring	When does this occur and is it via computer or brief discussions? What options are there if the client wants to drop out if his/her condition deteriorates?
Safety	How are suicide risk and adverse events identified? What happens to noncompleters?
Acceptability	How is acceptability to clients measured and when?
Satisfaction	How is treatment satisfaction measured and when?
Referral	Are program users self-referred or referred by a health care professional?

instruments are administered, and by whom, may also influence uptake and outcomes. Methods of screening reported in trials include the Programmable Questionnaire System (PROQSY) to diagnose depression used by Proudfoot et al. (2004) and the Kessler Psychological Distress Scale used by Christensen et al. (2004). Clarke et al. (2002, 2005) identified participants who had received medical services in the previous 30 days with a recorded diagnosis of depression. It is important to ask whether or not the method used to diagnose the disorder is appropriate and who is meant to administer the instrument.

Some software programmes include monitoring of symptoms, problem severity and risk. If suicide risk is identified, mechanisms must be in place to manage this. Monitoring may be at each session or regular intervals and may be via computer or through brief discussions with the therapist or other person. If clients try E-CBT and do not like it, other options must be made available to them. Likewise, the clients whose condition deteriorates must have other options made available to them.

Client Acceptability

Consideration needs to be given to how client acceptability and treatment satisfaction

will be measured and when. Acceptability may vary with different groups of people depending on age, sex, education, socioeconomic group, type of illness, experience with computers and preconceived ideas about effectiveness. Self-report measures, treatment uptake, continuation and dropout can be used as measures of treatment acceptability and satisfaction (Cavanagh et al., 2003; Waller & Gilbody, 2009).

ETHICAL CONSIDERATIONS

Many E-CBT software packages include some safety mechanisms. In evaluating any programme, it is important to note what mechanisms are included to monitor safety throughout the use of the programme. For example, Beating the Blues monitors suicide risk at the beginning of each session and generates a note to the person's doctor, informing him/her of the client's suicide risk. Very little information is reported on side effects or adverse events associated with E-CBT packages. These may include a worsening of symptoms or generation of additional symptoms. Clients who drop out of treatment are often not followed up and reasons for dropping out not identified. This may not be different from conventional treatment regimens and poses an ethical dilemma in research where partici-pants reserve the right to withdraw from treat-ment without giving any reason and pursuing this could invade this basic right. A consensus statement has been developed on how to define and measure possible negative effects associated with Internet interventions (Rozen-tal et al., 2014).

Some consideration needs to be given to how client data will be stored in order to pro-tect client privacy, including the question of who will have access to this data and how will it remain confidential. There are considerable privacy issues associated with programmes provided via the Internet.

LOGISTICAL CONSIDERATIONS

Clinical support may be provided in brief face-to-face sessions, or by phone, email or other media. The content and style of such support may significantly affect outcomes in ways that are as yet unclear from research evi-dence, although brief, regular, scheduled sup-port from a trained worker offered face-to-face or by phone has the strongest evidence base. Administrative support needs to be provided in order to ensure all necessary equipment is functioning, to answer client queries and to

alert staff to problems. Office space is often but not always necessary as some pro-grammes may be administered via the Inter-net at home, or in a library, community resource centre or Internet café. Implementa-tion will require training of staff and identifi-cation of sources of support.

It is crucial to assess the cost-effectiveness of E-CBT interventions if they are to be used widely. Costs of E-CBT programmes can vary considerably, and evaluation of costs may consider programme development costs and delivery costs, including clinical and technical support, as well as any direct com-mercial costs to the provider. It is to be ex-pected that costs of therapy itself are reduced by using E-CBT rather than (only) face-to-face therapy, but overall service costs may not necessarily be reduced. Clients receiving E-CBT may possibly still seek direct contact with health care professionals such as doctors, practice nurses and counsellors and therefore any evaluation needs to consider all service costs. To date, few studies have achieved this. McCrone et al. (2004) showed that compared to treatment as usual within a primary care setting, E-CBT resulted in slightly higher costs. Here though E-CBT was additional to usual care and did not substitute for other forms of psychological therapy. However,

Table 21.5
LOGISTICAL CONSIDERATIONS

Costs	What costs are there for hardware, software, administrative and technical support and office space? How many clients will be using the service? Relevant services used over a defined period can be recorded.
Hardware and software components	What is required and who sets up and services the components?
Administrative support	Who provides this and who will pay for it?
Office space	Will this be required, if so where? Room for a single user or multiple users? Only at home use?
Implementation	How will this be managed and paid for?
Training and supervision	What training and supervision is required for staff providing client guidance to the programme?

these additional costs were justified by the additional benefits achieved (reductions in symptoms of depression and anxiety and improved social functioning). Higher treatment costs may also be considered acceptable if savings are achieved elsewhere, for example in the form of reduced workloads. Therefore, evaluations need both to measure costs comprehensively and to combine costs with outcomes. Future evaluations need to incorporate full economic evaluations including established measures of quality-adjusted life years in order to make comparisons with interventions in other clinical areas.

CONCLUSION

In order to adequately evaluate an E-CBT package for depression and anxiety and be able to compare packages, a series of predefined criteria as described above should be considered. This enables informed comparisons between packages to be made and ensures that health care providers are able to offer optimal client care. The criteria can be applied to new programmes to assess suitability. These criteria can be used to ensure that E-CBT programmes providing optimal care for appropriately selected clients are chosen. Other relevant issues may become apparent so it is important that these issues are updated regularly.

REFERENCES

Andrews, G., Cuijpers, P., Craske, M. G., McEvoy, P., & Titov, N. (2010). Computer therapy for the anxiety and depressive disorders is effective, acceptable and practical health care: A meta-analysis. *PLoS One, 5*(10), e13196.

Cavanagh K., Shapiro D., & Zack J. (2003). The computer plays therapist: The challenges and opportunities of psychotherapeutic software. In S. Goss & K. Anthony (Eds.), *Technology in counselling and psychotherapy: A practitioner's guide.* Basingstoke: Palgrave/Macmillan.

Cavanagh, K., Shapiro, D., Van den Berg, S., Swain, S., Barkham, M., & Proudfoot, J. (2009). The acceptability of computer-aided behavioural therapy: A pragmatic study. *Cognitive Behavioural Therapy, 38*(4), 1–12.

Christensen, H., Griffiths, K. M., & Jorm, A. F. (2004). Delivering interventions for depression by using the Internet: Randomised controlled trial. *British Medical Journal, 328*(7449), 1200–1201.

Clarke, G., Eubanks, D., Reid, E., Kellerher, C., O'Connor, E., DeBar, L., Lynch, F., Nunley, S., & Gullion, C. (2005). Overcoming depression on the Internet (ODIN) (2): A randomized trial of a self-help depression skills program with reminders. *Journal of Medical Internet Research, 7*(2), e 16.

Clarke, G., Reid, E., Eubanks, D., O'Connor, E., DeBar, L., Kellerher, C., Lynch, F., & Nunley, S. (2002). Overcoming depression on the Internet (ODIN): A randomized controlled trial of an Internet depression skills intervention program. *Journal of Medical Internet Research, 4*(3), e 14. DoH. (2001). *Treatment choice in psychological therapies and counselling: Evidence based clinical practice guidelines.* London: Department of Health.

Eysenbach, G., & CONSORT-EHEALTH Group. (2011). CONSORT-EHEALTH: Improving and standardizing evaluation reports of web-based and mobile health interventions. *J Med Internet Res, 13*(4), e126.

Farrer, L., Christensen, H., Griffiths, K. M., & Mackinnon, A. (2011). Internet-based cbt for depression with and without telephone tracking in a national helpline: Randomized controlled trial. *PLoS One, 6*(11), e28099.

Foroushani, P. S., Schneider, J., & Assareh, N. (2011) Meta-review of the effectiveness of computerised CBT in treating depression. *BMC Psychiatry, 11*, 131.

Griffiths, K. M., Farrer, L., & Christensen, H. (2010) The efficacy of internet interventions for depression and anxiety disorders: A review of randomized controlled trials. *MJA, 192*, S4–S11.

Grist R., & Cavanagh, K. (2013). Computerised cognitive behavioural therapy for common mental health disorders, what works, for whom under what circumstances? A systematic review and meta-analysis. *Journal of Contemporary Psychotherapy, 43*, 243–251.

Hickie, I. B., Davenport, T. A., Luscombe, G. M., Moore, M., Griffiths, K. M., & Christensen, H. (2010). Practitioner-supported delivery of internet-based cognitive behavior therapy: Evaluation of the feasibility of conducting a cluster randomized trial. *MJA, 192*, S31–S35.

Horvath A. O., & Luborsky, L. (1993). The role of the therapeutic alliance in psychotherapy. *Journal of Consulting and Clinical Psychology, 61*(4), 561–573.

Kaltenthaler, E., Brazier, J. E., de Nigris, E., Tumur, I., Ferriter, M., Beverley, C., Parry, G., Rooney, G., & Sutcliffe, P. (2006). Computerised cognitive behaviour therapy for depression and anxiety update: A systematic review and economic evaluation. *Health Technology Assessment, 10*(33), All.

Kaltenthaler, E., Sutcliffe, P., Parry, G., Beverley, C., Rees, A., & Ferriter, M. (2008). The acceptability to patients of computerized cognitive behaviour therapy for depression: A systematic review. *Psychological Medicine, 38*(11), 1521–1530.

Khan, K. S., Kunz, R., Kleijnen, J., & Antes, G. (2003). *Systematic reviews to support evidence-based medicine: How to review and apply findings of healthcare research.* London: Royal Society of Medicine Press, Ltd.

Lal, S., & Adair, C. E. (2014). E-mental health: A rapid review of the literature. *Psychiatric Services, 65*(1), 24–32.

Lindner, P., Olsson, E. L., Johnsson, A., Dahlin, M., Andersson, G., & Carlbring, P. (2014). The impact of telephone versus e-mail therapist guidance on treatment outcomes, therapeutic alliance and treatment engagement in Internet-delivered CBT for depression: A randomized pilot trial. *Internet Interventions, 1*, 182–187.

McCrone, P., Knapp, M., Proudfoot, J., Ryden, C., Cavanagh, K., Shapiro, D., Illson, S., Gray, J., Goldberg, D., Mann, A., Marks, I. M., & Everitt, B. (2004). Cost-effectiveness of computerised cognitive behavioural therapy for anxiety and depression in primary care. *British Journal of Psychiatry, 185*(1), 55–62.

National Institute for Health and Care Excellence. (2009). *The treatment and management of depression in adults, CG90.* London: Author. http://www.nice.org.uk/guidance/cg90.

Newby, J. M., Mackenzie, A., Williams, A. D., McIntyre, K., Watts, S., Wong, N., & Andrews, G. (2013). Internet cognitive behavioural therapy for mixed anxiety and depression: A randomized controlled trial and evidence of effectiveness in primary care. *Psychological Medicine, 43*, 2635–2648.

Perini, S., Titov, N., & Andrews, G. (2009). Clinician-assisted internet-based treatment is effective for depression: Randomized controlled trial. *Australian and New Zealand Journal of Psychiatry, 43*, 571–578.

Proudfoot, J., Klein, B., Barak, A., Carlbring, P., Cuijpers, P., Lange, A., Ritterband, L., & Andersson, G. (2011). Establishing guidelines for executing and reporting internet intervention research. *Cognitive Behaviour Therapy, 40*, 82–97.

Proudfoot, J., Ryden, C., Everitt, B., Shapiro, D., Goldberg, D., Mann, A., Tylee, A., Marks, I., & Gray, J. (2004). Clinical effectiveness of computerized cognitive behavioural therapy for anxiety and depression in primary care. *British Journal of Psychiatry, 185*(1), 46–54.

Renton, T., Tang, T, Ennis, E., Cusimano, M. D., Bhalerao, S., Schweizer, T., & Topolovec-Vranic, J. (2014). Web-based intervention programs for depression: A scoping review and evaluation. *Journal of Medical Internet Research, 16*(9), e209.

Richards, D., & Richardson, T. (2012). Computer-based psychological treatments for depression: A systematic review and meta-analysis. *Clinical Psychological Review, 32*, 239–342.

Rozental, A., Andersson, G., Boettcher, J., Ebert, D. D., Cuijpers, P., Knaevelsrud, C., Ljotsson, B., Kaldo, V., Titov, N., & Carlbring, P. (2014). Consensus statement on defining and measuring negative effects of internet interventions. *Internet Interventions, 1*, 12–19.

So, M., Yamaguchi, S., Hashimoto, S., Sado, M., Furukawa, T. A., & McCrone, P. (2013). Is computerised cbt really helpful for adult depression? A meta-analytic re-evaluation of ccbt for adult depression in terms of clinical implementation and methodological validity. *BMC Psychiatry, 13*, 113.

Vernmark, K., Lenndin, J., Bjärahed, J., Carlsson, M., Karlsson, J., Örberg, J., Carlbring, P., Eriksson, T., & Andersson, G. (2010). Internet administered guided self-help versus individualized e-mail therapy: A randomized trial of two versions of CBT for major depression. Behaviour *Research and Therapy, 48*, 368–376.

Waller, R., & Gilbody, S. (2009). Barriers to the uptake of computerized cognitive behavioural therapy: A systematic review of the quantitative and qualitative evidence. *Psychological Medicine, 39*, 705–712.

Chapter 22

THE ROLE OF FILM AND MEDIA IN MENTAL HEALTH

Jean-Anne Sutherland

Oh My God, I Think I Understand This.
(Albee, 1962, *Who's Afraid of Virginia Woolf?*)

INTRODUCTION

For years, two lovers have struggled against and with their passion for one another. Their lives are such that they can't say it out loud – can't claim one another in their day-to-day lives. Separated, their thoughts turn to one another. Together they know a passion, a connection and a love they've yet to find with another. When they can, the lovers sneak away and renew their love. Years go by. Time does not heal or eradicate their love. Jack is ready to claim the relationship in his life, but Ennis remains locked in fear. His angst concerning social condemnation ensnares him in denial. Jack, aware that he can't push Ennis to a place he is unwilling to go, is reduced to anger and tears. Tired of their separation, emotionally depleted by the hopelessness of their passion, Jack says to Ennis, "I wish I knew how to quit you"

That line, "I wish I knew how to quit you," has become a kind of iconic symbol of a gnashing and seemingly impossible love. The movie (Brokeback Mountain, 2005) and the line struck a chord with audiences – tapping into feelings of loss, hopelessness and contradiction. According to cinematherapist Birgit Wolz (cinematherapy.com),

the main characters are incarnating the basic human needs for wholeness, fulfillment and a true love who accepts them as they really are. They struggle valiantly over the years to make their marriages, their children and their work sources of meaning, but neither man is able to fully engage with his life. Their story reveals the pain of living with hidden identities. (Wolz, 2009, p. 1)

Wolz then describes her work with Vince, a gay client who, after viewing the film, began an exploration into his lifelong attempts to repudiate his homosexuality. Gay or straight, viewers of this film have the opportunity to come face to face with relationship dynamics, the integration of identities, feelings of loss, heartbreak and a visual representation of the price of fear.

FILM AND THERAPY

Films provide an opportunity for clients in a therapeutic setting to recognize, struggle with and potentially identify with deep-seated

223

conflicts. Increasingly, mental health professions have turned to film in the therapeutic setting. In 1944, in an article entitled *Psychodrama and Therapeutic Motion Pictures*, Moreno argued that films could reveal behaviors similar to those of clients. Moreno had in mind the production of films specifically drawing from therapy sessions in order to offer viewers a dose of realism. A bit ahead of his time, Moreno predated the critically acclaimed television show *In Treatment* by some 60 years. In this show, Gabriel Byrne plays a psychotherapist who, while working with a series of clients, struggles with his own insecurities and losses. Praised as much for what this show doesn't say as for what it does, *In Treatment* allows viewers to read between the lines. As Simons (2009) notes, "No one needs to fully, linguistically explain human pain and rebound: we spot it when we see it" (p. 1). Moreno had the same idea – use the power of film to illustrate psychodramatic material.

While Solomon (1995) claims the title "Father of Cinematherapy," it appears that therapists' ideas about the usefulness of this medium stem from the early days of film. Since the publication of Solomon's first book, films have become increasingly accessible. Besides the cinema itself, movies can be found at video stores, public libraries, through the mail (e.g., Netflix), on pay-for-view television and as computer downloads. As the techniques of filmmaking have advanced, making images and sounds more "real," so too has the accessibility of movies become more sophisticated.

While mental health and therapy is a favorite topic in Hollywood films, it is often depicted with humor and distortion. Whether the inappropriate therapist (e.g., *Running with Scissors*, 2006) or the over-the-top client (e.g., *Analyze This*, 1999), psychotherapy and mental illness are crowd pleasers. Occasionally, depictions of mental health issues give us pause such as the schizophrenic portrayed by Russell Crowe in *A Beautiful Mind* (2001). Sometimes a serious condition is made light as was

Dudley Moore's loveable drunk in *Arthur* (1981). Considerably less funny was Nicolas Cage's performance as the writer who decides to drink himself to death in *Leaving Las Vegas* (1995). The question is, to what extent do these films matter? Can they "teach" us about our culture, ourselves, psychotherapy and mental health? Many argue that films are "just entertainment." However, louder is the argument that film, while a form of mass entertainment, instructs and informs audiences while both creating and reflecting culture (Giroux, 2002). Films are more than just entertainment; they can also be used to provide moral instruction or social observation, to offer a social context or to explore political judgment (Sutherland & Feltey, 2009).

Films tell stories. Myths once served to illustrate the beliefs, values and behaviors of its people. Today films provide us with glimpses into our culture. Like literature, movies instruct, entertain, offer principals and ideologies, values and life lessons. But, unlike literature, film does not rely on abstract symbols alone. Instead, films speak to us through images and sound (Boggs & Petrie, 2004). Films can both reinforce stereotypes and challenge viewers with new interpretations of old themes. Films show us the development of individuals as they struggle with identity and self-esteem. In movies, we watch characters interact within the contexts of relationships. Films are a new kind of "text" through which we are provided stories, frames, and representations of social life (Sutherland & Feltey, 2009). Just as mental health professionals have long integrated other media such as literature and music into counseling, films provide an opportunity for clients to view the representation of an otherwise abstract idea.

A REVIEW OF THE LITERATURE

The specifics of integrating film into therapy vary in the current literature. In their book,

Rent Two Films and Let's Talk in the Morning: Using Popular Movies in Psychotherapy, Hesley and Hesley (2001) outline the benefits of film in counseling sessions. They call it "Video Work," a process whereby therapists and clients "discuss themes and characters in popular film that relate to core issues of on-going therapy" (p. 4). The authors tell the story of a client struggling in her current relationship. Overeager to please her man, Hesley's client struggled with her own self-worth. Jan suggested she watch the movie *Singles* (1992). She asked her client to notice her emotions as she watched the film. Her client saw the connection between her struggles and the struggles of a woman in the film. Hesley notes that her client was also angry at having watched the film. What the client sees in a film often challenges personal constructions of reality. Helsey and Hesley stress that the use of films does not replace traditional therapy. Rather, this methodology "emphasize[s] the partnership of conventional therapy and film homework" (p. 5).

According to Hesley and Hesley, when a client is assigned a film to watch, seeds are planted for future sessions. Specifically, they assign a film, explaining to the client why that particular movie fits. Boundaries are established and clients are warned of offensive language or content. After a client views a film, the next session may or may not directly address it. Sometimes the client rejects the relevance of the movie, but still the session may take a turn that it otherwise would not. Hesley and Hesley do not suggest that films bring about change directly. Rather, having a client watch a particular film provides a focus and opens the possibility for self-understanding.

Other resources provide a "how-to" work with film and clients. In *Moving Therapy: Moving Therapy,* Ulus (2003) provides instructions to become a movie group therapist (he even offers suggestions regarding proper billing of clients for movie therapy). Ulus acknowledges the increased use of films by psychologists and educators, reviewing the concept of film use in group settings. In *Movies and Mental Illness: Using Films to Understand Psychopathology,* Wedding et al. (2005) regard films as the social mirror in which we are projected. The authors see films as significant teaching tools to augment students' understandings of psychopathology. Their book is organized by particular disorders, with suggested films that serve as illustrations. Both texts offer readers justification for the use of movies while providing a rich index of films to draw upon.

For a specific link between film and the psychoanalytic perspective, see Sabbadini's edited text, *Projected Shadows: Psychoanalytic Reflections on the Representation of Loss in European Cinema* (2007). In this work, film scholars and psychoanalysts explore film and Oedipal crises, representations of pathology, dreams, and fantasies. Less a "how to" book than those previously noted, these essays provide a more academic grounding to the relationship between film and psychotherapy.

A visit to Wolz's website provides individuals with the tools for exploring one's inner life (emotionpicture.com; cinematherapy.com). At Wolz's site, one can skip the therapist and work alone. Wolz offers a list of films associated with particular struggles. After viewing, individuals are encouraged to ask themselves a number of questions such as: how did you feel when you observed; how and where in your life could you adopt this attitude; can you remember one situation in your life when you faced a fear? According to Wolz, movies can heal and help an individual in their "transformation." Wolz's model, outside of the context of therapy, lacks the give and take which stems from dialogue. As Hesley and Hesley note, the client may or may not make the immediate connection between the film and their personal lives. Certainly films can be viewed and explored by individuals outside of therapy with persons fully capable of reflection. However, oftentimes the temptation with film is to take literally that which can also be read symbolically. Dialogue with another provides the opportunity to steer clear of generalizations and arrive at meaningful connections.

Brown (2003) found that films were successful for use with female adolescent offenders. Acknowledging that films play an important role in the lives of adolescent girls, Brown developed a manual for use in treatment that centers on representations of sexism, racism, abuse/trauma, depression, and substance abuse in film. In a full session, the girls watch a particular film. Subsequent sessions allow the adolescents to discuss relevant scenes. In this way, group leaders utilize film as a means of stimulating discussions of potentially difficult topics.

When discussed as a scene in a film, sensitive topics (e.g., abuse, depression) can feel more accessible to clients. After all, it is happening to someone else. Watching something "happen" to someone else can offer validation to clients who might have otherwise felt alone with their experiences. And subsequent discussions can allow clients to make connections between what they see as "film moments" and what they experience in their lives. That is, film has the potential to make clear the abstract – to bring into view what was otherwise distant and vague.

Also of significance is the body of literature addressing the usefulness of film in counselor student training. As Toman and Rak (2000) noted, "the use of motion pictures as a teaching tool can bring the personable and intimate study of human issues directly into the classroom, providing dialogue in the context of film characters' life circumstances." Between 1994 and 1998, Toman and Rak evaluated the use of film across four courses (teaching diagnosis, counseling theories, counseling interventions, and ethics). Their overall results, based on the administration of a student survey, demonstrated positive responses from students. The use of film in classes was successful in "providing visual case examples for role plays, serving as catalysts for class discussions, bringing the tenets of theory to life, giving students the opportunity to rewrite ethical endings to replace unethical depictions and bringing dialogue and context into the classroom." The authors note concerns and considerations that must be addressed when using film in the classroom. Did the viewing of films actually increase knowledge of the material? To what extent are instructors offered a pedagogical tool for teaching with film?

As more therapists and course instructors integrate film into counseling and counseling training, the question of pedagogy becomes essential. Who is teaching us how to teach through film? While numerous works point out the advantages that film offers, fewer studies discuss the specifics of the pedagogical process. Higgins and Dermer (2001) go beyond a discussion of the advantages and offer detailed strategies for use in the classroom. These include: evaluating films from different theoretical orientations; evaluating films from different characters' perspectives; watching a film clip with no sound; analysis of student reactions; developing hypotheses and demonstrating how they were generated; development of treatment plans (for the characters in the film); evaluating development; film used as exam replacement or supplement. Part of building a film pedagogy involves thorough development of exercises and assessment of the effectiveness of such tools. Future work with film should consider not only the abundant advantages for the use of film, but also the intended objectives and outcomes.

CAUTIONS AND CONSIDERATIONS

A general caution must be considered when working with film. As we know, films, even when they look "real" and, even if they might be "inspired by a true story," are produced within the power structure of Hollywood or, at least, of a film production company. Problems can arise when films are accepted at face value without critical analysis. Issues of sexism, racism, classism, ageism (all of the "isms") are potentially missed without careful deliberation.

Unlike a novel which is usually the work of an individual, a film comes to us via a plethora of artists. The producers, screenwriters, directors, editors, cinematographer, sound crew, and, of course, the actors all participate in the telling of the story. Each of those contributors brings something to the project. Each stands in a particular place that will impact the final story that we see and hear on the screen. Also, unlike works of literature, film production (particularly Hollywood films) almost always occurs under the umbrella of capitalism. Will the film profit financially? Will young men want to see it (movie makers know the importance of this demographic)? Thus, when a subject as sensitive as mental illness, or as complicated as human emotions, is approached in a film, it will take on drama and absurdities not necessarily "real." For example, when telling the tale of domestic violence, it is much more "interesting" to watch Jennifer Lopez pump iron so that her body is strong enough to beat the hell out her husband than to depict the usual methods by which a battered woman typically escapes (*Enough*, 2002). Issues of community, reliance on social networks – these are the resources needed for escaping an abusive home. But, that would make a boring film (or so Hollywood has trained us). Thus, while the film might motivate a woman to find some internal strength to "fight back," it is hopeful that the "fighting back" will seem as much symbolic as literal.

I am not suggesting that clients (or anyone for that matter) are passive participants in film viewing. While we once regarded audiences as sponge-like and vulnerable, we now understand that viewers participate in film viewing through processes of interpretation (Sutherland & Feltey, 2009). Even as we are inundated with movies, individuals sustain a kind of dialogue with films – dismissing parts that do not fit cognitively and embracing other parts. Even so, any discussion of film benefits by placing it into historical and social contexts. Consideration of the multiple layers of sexism, racism, and classism allows us to see more clearly the perils the characters in this film face. Moreover, consideration of "isms" allow the film to speak to those layers of a client's life. That is, for example, how might the outcomes of the character be different if she were African-American and not Caucasian? Or: what does this film *not* say in terms of social class limitations?

While we acknowledge that audiences are not passive, we also grant that movies tend to be utilized far more for escapism than for reflection. Miller (1999) noted that most moviegoers "see films as a means to get away from moral arguments, not to get into them" (p. 1). Most audience members are not searching a film for a theory or even a "lesson" for that matter – that is not how we are culturally oriented towards movies. Thus, while films stimulate dialogue and offer opportunities for contemplation, the "skill" for such musings is not necessarily intuitive. Guiding clients through a "reading" of film requires cognizance of film pedagogy. Giroux (2002) warns us against "textual essentialism," and the temptation to read films as sites of particular meanings and interpretations. Rather, when using film, we must remember to place our readings within the larger social contexts of dominant discourse, ideology, and capitalism. *Who* has the power to tell the stories of love, loss, hopelessness, abuse, addiction, and mental illness? From where did the dominant ideas of human struggling emerge? As we offer clients or students film in order to illustrate a concept, we must remember how representation itself works within the relations of power.

CONCLUSION

Increasingly, films are employed in therapy in order to illustrate behaviors, circumstances, disorders and distractions. Therapists know that people are more likely to view a movie about addiction than to read a text about the subject.

At present, there are multiple texts and websites for specific instruction concerning film and therapy. Resources range from the specific "how-to" to the theoretical. It follows that as access to films expands, use of film in therapeutic settings will increase. Important considerations involve appropriate "readings" of films – placing them within the larger social and historical context in which they are produced. While films strike at the heart of issues, they don't themselves capture the complexity of the issue. Films are an ideal tool for illustrating life, pain, loss, and joy. The work of the therapist is to frame those representations in such as way as to provide meaningful analysis for the client. As Buddy (played by Kevin Spacey) reminds us in *Swimming with Sharks* (1994), "Life is not a movie. Good guys lose, everybody lies and love . . . does not conquer all."

REFERENCES

Albee, E. (1962). *Who's afraid of Virginia Woolf?* New York: Signet.

Boggs, J. M., & Petrie, D. W. (2004). *The art of watching films* (6th ed.). New York: McGraw-Hill.

Brown, T. K. S. (2003). *Therapeutic use of media with female adolescent offenders: A group treatment manual.* Thesis (Psy. D.). Alliant International University, California School of Professional Psychology, San Francisco Bay.

Giroux, H. (2002). *Breaking in to the movies.* Malden, MA: Blackwell.

Hesley, J. W., & Hesley, J. G. (2001). *Rent two films and let's talk in the morning: Using popular movies in psychotherapy.* New York: John Wiley and Sons.

Higgins, J. A., & Dermer, S. (2001). The use of film in marriage and family counselor education. *Counselor Education and Supervision, 40*(3), 182–193.

Miller, B. (1999). The work of interpretation: A theoretical defence of film theory and criticism. *Kinema: A journal for film and audiovisual media* [online]. [Accessed December 3, 2009]. Available from: http://www.kinema.uwaterloo.ca/article.php?id=209&feature.

Moreno, J. L. (1944). Psychodrama and therapeutic motion pictures. *Sociometry, 7*(2), 230–244.

Sabbadini, A. (2007). *Projected shadows: Psychoanalytic reflections on the representation of loss.* New York: Routledge Press.

Simons, I. (2009). HBO's 'In Treatment'. *Psychology Today* [online]. [Accessed December 3, 2009]. Available from: http://www.psychologytoday.com/blog/ the-literary-mind/2009 04/hbo s-in-treatment.

Soloman, G. (1995). *The motion picture prescription: Watch this movie and call me in the morning.* Santa Rosa, CA: Aslan.

Sutherland, J. A., & Feltey, K. (2009). *Cinematic sociology: Social life in film.* Pine Forge, CA: Sage.

Toman, S. M., & Rak, C. F. (2000). The use of cinema in the counselor education curriculum: Strategies and outcomes. *Counselor Education and Supervision, 40*(2), 105–115.

Ulus, F. (2003). *Move therapy: Moving therapy.* Victoria, BC: Trafford.

Wedding, D., Boyd, M. A., & Niemec, R. M. (2005). *Movies and mental illness: Using films to understand psychopathology.* Göttingen: Hogrefe and Huber.

Wolz, B. (2009). Therapeutic movie review column. Cinematherapy.com [online]. [Accessed February 2, 2009]. Available from: http://www.cinematherapy.com/birgitarticles/brokeback-mountain.html.

Part Two

THE USE OF TECHNOLOGY
IN TRAINING AND SUPERVISION

Chapter 23

AN APPROACH TO THE TRAINING AND SUPERVISION OF ONLINE COUNSELLORS

Cedric Speyer and John Yaphe

INTRODUCTION

The growth of online counselling as an effective therapeutic modality has created the need for ongoing supervision of e-counsellors. This chapter will describe one model of online supervision as it applies to asynchronous communication, as well as reviewing practices that have emerged within the framework of an established e-counselling service. It will present the principles of online supervision used in this service, discuss common challenges faced by counsellors and present some online supervisory interventions using composite case excerpts. It will conclude with reflections on future developments for Internet supervision of distance counselling.

Online supervision is defined as the provision of supervision to e-counsellors delivering online clinical service. It is intended to assure the quality of online counselling and the effectiveness of therapeutic outcomes. It also promotes the knowledge, skills and clinical attributes required by e-counsellors who are making the transition to text-based counselling. Supervision supports their online professional development. Nagel et al. (2009) include a discussion of the historical development of online counselling in their review of the influence of new technologies in the practice of clinical supervision.

Recently published studies on the effectiveness of electronic counselling refer to the importance of the supervision of counsellors. Gulec's report (2014) of an online program for patients with eating disorders in Germany mentions supervision of doctoral students by senior clinicians. Kivi's study (2014) of Internet-based CBT for patients with depression in Sweden reports that all the licensed counsellors and psychotherapists providing online counselling in their survey group received continuous supervision by senior researchers. Dear's research (2015) on CBT-based online interventions for patients with anxiety disorders in Australia included weekly supervision of counsellors provided by senior members of the research team. In these three studies it is not specified if the supervision was provided online or in-person.

Clinicians recognize the need for adequate supervision when providing online counselling. In Schnur's study (2012) of 120 oncologists, over 80% affirmed that online counselling would be appropriate for their patients and their families; almost all wished that skilled supervision were available, but few had access to it. Online supervision might resolve this issue for counsellors eager to expand their range of services.

Using email exchanges in conjunction with phone sessions as necessary (for risk situations, etc.) has proven to be an effective way to supervise e-counsellors. Asynchronous communication via email does not take place in 'real time,' but rather whenever the participants have a chance to respond to one another (Rochen et al., 2004). Asynchronicity allows reflection, but as with online counselling between client and counsellor, it is not immune from misunderstandings. As is the case with online counsellors, online supervisors must be aware of the lack of spontaneous clarification (Speyer & Zack, 2003). Nevertheless, the raw material of case management (transcripts of the correspondence when ethically appropriate) is readily available to the supervisor; therefore quality assurance can be hands-on. Supervision is more directly accessible. It is not based solely on the therapist's perception and report of the therapeutic interchange. Supervisors can offer guidance by reading the client's text independently of the e-counsellor's response and review the e-counsellor's clinical process before, during, or after the asynchronous session.

IN-SERVICE SUPERVISION

Counsellors in the service described here, an e-counselling program of a major Canadian Employee and Family Assistance Program (EFAP) provider, are drawn mainly from the fields of social work, counselling and psychology with a Master's degree and a minimum of five years of counselling experience as minimal requirements. There is also a family physician on staff. Counsellors pass through three stages of screening to assess the level of integration of their writing and therapeutic skills and are subsequently provided with extensive on-the-job training and ongoing supervision. In a more recent development, telephone counsellors based in the EFAP Care Access Centre (CAC) have been

receiving intensive training and supervision for online case assignments, to enhance their increasingly multimodal skill sets.

The founder of the service (Cedric Speyer) serves as clinical supervisor for case management challenges of all kinds and as an on-going mentor for e-counsellors. Practical training for the short-term approach uses a template known as the *CARE* model for e-counsellors to follow as a framework for case management. The acronym stands for Connect and Contain (*"your challenge is human and manageable"*); Assess and Affirm (*"you've got what it takes to get through this"*); Reorient and Reaffirm (*"you are not defined by your life situation"*); and Encourage and Empower (*"keep going, one step at a time"*) (Speyer, 2010).

A second experienced e-counsellor fulfills the role of clinical cosupervisor for counsellor management and extended training, addressing the need for the application of specialized skills and best practices, given the overall challenges of the modality. Some examples of these case management challenges are presented below. The family medicine specialist on the e-team (John Yaphe), with experience supervising the clinical work of medical residents and students, has served as a consultant for online case conferences and has also conducted an in-service training workshop. In principle, supervision follows the general guidelines established for the practice and protocols of online clinical supervision by the British Association for Counselling and Psychotherapy (Anthony & Goss, 2009).

E-counsellors benefit from both individual and group supervision. Individual supervision occurs as the need arises at the counsellor's initiative, at regularly scheduled intervals or at the initiative of the supervisor, using selected cases as teaching vehicles and following up on feedback from clients. Counsellors can receive individual supervisory guidance upon request at any time before, during, or after case exchanges. Supervision is mandatory for high-risk cases needing offline intervention, including suicidal or homicidal intent, domestic abuse/violence of any kind, risk to children (reportable issues) severe addiction or mental health issues, and other crises requiring immediate support.

Continued collaboration, consultation and training occur online via ongoing discussion on a listserv and by webinar at quarterly in-service training workshops. ViewPoint (the listserv) is a professional development forum for E-team networking and sharing. Participation is authorized by the Clinical Supervisor. Discussions pertain to the quality, effectiveness and influence of online counselling in an EFAP setting. Members offer support, encouragement and resources to each other in the interests of team-building.

CASE MANAGEMENT CHALLENGES

In the following section we present clinical material to illustrate best practices and common challenges encountered in e-counselling. The material has been modified to preserve the anonymity of counsellors and clients and uses composite case excerpts to illustrate key principles.

Close Attention to the Client's Text

The client in the following example is a 40-year-old woman who requested help in dealing with sources of stress in her life.

Client (intake form): This is all absorbing. I'm avoiding social occasions, not in the mood. I stopped going to tango nights, my dance partner senses my stress, which just escalates his, and that spoils the fun, plus I can't really concentrate and when you're really into tango, you need to.

The e-counsellor replied to the client in the first exchange using the following formula in order to elicit more about the client's interests

and activities in a solution-oriented way, despite already knowing about one of client's passions, namely dancing the tango.

E-Counsellor (first exchange): I am curious to know what your life outside of work is like at this time. What sort of life-work balance do you have at this time? Who are the significant people in your life? What sort of activities do you participate in outside of work? What do you do to relax/de-stress? Taking care of yourself during an emotionally stressful time like this is very important. What can you do at this time to take care of you?

The counsellor continues with psychoeducation and the following homework assignment for the client.

E-counsellor: During emotionally stressful times there is a tendency for thoughts and feelings to be chaotic. Journaling is a wonderful way of releasing the thoughts and feelings onto paper. You can also type them into your computer, if you feel more comfortable doing that.

During case consultation, the supervisor reminded the counsellor that during the intake process, the client had already told part of her story online, thereby answering some of the counsellor's subsequent questions. A generic response recommending homework also misses the opportunity to reinforce what the client is already doing in the context of her text-based relationship with the counsellor. The supervisor emphasized the importance of building upon existing disclosures and client engagement at intake.

Person-Centred vs. Problem-Saturated Approach

Clients usually present their issues in a problem-saturated manner. E-counsellors in this service are encouraged to "find out what's right with the client" rather than engage in discussion of dysfunction as the central theme of the online dialogue (in the name of removing blocks to the client's happiness and well-being). In this short-term approach, e-counsellors are coached to focus on the "person behind the problem" and draw upon inner resources that will enable the client to choose a response to their life situation, rather than to continue to feel victimized by it.

In the following example, a 24-year-old woman requested help in dealing with the many challenges of her daily life.

> Client: I am really stressed out with many family issues such as father possibly having MS . . . brother on crystal meth . . . guilt that my grandparents are barely keeping a roof over their heads . . . me having money problems . . . missing sister who is in another country . . . weight issues . . . lonely and depressed. I wish I would not want to cry all the time. I would be skinny lol I would want to be out there having fun rather than sitting at home.

The counsellor, who was a novice, responded in her first exchange as follows.

> E-Counsellor: Hi Louise and welcome to e-counselling which is a place that you can feel free to share your feelings and thoughts without having to worry about what you should or should not say. My name is Johanna and I will be your e-counselor. I look forward to having a few back and forth exchanges with you to help you try and figure out what has you feeling so unhappy.

She continued with the following synopsis . . .

> E-Counsellor: From reading your email I see that you are feeling pretty unhappy

and seem to be lacking in energy and motivation – kinda' like your get up and go has got up and went?

The supervisor picked up on this problem-centered approach and suggested a more person-centered approach:

> Supervisor: Instead of leading with the negative as a goal and buying into client's depressive line of thinking when you say, "I am here to help you try to figure out what it is that has you feeling so unhappy," you might try relating to the person behind the problem. You could lead with a capsule summary of the life situation in positive terms. For example: "You are coping with many family concerns including your father's illness, brother's addiction, grandparent's needs, not to mention your own money and weight issues. Yet I also see you have a clear idea of who you could be when you say: "I would not want to cry all the time, I would be skinny, I would want to be out having fun rather than sitting at home." I wonder what kind of fun that would be, Louise, and what it would take to bring a little more of what you want into your life?"
>
> You have a good upbeat, conversational tone and offer some excellent guidance. Now you need to instill the feeling that depression doesn't define her and transmit that along with the empathy of the first exchange by connecting with the person who was able to write "lol" in the midst of listing her burdens.

Positive Core Issue: The Glare and the Gaze

When e-counsellors apply the full scope of their clinical expertise to the etiology of the negative core issue, this is the necessary *glare* of the assessment phase. Yet the tone of the online dialogue is the antidote to client discouragement. E-counselling exchanges are characterized by a positive *gaze* on client strengths. While the 'glare' provides valuable insight into self-defeating attitudes and patterns, the 'gaze' is focused squarely on the inherent capacity to overcome, transform, or transcend painful life predicaments.

> E-supervisor: I am talking about listening to the client in a solution-focused way, by acknowledging that she is a survivor of sexual abuse, in response to her disclosures. You can also ask her if it is something she had received help with in the various forms of therapy she has undergone. We are not looking for cause and effects in any clinical way, because we are not using the medical diagnostic model in this short-term EFAP service, nor actively revisiting past trauma.

There has been much clinical discussion at all levels, as well as trial and error on the ground among numerous e-counsellors, and the perspective presented here has emerged as perhaps the best way to field revelations of past abuse, in the authors' view. In the short-term online process, it is not best practice to invite clients to revisit past abuse in the name of 'abreaction,' yet we also need to honour the trust clients place in us when they reveal painful episodes of the past. There is a generic way to acknowledge and reframe past abuse, as an integral part of addressing current client scenarios. This following essential message to the client serves as a template for the therapeutic approach we recommend when clients disclose a history of past abuse.

> E-Counsellor: The good qualities that came to the surface as a result of childhood abuse and still do, enabled you to survive at the time and continue to build a life for yourself in which you can thrive. Those strengths say more about who you

are than how the original trauma made you feel, which is powerless and of no value.

> As an adult, you have the power to experience yourself with compassion as someone susceptible to feelings which may lead you to believe something is wrong with you. However, those feelings can cue what is most right with you; the ability to take care of yourself in exactly the ways your caretakers failed to do.

Online Guidance without Pen-Pal Dependence

Clients are encouraged to view their e-counsellor as a guide at the crossroads who is trained to point them in the right direction (for them), rather than serve as a virtual companion or penpal. E-counsellors encourage clients to be emotionally self-sufficient, rather than position themselves as helpers who will 'be there for them' on an on-going basis. The general goal, as much as possible, is to cut to the chase of the client's essential qualities, values, and strengths.

In this example, the counsellor consulted with the supervisor because of difficulties in achieving closure with a client.

> Client: Gotta go now . . . hope to chat soon . . . thanks for being there . . . getting your take on things is the highlight of my day!

The supervisor responded in this manner.

> E-supervisor: It is a challenge to set parameters for certain clients, with no perceived loss of compassion. As in all forms of therapy, you need to stay in charge of the process (not the person) by keeping control over the framework. Otherwise, some clients will just keep coming back to the well, as thirsty as ever. What we mean by client centred case management is the

ability to support clients without propping them up; that means clearly leaving the responsibility for their health and wholeness with them, again with no loss of compassion. The general goal is to leave clients with confidence in their own resources. So be explicit about how you are a guide for a short while on the journey; it's all about which direction to take at the crossroads. You're a guide, not a companion, so every case is about handing the compass to the client so they can find the direction (inner and outer) that's right for them. Keep the clinical goal of closure in mind from the beginning: guiding, advising and concluding in the spirit of "My voice will go with you." (Rosen, 1982)

This counsellor adopted the supervisor's advice during the last exchange:

E-counsellor: I am often a little sad when I come to the end of a brief journey with people I meet in counselling. It has been a pleasure and a privilege to correspond with you and I admire the way you have faced your difficulties and dealt with them. You are now on your way! Sometimes I see my job like that of a guide who helps people across a swift-flowing river. It's tricky but it helps if someone shows you where the solid stones are so you can get firm footing. Now it's time for me to go back and help someone else across.

Finding Out What's Right with the Client

In our short-term approach, e-counsellors encourage clients to separate their sense and source of identity or self-fulfillment from their life circumstances (at first by simply witnessing their predicament with borrowed functioning coming from the e-counsellor's compassion and loving-kindness). When we see through the self-concept shell of damaged goods that many clients present at intake, we discover essential qualities at the heart and core of client personhood that allow us to reframe the challenging crux of their issues in terms of personal hope and faith already accessible to the client's essential self.

E-supervisor: I hear a tone of bitter resignation in the client's sign-off to you and that goes with the territory of what she's been through lately. You can understand the conclusions she comes to without buying into the spirit of them; just the opposite. You started this case off well but the problem-saturated story took over, with you in the more traditionally therapeutic role of uncovering layers of her distress. You tried to get at her underlying positive values as an entry point for believing in herself, yet she succeeded in steering the dialogue back to her grievances. You need to keep your gaze on the redemptive aspects of her personhood and attune the client to the vision of her strengths, which you steadfastly hold on the client's behalf (which is different than any facile praising or 'cheerleading' of good traits).

The clinical microscope revealing the deep-seated roots of her flaws and failings needs to be put aside in favour of the magnifying glass applied to what's right with the client; not what's wrong with her. You're the role model for those perceptions.

E-counsellor (practicing recommendations): When I first read your letter, a number of thoughts and feelings surfaced in me and I would like to share them with you to see how that can help us get started. The first thought was a question. "Who is Shannon?" I read about diagnoses, medications and doctors, but I don't think that gives me a good picture of you. I don't see you as a patient in need of treatment. I read a little more and I learned about a wife, a daughter, a worker with lots of experience in a responsible position and felt "that's more like it!" Then I heard about someone who is looking for a new way to make progress in the personal, family, work, and social spheres. This sounds like a person who is ready to work with me and move forward. That is the person I want to get to know better.

E-supervisor (responding to another case consultation): Meanwhile, if your role is not to diagnose any condition or treat any mental illness, then guess what? You can explore what's right with her – by writing a full, compassionate, soul-making first exchange inviting her to explore the personhood that is not defined by "severe anxiety/depression/stress issues" but instead highlights the following:

Client (at intake): I still value life and my family really matters to me. I want to do work that gives me a reason to get up in the morning. I need an emotional boost and could use some advice on how to stop hating my ex. I'd be able to walk into the lawyer's office to complete the divorce settlement with confidence and have nothing to fear.

Letting Go of Outcomes ("Don't Work Harder Than Your Client")

After supervised practice, experienced e-counsellors may become adept at sensing potential healing for the client at whatever point in their life they may be ready to own it. This is the big picture or view from the mountaintop. When guiding the client through the valley of their present predicament, e-counsellors can see the forest for the trees and pace themselves accordingly; they can walk their client towards the nearest clearing without necessarily taking them through all the tangled thickets of the negative core issue.

One e-counselor was advised as follows:

A, B, C's of "not working harder than the client":

A. Hold the vision of healing and enjoy the soul-restoring effect of writing accordingly, without disregarding the client's pain ('where it hurts').
B. Pace and lead the client one or two steps further than where they are, while encouraging their progress, no matter how minimal.
C. Watch out for feelings related to taking on too much responsibility for the outcome. Counsellor impatience, irritation, or anger at the lack of client movement can all be clues.

Increasingly, e-counsellors are facing situations in which online clients are at apparent risk of harm to themselves or others. A counselor who consulted on a potential high-risk case was advised:

E-supervisor: The first exchange serves as a context in which to connect with the whole person. The clients usually initiate a dialogue organized around the problem. Without minimizing their pain, we do not have to do the same. The empathy and compassion for what clients are going through, no matter how extreme, needs to be accompanied by great interest in the life in which this life situation is taking place. *Where attention goes, energy flows . . .* that's why you don't want to focus the first exchange exclusively on the pain that leads to "thoughts of hurting yourself." More importantly, the contracting for safety (which needs to be *part* of the first exchange and not set the whole tone) is counter-productive if it displaces connecting with the client on the basis of your confidence in them.

Intuitive Assessment without Diagnostic Questioning

E-supervisor: Every intake comes with a

feeling tone to it and a core issue behind that feeling. In this case, there is a tone of insecurity and vulnerability. Connecting on a feeling level always comes first, before the psycho-education starts to build on the (positive) core issue. It appears the client could be ready to grow in the direction of self-validation. Strengthening her own emotional 'container' could help with the mutual boundary-setting that helps make the marriage a safe place. All this needs to be addressed by creating an alliance with the client on the basis of what she's already shared rather than asking 'further assessment' questions about the problems in her marriage.

Prepare your response in a way that signifies to the client that you have carefully read and understood the presenting issues. This can be achieved through validating the client's experience, reflecting what the client is communicating 'between the lines' and extending unconditional positive regard, with a minimum of strategic questions to move the dialogue forward.

Search for client strengths and refer to these often in the context of the presenting problem, quoting the client's words to illustrate themes.

In the text of the correspondence, there is often a subtext, or underlying issues that need to be addressed. As long as you are making educated guesses and resonating with the client's agenda, rather than assuming hidden issues, it is an important part of the assessment process to follow hunches, trust gut feelings and lead with an intuitive sense of the person on the other side of the computer.

Client-Friendly Language and 'Voice'

A counsellor consulted with the supervisor regarding the tone or 'voice' to be used in first exchanges.

E-supervisor: In the process of bonding with the client, keep in mind both the purpose and the overall goal of the exchanges, which is to reinforce what is right with the client rather than diagnose and treat what is wrong with them. To that end, write in the tone of a close friend, without being presumptuous about it, especially at the beginning.

Be aware that the most important goal is to create a therapeutic bond with the client which has the tone of warm, respectful, caring, letter writing.

Validate the client's experience within the client's frame of reference. Comment often on the progress being made. Express appreciation for the depth of honesty in the person as it emerges through the correspondence. Be transparent about your thoughts and feelings as they arise, to avoid a 'canned' effect in text.

Maintaining Consistent Online Framework and Parameters

The e-counsellor sets the parameters for short-term correspondence. This spells out the pace, momentum and rate of replies on both sides and the need for a theme, in order to take charge of the case management. Initial parameter-setting sends the message that clients have a few focused back-and-forth exchanges to work with over a limited period of time. In the short-term model, the window clients have to communicate with a counsellor does not stay open indefinitely. Files are opened when clients register and closed when the correspondence concludes, within a flexible timeframe. Short-term asynchronous cases are not designed for periodic contact. Clients need to perceive their e-counselor as a guide who is trained to point them in a self-sustaining direction and make sure that they are equipped for their own journey, rather than someone who is there for ongoing consultation or an on-call consultant who they can turn to during the drama of each new difficult episode.

E-supervisor: The emphasis is always on the perspective or direction that the client needs to move forward and the 'remaining exchanges' invoked in the context of the positive core issue. Sometimes you have to explicitly orient the client on how to make the most of the medium and short-term nature of the service.

Reading Between the Lines for Feeling Tone

Writing can reflect the thought processes and emotional state of the client, even when the personality or attitude behind the core issue is not directly expressed. Experienced e-counsellors learn to intuitively assess the nature of their correspondent by paying close attention to their idiosyncratic use of language. Consider the difference between these two ways of presenting the same marital issue and what it says about the personality behind the words.

Client A: I am seeking professional assistance for marital difficulties that have led to temporary separation from my spouse.
Client B: Hope someone there can help me! My husband just walked out on me and I don't know what I'm going to do. I knew there were some problems, doesn't everyone have them? But this feels like a kind of amputation. I feel cut off and torn in half!
E-supervisor: When you read an intake, you really have to sit with it for awhile, so you can enter into the client's world and get a sense of their felt presence through paying close attention to what they're saying as well as feeling; making the connection warm, close, empathic and heartfelt.

Mastering the Nuances of Tele-Presence

Since the writing process mirrors a person's thought process, it can provide opportunities to explore the client's irrational beliefs and distorted perceptions through text-based input alone. Writing style can be as revealing as body language. It's a way of 'composing oneself' in more ways than one, revealed in writing as visible 'self-talk.' There is also an intangible *attunement* as Suler (2004) observed: "There is a special type of interpersonal empathy that is unique to text relationships. Some claim that text-only talk carries you past the distracting, superficial aspects of a person's existence and connects you more directly to the other's psyche."

E-supervisor: There are three ways of writing to a client. The first and least attuned is when we write *at* the person with all our expertise on the issue in mind. The second is when we write *to* the person – however, it is still the person who has the problem, while we have possible solutions. The third and most effective form of e-counselling is when we are writing *with* the person by entering their world from our side of the computer. Then psychological shifts take place as a result of the layered intersection of perspectives, from which new possibilities and creative alternatives can emerge.

Client feedback: While the traditional therapeutic relationship is ideally a collaborative process, I felt that this medium moved things in that direction much more quickly. It seemed that we were both beginning on the same level with no preconceived notions. By this I mean that there was no room for outside influences – for example, the physical characteristics of either of us, the office, other people, tones of voice, etc. . . . These were not present and as such, allowed for the pureness of the words to be heard. The true content of our discussions is the focus, not the other stuff that can often impede effective communication. I had no idea it was possible to form a bond and a trust with someone based solely on the written word. Thoughts and feelings just seemed to flow out of me in a way I never could have imagined. My e-counsellor helped me put things in perspective and look at things going on in my life in a whole different light. I was apprehensive about trying e-counselling but find it was the best move I ever made.

Leading the Process without Imposing an Agenda

E-counsellors are trained to focus on client strengths and resources. From that point of view, they are able to reframe significant stressors and conflicts. The problem and its consequences are then situated within a more meaningful story, allowing choices to be made in freedom and out of self-love. Yet it all starts with the *joining* and the client's gut feeling that no matter what else is being discussed, the counsellor is saying, in effect, *I am with you, I sense your pain, I know what's wrong, but I also know it's not bigger than you; so let's walk through this together and discover all the inner and outer resources pointing the way forward.* That allows for a "cut to the chase"effect when it comes to the (positive) core issue, i.e., what will be life-giving for the client.

E-supervisor: Your assessment of the core issue still needs some fine-tuning, in that you tend to use a wide-angle lens in the first exchange due to good in-person, client-centered training in which there's an open-ended unconditional positive regard. In this short-term approach we keep the unconditional positive regard, yet it is not as open-ended as in face-to-face counselling. In this case, for example, you can explore how and when the client feels loved by her husband. In a few exchanges you

can plant the seeds of what she needs to achieve more emotional intimacy in her marriage. It's a matter of getting to know her preferred state first; what true intimacy means to her. The first exchange also sets the theme and this is where you need a working hypothesis that contains a vision of her healing, or what the antidote would be to: "I can't really figure out what is wrong lately but I'm not happy." What exactly will happiness look like for this client?

CONCLUSION

The growth and development of e-counselling and online supervision have presented many challenges and opportunities for creative solutions. Ongoing research published since the first edition of this book has provided evidence of the benefits of the approach presented above as well as the effectiveness of the methods described. Both quantitative and qualitative measures have been applied to study the efficacy of e-counselling and e-supervision. More research is needed. We continue to explore the full range of issues that can be effectively dealt with in this format. We are getting a better sense of the kinds of counsellors who are best suited to work in this modality, yet standardized screening systems have yet to be fully developed. We also need to clarify the approaches to supervision which will be most effective in training and guiding online counsellors. How will these methods be incorporated into the traditional repertoire of skills taught to professionals who use counselling methods in their daily work? We look forward to further development in these directions, as Internet-mediated mental health services become an increasingly mainstream mode of service delivery.

REFERENCES

Anthony, K., & Goss, S. (2009). *Guidelines for online counselling and psychotherapy including guidelines for online supervision* (3rd ed.). Lutterworth: BACP.

Dear B. F., Zou J. B., Ali, S., Lorian, C. N., Johnston, L., Sheehan, J., Staples, L. G., Gandy, M., Fogliati, V. J., Klein, B., & Titov, N. (2015) Clinical and cost-effectiveness of therapist-guided Internet-delivered cognitive behavior therapy for older adults with symptoms of anxiety: A randomized controlled trial. *Behavioral Therapy, 46*(2), 206–217.

Gulec, H., Moessner, M., Túry, F., Fiedler, P., Mezei, A., & Bauer, S. (2014). A randomized controlled trial of an Internet-based posttreatment care for patients with eating disorders. *Telemedicine Journal of E Health, 20*(10), 916–922.

Kivi, M., Eriksson, M. C., Hange, D., Petersson, E. L., Vernmark, K., Johansson, B., & Björkelund, C. (2014). Internet-based therapy for mild to moderate depression in Swedish primary care: Short term results from the PRIM-NET randomized controlled trial. *Cognitive Behavioral Therapy, 43*(4), 289–298. Nagel, D. M., Goss, S., & Anthony, K. (2009). The use of technology in supervision. In N. Pelling, J. Barletta, & P. Armstrong (Eds.), *The practice of clinical supervision.* Bowen Hills, Qld.: Australian Academic Press.

Rochlen, A. B., Zack, J. S., & Speyer, C. (2004). Online therapy: Review of relevant definitions, debates, and current empirical support. *Journal of Clinical Psychology, 60*(3), 269–283.

Rosen, S. (Ed.). (1982). *My voice will go with you: The teaching tales of Milton H. Erickson.* New York: W. W. Norton.

Schnur, J. B., & Montgomery, G. H. (2012). E-counselling in psychosocial cancer care: A survey of practice, attitudes, and training among providers. *Telemedicine Journal of E Health, 18*(4), 305–308.

Speyer, C., Zack, J., & Suler, J. R. (2004). The psychology of text relationships. In R. Kraus, J. Zack & G. Stricker (Eds.), *Online counselling: A handbook for mental health professionals.* San Diego, CA: Elsevier Academic Press.

Chapter 24

USING CHAT AND INSTANT MESSAGING (IM) TO ENRICH COUNSELOR TRAINING AND SUPERVISION

DeeAnna Merz Nagel and Kate Anthony

INTRODUCTION

Using text-based, real-time chat to conduct supervision is quickly becoming an integral part of many educational, organizational and employment settings. This chapter will describe the use of chat and instant messaging in a work setting, offering the reader an opportunity to envision how this particular use of technology may be incorporated into various controls.

We will begin by defining the following four terms:

- online chat
- clinical supervision
- peer supervision
- field supervision

Wikipedia states that:

Online chat may refer to any kind of communication over the Internet that offers a real-time transmission of text messages from sender to receiver. Chat messages are generally short in order to enable other participants to respond quickly. Thereby, a feeling similar to a spoken conversation is created, which distinguishes chatting from other text-based online communication forms such as Internet forums and email.

Online chat may address point-to-point communications as well as multicast communications from one sender to many receivers and voice and video chat, or may be a feature of a web conferencing service. (Wikipedia, 2015)

This is a process whereby users of the Internet engage in real-time or synchronous conversations using their computers. Online chat consists of these users exchanging text messages. In order to engage in online chat, a chat client must log-in to a chat channel and contact a chat server. There are a large number of chat channels, ranging from those that support general conversations to those that are devoted to a specific topic. Other terms include Internet Relay Chat (IRC), instant messaging and private chat (Ince, 2001).

Clinical supervision is,

an intervention provided by a more senior member of a profession to a more junior member or members of that same profession. This relationship is evaluative and hierarchical, extends over time and has the simultaneous purposes of enhancing the professional functioning of the more junior person(s), monitoring the quality of

242

professional services offered to the clients, she, he, or they see . . . and serving as a gatekeeper for those who are to enter the particular profession. (Bernard & Goodyear, 2009, p. 7)

Peer supervision, also referred to as peer consultation, has been proposed as a potentially effective approach to increasing the frequency and/or quality of supervision available to a counselor (Benshoff, 1989; Remley et al., 1987). Peer supervision may also be defined as a process that allows counselors to assist one another in becoming more effective and skillful helpers by using their relationships and professional skills with each other. Counselors can develop their own peer consultation relationships to fill a "supervision void" or to augment traditional supervision by providing a means of getting additional feedback from their peers (Wagner & Smith, 1979).

Field supervision is also referred to as field education and the term is often associated with the social work profession. In addition, the term is used in counselor and social work education to refer to the student's placement in the field and resulting supervision of field work. Field supervision may also be referred to as "direction." For instance, direction can be defined as

the ongoing administrative overseeing by an employer or superior of a Professional Counselor's work by a director. The director shall be responsible for assuring the quality of the services rendered by that practitioner and shall ensure that qualified supervision or intervention occurs in situations which require expertise beyond that of the practitioner. (Georgia Composite Board of Professional Counselors, Social Workers and Marriage and Family Therapists, 2003, p. 8)

The field supervisor may be external or internal from the organization. Depending on the geographic region, internal and external supervisors, whether clinical or field, supervisors may be assigned different roles and expectations (Franséhn, 2007).

Regardless of the particular role a supervisor plays, supervision generally involves consultation about specific client information including background and presenting issues. The supervisor may be an employer, a peer, a professor, or a clinician. The role of supervision may be to satisfy the coursework necessary to complete a degree, or to satisfy requirements toward certification or licensure. Supervision may also be considered a professional growth endeavor that is neither required nor expected.

THE CASE FOR SUPERVISION VIA CHAT

The age of the portable laptop and response on demand has arrived (Reisch & Jarman-Rohde, 2000). It is easier for some to sit in front of their computers and schedule appointments, confirm dates, times, locations and/or discuss cases with peers. Online forums, chat rooms and instant messaging give professionals other options for communication that deviate from the traditional face-to-face and telephone encounters. As with any supervisory relationship, this connectivity via chat warrants several considerations to include informed consent, confidentiality, crisis situations, jurisdiction and technical competence (Fenichel, 2000; Paiios et al., 2002; Watson, 2003).

Supervisees and supervisors should be aware of the limitations of online consultation and supervision. Confidentiality is paramount. Depending on the particular setting, actual names and identifying information may be blinded to further protect the client's record. For instance, in the case of peer supervision, it is advised that identifying information such as name, demographics, or details of the case be avoided so that the actual client identity is not revealed to peer professionals. This would apply to educational settings or group supervision in which all of the participants are not part of the same organization. If the supervision occurs within a work setting, client information may be revealed, assuming the employer is the owner of the record and employees take on various roles within the organization as is the case in the illustration that follows. To further ensure that all communication is as confidential as possible, chat and IM dialogue online should always be encrypted (Anthony & Goss, 2009). Encryption is no longer cost prohibitive and can be achieved with relative ease. Formal platforms are available, offering organizational branding, email and file storage options. Supervisors who are interested in incorporating encrypted chat should be sure to use a service, program or platform that is encrypted. Supervisors should take extra steps towards protecting the process and effectiveness of their supervision. Supervisors have a professional, ethical and legal responsibility to monitor the quality of care that is being delivered to their supervisees' clients (Vaccaro & Lambie, 2007).

At many times, professionals feel isolated, struggling with written documentation, direction of treatment, appropriate referral(s), or an ethical or professional dilemma. It is now accepted, respected and expected to seek professional connectedness through the Internet. It is easy to instantly chat with a peer, a supervisor, a supervisee, or a group to assist with a case that may benefit from a variety of insight and objective input. Supervision is critical in the development of a counselor (Gladding, 2002).

CASE SCENARIO

The authors of the first edition of this chapter, DeeAnna Nagel and Sarah Riley, worked together for a period of several years in an agency setting that offered in-home counseling and evaluation services to clients in several rural and remote parts of Georgia, USA. The agency served 20 counties in the southernmost and northern-most areas of the state. While the agency had offices in both northern and southern locations, the office was still a two-hour drive for some employees. It became crucial to create an online environment that allowed communication between manager and supervisors and their employees and supervisees. Field work was conducted by a constellation of people comprising a team of parent educators, mental health professionals and supervisors. Mental health professionals held varying degrees and were either fully licensed or working toward licensure. While it is not considered ideal for a clinical supervisor to fill the role of both supervisor and employer, because of the rural and remote nature of the work, the clinical supervisor was sometimes also the employer. Other supervisors also offered clinical input and direction to workers in the field. The owners of the agency were fully licensed and qualified clinical supervisors and often filled the role of clinical supervisor for employees who would not have otherwise had access to clinical supervision under the rules of the state licensing board.

While the clinical supervisor offered therapeutic and clinical input online via chat in real-time, that time did not meet the requirement for supervision hours needed for licensure. Clinical supervision was, at that time, interpreted as occurring face-to-face. To further meet the requirements of the state and despite the distance and inconvenience, face-to-face clinical supervision was also offered.

In between face-to-face opportunities for further training, professional development and clinical supervision, the day-to-day "operations" were conducted online. The agency utilized a platform that offered email, chat and file storage options. Email worked much like standard email programs such as Eudora or Outlook, but the platform was web-based. All emails sent within the agency were encrypted.

All emails sent outside the agency were not encrypted. At any given time, once logged in, an employee could see everyone online at the same time. Anyone online and showing "available" could engage in chat with one or more employees. Since the owners and supervisors of the agency were hundreds of miles apart and employees numbered up to 70 at the agency's peak, the ability to reach out online became the essence of clinical operations.

Formal times were sometimes set aside for chats online but, often, "chatting" became the preferred method for communicating about cases when the employee or clinician had a specific question or needed direction. Because many of the employees used cell phones and often did not have a land-line phone at home, case consultation was not conducted on the phone. Employees were instructed to use cell phones to communicate with or on behalf of a client only in cases of scheduling or cancelling appointments or in times of client crisis. When the employee returned home or to the office, he or she would often log in, check email and chat any necessary information or questions resulting from the day's work.

In addition, the chat platform served as a way for employees to gain a strong sense of community within the agency. Often, employees could rely on each other for support as well as answers to administrative questions. Employees in the field had instant access to administrative employees who worked from the office. Clinicians and paraprofessionals worked from home, writing progress notes, reports and other clinical documentation. While using, say, Microsoft Word, an employee could move quickly to the online chat platform and ask a question of his or her supervisor if necessary. The employee was able to avoid a break in concentration avoiding the shift to aural input that a phone call would require. Since chat is in real-time, the employee did not have to wait for an email response.

Sometimes a clinician and paraprofessional were both assigned to a case. Chat made it convenient for both to discuss the case and when necessary a supervisor could open a chat with two or more people creating a group discussion. This real-time collaboration allowed for open discussion about possible interventions. Employees were often more responsive online than on the phone or face-to-face because the intervention was immediate and offered a level of anonymity which was not afforded in-person or on the phone. Text-based communication would allow the disinhibition effect to work in favor of the case consultation, leveling out authority of positions within the agency, and allowing all parties to participate with equal weight (Suler, 2004). Employees, whether administrative, paraprofessional or clinical, also benefited from having ready access to supervisors. Despite the lack of face-to-face interaction in this rural agency setting, employees could often seek immediate consultation.

While chat was but one way in which communication was delivered, it allowed for everyone to be able to maintain a constant presence within the agency and offered a connection to clinicians and employees in the field. Supervisors, clinicians and paraprofessionals often reported that communicating through chat was as effective as communicating in-person or on the phone. While this is anecdotal information, it does speak to the power of the written word offered in real-time. Supervision offered through chat, whether as stand-alone or as adjunct to in-person and other technological delivery methods, is an effective way to process clinical supervision issues (Nagel et al., 2009).

CONCLUSION

It should be noted that scheduled online clinical supervision should be revered in the same way as a scheduled online therapy session. Whether the supervision is within a work setting, or an external and contracted clinical supervision relationship, parameters should be set that suit the particular purpose of the interaction. Clinical supervision often relies on the supervisee's disclosure about his or her interpersonal and psychodynamic experience within the client/therapist relationship. As is the case with an online chat therapy session, when working online in a scheduled clinical supervision session, attention should be paid to the virtual consultation room, allowing complete focus on the supervisory process and to the supervisee (Nagel, 2009). If the supervisory interaction is impromptu, attention should be paid to the pace of the online conversation and the effect on the supervisee. Particular awareness of emotional content is necessary so that the supervisee feels heard and validated. The supervisor, while not in a scheduled session, should still remain cognizant of the client/therapist relationship even within the context of answering what appear to be administrative or logistical inquiries about the case and intervene as necessary if it appears that the supervisee requires processing of emotional content.

Controversy exists about whether or not online supervision is valid and some professionals state that ideally supervision should be face-to-face with technology only being utilized in an adjunct role (Borders & Brown, 2005). The agency scenario delineated here, because of remote and rural geographical logistics, utilized online supervision as a primary process while face-to-face supervision and interaction remained secondary. The availability of online supervision through chat and instant message allowed the organization to remain vibrant, offering quality services in areas of the state that were not otherwise easily accessible. Many of the reasons for accessing online therapy are valid for accessing online supervision. Another scenario offered for validating the use of distance supervision via technology is offered by Wood et al. (2005). Distance, travel and mountainous roads were but a few of the difficulties supervisors

encountered in providing weekly supervision. The authors believe that more and more rural areas of the world will embrace online supervision. Online supervision should not be viewed as inferior. On the contrary, distance supervision via technology will allow access to skilled experts and clinical supervisors across the globe.

This chapter has summarized how online supervision can work within an agency setting that offers community-based in-home services. These concepts can be applied to other settings including organizations that offer traditional face-to-face therapy and online therapy services. E-clinics offering online therapy exclusively can easily add chat supervision or consultation and other groups of peers can choose to work together online one-to-one and in group chats. Chat supervision can be used as a stand-alone method of delivery or it can be combined with other technology and face-to-face supervision, enriching any supervisory experience.

REFERENCES

Anthony, K., & Goss, S. (2009). *Guidelines for online counselling and psychotherapy including guidelines for online supervision* (3rd ed.). Lutterworth: BACP.

Benshoff, J. M. (1989). *The effects of the structured peer supervision model on overall supervised counseling effectiveness ratings of advanced counselors in training.* PhD Thesis. The American University.

Bernard, J. M., & Goodyear, R. K. (2009). *Fundamentals of clinical supervision.* London: Pearson.

Borders, L. D., & Brown, L. L. (2005). *The new handbook of counseling and supervision.* Mahwah, NJ: Lawrence Erlbaum.

Fenichel, M. (2000). *Online psychotherapy: Technical difficulties, formulations and processes* [online]. [Accessed December 19, 2009]. Available from: http://www.fenichel .com/

technical.shtml.

Franséhn, M. (2007). The importance of supervision in social work – the example of Sweden. *SP Sociálni Práce, 4*, 72–78.

Georgia Composite Board of Professional Counselors, Social Workers and Marriage and Family Therapists. (2003). *Rules of Georgia Composite Board of Professional Counselors, Social Workers and Marriage and Family Therapists* [online]. [Accessed December 19, 2009]. Available from: http://sos.georgia.gov/acrobat/PLB/Rules/chapt135.pdf.

Gladding, S. T. (2002). *Counseling: A comprehensive profession* (4th ed.). Upper Saddle River, NJ: Prentice Hall.

Ince, D. (2001). Online chat. Encyclopedia. com [online]. [Accessed December 19, 2009]. Available from: http://www.encyclopedia.com/doc/1O12-onlinechat.html.

Nagel, D. M. (2009). Filling the void in the virtual consultation room. *Voices: The art and science of psychotherapy, 44*(1), 98–101.

Nagel, D. M., Goss, S., & Anthony, K. (2009). The use of technology in supervision. In N. Pelling, J. Barletta, & P. Armstrong (Eds.), *The practice of supervision.* Bowen Hills, Qld: Australian Academic Press.

Paños, P. T., Paños, A., Cox, S. E., Roby, J. L., & Matheson, K. W. (2002). Ethical issues concerning the use of videoconferencing to supervise international social work field practicum students. *Journal of Social Work Education, 38*(3), 421–437.

Reisch, M., & Jarman-Rohde, L. (2000). The future of social work in the United States: Implications for field education. *Journal of Social Work Education, 36*(2), 201–214.

Remley, T. P., Benshoff, J. M., & Mowbray, C. (1987). A proposed model for peer supervision. *Counselor Education and Supervision, 27*(1), 53–60.

Suler, J. R. (2004). The online disinhibition effect. *Cyberpsychology and Behavior, 7*(3), 321–326.

Vaccaro, N., & Lambie, G. W. (2007). Computer based counselors in training supervision: Ethical and practical implications for counselor educators and supervisors. *Counselor Education and Supervision, 47*(1), 46–57.

Wagner, C. A., & Smith, J. P. (1979). Peer supervision: Toward more effective training. *Counselor Education and Supervision, 18*(4), 288–293.

Watson, J. (2003). Implementing computer technology into the delivery of counseling supervision. *Journal of Technology in Counseling, 3*(1) [online]. [Accessed December 19, 2009]. Available from: http://jtc.col-state.edu./Vol3-1/Watson/Watson.htm.

Wikipedia. (2009). *Online chat* [online]. [Accessed December 21, 2009]. Available from: http://en.wikipedia.org/wiki/Onlinechat.

Wood, J. A. V., Miller, T. W., & Hargrove, D. S. (2005). Clinical supervision in rural settings: A telehealth model. *Professional Psychology: Research and Practice, 36*(2), 173–179.

Chapter 25

USING FORUMS TO ENRICH COUNSELOR TRAINING AND SUPERVISION

Linnea Carlson-Sabelli

INTRODUCTION AND DEFINITIONS

This chapter is designed to introduce you to technical developments that are being used to enhance clinical supervision for Psychiatric Mental Health-Nurse Practitioner students and professionals and to discuss the impact that asynchronous forums have had on the way we are able to supervise psychotherapy interventions.

Our goals are to provide definitions, applications, ethical considerations, illustrations of supervision techniques and speculation on the future of online text-based clinical supervision based on our extensive experience supervising graduate level Psychiatric Mental Health-Nurse Practitioner students at a major medical center university located in the Midwest, United States.

Through "Project Aha!" we designed and implemented the Aha Center for Clinical Reasoning, a virtual networking community for advanced practice psychiatric nurses. Project Aha! was initially designed to overcome practical difficulties of delivering online clinical practicum supervision for Psychiatric Mental Health-Nurse Practitioners (PMH-NP) for whom on-campus participation would never be possible. Through this program we develop innovative asynchronous tools useful in delivering online psychotherapy supervision to PMH-NP students at distant clinical practicum sites.

Our clinical supervision program is competency based. It is asynchronous and is conducted within a fully accredited university where registered nurses are earning an advanced practice degree or advanced practice nurses are earning a postmasters certificate in psychiatric mental health nursing. Graduates of our program are eligible to take the American Nurses Credentialing Center (ANCC) national certification exams for PMHNPs. The techniques we will describe here are text-based and are suitable for long-distance supervision that is conducted in online forums used by the faculty and onsite supervisors and student *supervisees*.

Because the techniques are asynchronous forums, they support 24-7 student access, allowing students to work at the times that are most convenient. Responses can be given more thought encouraging reflection. Group supervision is possible as students can post and discuss their assignments with each other. Copies of selected assignments and assessments can be compiled into a student-controlled portfolio. Students can share clinical stories with one another, ask and answer questions, and role play "what if" scenarios with faculty supervisors. These are some of the ways that we have improved the way we are able to supervise psychotherapy interventions. We can replace tape-recorded therapy sessions with process recordings where students not only recreate the dialogue, but also type in what they might have been thinking and feeling and saying or showing. The rationale for interventions can be interspersed within dialogue snippets. Assignments can be selectively released to provide additional competency practice, student by student, based on the quality of previous work. In these ways, text-based online forums provide methods for overcoming challenging aspects of a providing a competency-based curriculum for advanced practice nursing students of diverse backgrounds and experience, living in underserved and rural locations.

Within our program, we have two types of clinical supervisors – faculty clinical supervisors who are based at the university and onsite clinical preceptors who are based at the clinical site. All faculty clinical supervisors are doctorally prepared and are certified nurse practitioners or clinical specialists. Faculty supervisors have extensive practice experience and are currently in practice roles as well as educator roles. The third year of our part-time program is a clinical practicum. During the clinical year, each student does a 500-hour clinical practicum and residency with an additional 120 hour clinical supervision component. For this experience, each student is assigned to a clinical site near where they live. The site must have an onsite "clinical preceptor," whose role is to facilitate students' learning as mentor, teacher, and supervisor. The onsite clinical preceptor must be credentialed as a certified advanced practice nurse in psychiatric mental health, or be a board certified psychiatrist.

CLINICAL SUPERVISION

The onsite preceptor provides mentoring and direct supervision in a number of competencies, including psychotherapy and medication management and may bring in other mental health professionals to model and mentor the student in specific modalities such as group psychotherapy. The preceptor compiles evaluations across multiple experiences when needed and rates the student's progress on a Competency Development System (CDS), described further below. During the first week of the quarter, the preceptor and student discuss competencies and corresponding clinical experiences needed to practice them. They also identify competencies that will be difficult to complete within the setting. Later discussion is about congruency of student and preceptor ratings to guide the student toward the development of an action plan, to maximize strengths and overcome weaknesses.

Onsite preceptors evaluate development in psychotherapy competencies through direct supervision, viewing the student's clinical notes on individual patient interactions which are recorded onsite and in specialist "Typhon" software (described in more detail below) and through reviewing student "moment map" assignments (also described further below) and comments from faculty staff. They post numerical scores in the CDS software as the student progresses through the course. Faculty supervisors evaluate students based on the Typhon clinical note entries, assignments, and an analogue rating scale based on student postings, clinical stories, and participation in online clinical supervision. "Learn More" activities are developed by faculty supervisors for students who are unable to meet a particular competency at their site. One type of activity is the "Branching Story Simulation." We will now introduce you to the application of these technical developments in providing online clinical supervision.

APPLICATION OF THE TECHNOLOGY IN PROVIDING ONLINE CLINICAL SUPERVISION

Discussion Forums/Groups

The majority of supervisory interaction among students takes place in discussion forums. To keep discussions organized and focused, we divide them into a variety of topics such as announcements, ice breaker, questions and answers, folders for each assignment with due date, private discussion topics for each student, private discussion topic for faculty and a topic for socializing. The discussions are used to post up-to-the-minute faculty announcements, ask and answer questions about the course, share and discuss assignments among classmates and faculty, keep social conversations in one place and provide private feedback. We always include an introductory message in each discussion topic in which we detail what the discussion topic is about, directions for posting, and sometimes the rationale for the topic. We socialize the students into posting within this scheme by moving postings to the correct place if students post in the wrong topic. We try to engender lively discussions by breaking students into groups of 12 or less to prevent overwhelming a discussion. We give feedback more frequently at the beginning of the course, model what we want the students to do and give specific praise.

We organize the course by weekly assignments. The assignments are then posted by students in a discussion topic and shared with each other. Students are taught to become the discussion facilitators of their own assignments to engender the kind of feedback that is most useful to them from their classmates. In addition to the assignment discussions we use clinical stories as a springboard for weekly here and now discussions.

Clinical Stories

We ask students to share clinical stories with each other throughout the clinical year. We prescribe the type of story that is to be told on a weekly basis. We modify the type of story we request based on the learning that we are supporting in the management courses that accompany clinical practice.

We start out with stories about forming therapeutic relationships and move into stories of "Wow!" experiences. These stories include moments where students learned something new. We also ask students to relay stories of therapy that illustrate how they use various modalities such as cognitive, narrative, motivational interviewing, dialectic behavioral and process therapy. Next we move into evidenced based stories – where students present clinical questions that arose in the course of clinical practice and the process by which the student explored the answer. Classmates invite each other to address their clinical questions with evidenced-based responses. The guidelines for clinical stories are that they are to be in story format. Students are encouraged to respond with another story, whenever possible, rather than give advice. Stories are posted in asynchronous discussion topics and students are required to respond to at least one or two other stories each week. Faculty staff moderate the story discussions as needed. While we use asynchronous discussions for clinical stories, this activity could also take place in a blog.

Here is a short discussion thread illustrating faculty moderated clinical story discussion.

Title: Swap Clinical Stories – "Being with" a Patient

Initial faculty posting with discussion topic instructions:

This is a weekly activity

As you are in your clinical sites, you have many opportunities for "being with" patients.

Each week we want you to tell us a story of a meaningful interaction that you have with a patient. In the story, detail the aspects of the interaction.

The main purpose for these stories is to continuously focus your awareness on "being with" a patient and exploring ways of being an active participant in helping the patient create meaning in their continuing life story. This involves cultivating reflection, mindfulness, and patience.

It can be helpful to include in your stories some of the thoughts you were thinking about, but not saying.

The expectation is that you will read everyone else's stories and respond to at least one other story per week.

Rationale for the Assignment

As you progress through the supervision, it is expected that the quality of your contributed stories will increase enabling you to build a repository of narratives that can be adapted for use as formative peer teaching-learning activities.

In this way, you are socialized into the process of clinical reasoning and into the role of a facilitator of reflection. This provides you excellent experience in guiding reflective practice in others which will be useful to you as you later serve to facilitate the clinical growth of other nurses, and is a crucial role of the expert psychiatric nurse.

We will organize feedback toward helping you develop increasing skills in three areas:

Reflection on Practice
Clinical Reasoning
Engagement in Supervision.

Posting 1 Title: "Being with" the Family Member of a Patient

Mary Student's Initial Story Posting.

I have repeated this conversation with just minor variations four times in the past three weeks. This is about "being with" the family member of a patient.

LC is a 75-year-old married male admitted to our unit from the nursing home where he has been a resident for one month. He was placed in the nursing home after he became unable to ambulate and was incontinent. He has a history of strokes and had been cared for at home by his wife until his admission to the nursing home. The patient's wife requested the patient be admitted to this unit for a medication evaluation and to assess his behavior. Problematic behaviors include restlessness at night with poor sleep, a.m. somnolence with poor intake at breakfast and inability to feed himself, pushing staff away that attempt to feed him, resistance to taking medication, combativeness with staff with personal care and raising his fist at his wife. The patient had orders for Valium severe agitation, Tylenol and Lunesta. Psychiatric medications in place included: Seroquel, Zoloft, and Xanax. The patient's wife believes he has been on Zoloft for about one year. All other psychotropic medications were initiated within the past month.

The patient's admission MMSE (Mini-Mental State Examination) was 9/30. His MSE showed him to be restless, alert, but oriented only to self, with poor concentration, poor recall, and poor short-term and long-term memory.

I visited with the patient's brother while the patient's wife was talking with the social worker. He lives across the street from the patient and is eager for his brother to return home. Later I visited with the patient's wife and asked her about her plans for her husband after he is discharged from the hospital. She said, "I know I can't take care of him at home anymore, but his kids and brother think I should." I felt empathy for this elderly woman who has been the sole care-provider for this man for many years as his health has declined. She has endured lack of sleep, back breaking work of caring for a man twice her size, and emotional strain. I hypothesized that she might feel guilty for being unable to continue homecare and would benefit from support in her decision. I explained to her that we often see family members who are not involved in the day-to-day care of patients insist that they can be cared for at home. I assured her that she had made the right decision. Based on her husband's cognitive functioning and physical limitations, he was no longer a candidate for homecare. I also supported her decision for evaluation of her husband's medication in this setting as I believed we could address his sleep, appetite, daytime somnolence, restlessness, and agitation with medication adjustments. She was not surprised to hear that her husband's cognitive function would not improve dramatically and that his physical improvement would most likely be modest in that he should improve in his ability to feed himself and follow directions.

Most importantly, I assured the patient's wife that we supported her decision and would be happy to talk with any family members who needed information as to why nursing home placement was the best decision for her and the patient's well-being. I told her that there was no need for guilt in this situation and that she had done an admirable job in caring for her husband and continuing to oversee his care.

This woman seemed relieved after we visited. I believed she benefited from professional support in her decision making and a sense of hope that her husband would make some improvement.

Mary

Posting 2 Title: "I Vowed I'd Never Do This [Nursing Home Placement] to Any of My Loved Ones"

Peter Classmate's Response
Mary,

I like what you're doing! We need to see that often our treatments are not "just for the patient" but include the entire family – therefore you're treating the entire family in this case – this will impact the outcomes for the patient.

Family dynamics are very interesting. There's so much guilt about nursing home placement. I can't tell you the number of times I've had family members tell me, "I vowed I'd never do this [nursing home placement] to any of my loved ones." "Family Rules" about caring for and not abandoning are all so very real and part of the discourse – but this is where psychoeducation comes in. Often I find myself having to "reframe" their beliefs and have them look at the "big picture" asking, "what's this doing to you [having the loved one at home]?" Directly addressing the "guilt" is important as they won't talk about it often unless it is directly addressed. Then "reframing" the situation to a realistic context saying, "you're needing help . . . the nursing home is one way that you can help him . . . they can be a support . . . you're not giving up so much as you are finding new ways of helping him and taking care of yourself as well . . . you're not giving up on caring . . ."

Regardless, this is a "gut wrenching" decision on the part of families who are entrenched with beliefs/guilt about the thought of abandoning someone – like the nursing home is a "death sentence" – it doesn't have to be – it can be what is needed.

The vast majority of families are relieved after the move. They have to "work through" the emotional issues – but ultimately they begin to see the wisdom with their decision and find they are able to be "better involved" (if they choose to be). Nevertheless, it's rough.

Peter Classmate

Posting 3 Title: Amazing Things Have Happened

Mary Student's Response to Peter Classmate:
Thanks for your feedback, Peter. . . . And now, for the rest of the story!

Amazing things have happened since we took this patient off all the psychotropic medicines and got his sleep stabilized! It took a combination of Trazodone 100 mg and Ambien 10 mg, given together, to assist his sleep. Now that he is rested and eating well, he is gaining strength and began walking by himself today! When I expressed my surprise at seeing him walking independently, he said, "What's the big deal? I've been doing this all my life." Also, when his family visited him today and started playing the guitar, he really did a great job of singing! What a comeback for this man who was having so many problems on admission!

I celebrated with this patient's wife! I reminded her that this is the benefit of not having to be the constant caregiver. You can enjoy the visit, bring people in with you that your spouse enjoys, and then go home and get a good night's sleep!

Mary Student

Posting 4 Title: I'd Celebrate Too!

Theresa Classmate's Response to Mary's Second Posting:

Mary,

Wonderful story! I was wondering about some of the med combo's that you had described in the previous post. Elderly folks don't do so well with a lot of the medications and dosing that you had described – kind of made him a bit of a "zombie" – never-the-less I've seen weaning people off meds – especially those that exacerbate dementia (or delirium symptoms) who make remarkable recoveries. I'd celebrate too!

Theresa Classmate

Posting 5 Title: A Long-range Perspective

Clara Faculty's Response:

This is indeed one of the happier endings of this story set.

It may become difficult for this woman if her husband keeps improving. She may be back into the dilemma of "Can I care for him?" But as you state, this story is an excellent example of "being with" a patient.

I'm curious to know what the literature has to say about best practice and withdrawing patient's from psychotropic drugs to reassess baseline symptoms and behaviors.

Cara Faculty

Posting 6 Title: Lewy Body Dementia? An Evidence-based Inquiry

Anita Classmate's response:

Mary and others,

I typed "Prescribing psychotroic drugs for the elderly" into a google search box and found two interesting articles. The first article is from 1994, but indicates several key learning points at that time: One of them is: "patients with Lewy body dementia are particular sensitive to neuroleptics" http://apt.rcpsych.org/cgi/reprint/1/1/23.pdf.

Do you know if the patient you were talking about had Lewy body dementia?

Anita Classmate

Posting 7 Title: Good Question

Mary Student's Reply:

Anita, you have a good point. I will have to check on this.

Mary

Posting 8 Title: Inappropriate Prescribing of Psychotropic Medication in the Elderly

Sally Classmate's response:

I found another interesting research article (1999) which suggests that inappropriate prescribing of psychotropic medication in the elderly has become a public health concern. The study polls physicians about their practices and attitudes in prescribing psychiatric medications (http://www.cmaj.ca/cgi/content/full/161/2/143).

An interesting finding of this study was that physicians often had patients who had been taking psychiatric medications for years, medications they didn't initially prescribe. They overwhelmingly decided to keep prescribing these, because they reported having difficulty dealing with the suffering they witness without prescribing medication. They were also afraid the patient's would change doctors.

Sally Classmate

Posting 9 Title: Wrap-up

Clara Faculty's second response:
What are the some of the learning points to consider as we wrap up this particular story discussion thread? "Being with" a patient means "being with the family," as well.

Psychotropic medication can cause side effects that impair cognition and behavior.

As patients grow older and their metabolism changes, their psychotropic medications and dosages may need to change, too.

Things change and it may be that this woman will want to bring her husband home and it is ok to support this decision as well.

There is a rich literature available to guide clinical practice, which we encourage you to share with us as the clinical year progresses.

Clara Faculty

Posting 10 Title: Thanks for the Lead

Mary Student's final posting:
Anita and classmates. I mentioned Lewy Body Dementia to my preceptor. She thinks it is a distinct possibility. We will follow-up on this. Perhaps it was removing the Seroquel that was most effective? Wow! I really learned a lot from this experience.

This example from a discussion forum is a single thread of a student's posting of a weekly clinical story and corresponding classmate and faculty comments. Since each student posts and facilitates their own thread,

the discussion topic is rich, interactive and allows issues that are relevant to the students to emerge. Students learn what their classmates are doing, serve as mentors for each other and have experience facilitating discussions. A major goal of our online clinical supervision program is to guide our students to learn how to think, to problem solve and to base their responses on evidence beyond personal experience. Faculty monitor the discussions and attempt to focus or deepen a discussion, while allowing most of the material to emerge from the students.

While the purpose of this chapter is primarily focused on discussion forums, the Aha! platform offers additional applications to enhance the supervision process.

Competency Development System (CDS) Evaluation

The Competency Development System described here is a work in progress. It is designed to personalize competency development to fit each particular student's individual needs. It serves both as an evaluation system for students to self-evaluate and for preceptors to evaluate students. It is administered online and can be accessed by enrolled students, assigned preceptors and university faculty anywhere there is Internet access. The current version records and tracks an initial student self-assessment and from this data, prioritizes competencies according to importance for the role and the student's level of experience with the competency in the past. Students are required to discuss the self-assessment report with their preceptors at the beginning of each clinical quarter as a tool to facilitate planning of clinical experiences. The tool also provides a method for continuous self- and preceptor assessment. It contains a feature where students who are not progressing on specific competencies are prompted to create action plans for demonstrating the competency. It also contains "Learn More" simulations, such as branching stories, that can be used to fill gaps. It is only available for students enrolled in our university. Plans are being made to make it more widely available for use in other competency-based nursing programs.

The CDS is divided into domains. Delineated domains are based on nationally recognized core and specialty guidelines – National Organization of Nurse Practitioner Faculties (NONPF). Each domain is divided into related competencies and cues integrated from the professional psychiatric nursing associations that guide nursing practice and education in the USA. In addition, competencies within domains are weighted according to the 2003 ANCC Role Delineation Report.

Psychotherapy Competencies Are Integrated Within All of the Domains

Students can easily access the CDS through any learning management system by an imbedded link to the Internet. Access to individual rating entry and reports is password protected. Clinical preceptors can access only the information for their assigned student.

When a self- or preceptor rating is requested, the rater can access a series of drop down cues for each competency to be rated.

Drop Down Cues Are Available for Every Competency

Self and preceptor ratings are requested on a five-point scale, which assess the degree to which the student is meeting a competency. These ratings are:

1=Does not meet objective,
2=Routinely needs continual guidance to meet objective,
3=Demonstrates progress toward meeting the objective,
4=Meets specific objective frequently,

5=Meets specific objective consistently
NA=Not applicable. Student action was not evaluated.

Faculty staff can print reports of all student and preceptor ratings for the permanent student file. Students and preceptors can print all reports to which they contribute.

The CDS tracks skill development toward meeting clinical competencies, identifies substandard areas of performance, highlights gaps in clinical site experiences, and promotes reflection by students on the core competencies, weekly.

The responsibility is with the student to negotiate competency experiences through the initial discussion with the preceptor and student generated-action plans. The student-generated action report is another feature of the CDS.

Student-Generated Action Plan

The CDS also provides "Learn More" activities through which the student can gain competency experience.

If a student receives a rating less than three from the preceptor, or receives an NA rating indicating that competency practice was not available at the clinical site, a call for an action plan is generated by the software. The student is notified, fills out the form indicating how they have met or will meet the competency and submits the plan. The preceptor is prompted to review and sign off on the plan. One way a student can meet a competency is by completing a "Learn More" activity.

"Learn More" Activities

Based on Shulman's (2002) table of learning, integrated with Sabelli's bios theory (Sabelli, 1989; Sabelli & CarlsonSabelli, 2006), the conceptual model for development of online clinical supervision components focuses on three sets of interacting opposites.

We strive to move students from engagement in our learning program to commitment to an advanced practice role. We help students translate knowledge into clinical judgment. Finally we emphasize a continuous cycling between reflection and action. Reflection on practice is necessary for skills to develop. The CDS started off as a reflection tool but has expanded to incorporate judgment building "Learn More" activities as well.

Branching Story Simulations

Branching story simulations provide a student with an imaginary role that allows them to try out new behaviors in a "mistakes allowed atmosphere" where consequences are experienced, but no one gets hurt. In this way we connect reflection on action with clinical reasoning, building judgment.

The branching story is an "as if" simulated clinical practice reasoning experience that requires the student to make judgments, take actions, experience consequences and report progress. Branching stories are asynchronous, text-based activities that allow students to practice and demonstrate core competencies that might otherwise not be accessible in their particular clinical area. They are ideal for helping students to grapple with common misconceptions related to psychotherapy and avoid some of the problems that are likely to encounter in actual practice. One of our branching stories lures students into making mistakes during a therapy session with a potentially suicidal patient. Those students who act on a misconception, experience consequences of the mistakes and are guided to find additional information to change their course of action. They are able to revisit the point where the mistake was made and try another path. A sample of a branching story can be found at the URL http://demo.knowledgeanywhere.com/Rush/by using the username: student and password: test.

Moment Maps

The moment map is another asynchronous, text-based tool that we have pioneered for psychotherapy supervision. The moment map is an advanced level process recording that the student prepares in PowerPoint. The task is to present various elements of a clinical therapy session in a formalized way using a template. The purpose of the moment map is to promote development of self as a therapeutic instrument; provide the student with a format with which to present, analyze and discuss a meaningful psychotherapeutic intervention; and to organize thinking in the context of the patient's life story. The moment map is similar to a process recording but with additional elements. It was designed to replace taped recordings of a session – which most of our clinical sites no longer allow. Before constructing the first moment map, students are provided with a PowerPoint template, the grading rubric and samples of mediocre, good and excellent examples of moment maps prepared by previous students. It is a required activity several times during the clinical year. The moment map is shared among all students in a clinical cohort for feedback and discussion. Discussion is monitored by the university supervisor. For the initial moment map, we assign a case study of a standardized patient scenario. Students read the case material and then create the moment map. For this assignment they create the dialogue for a therapy session, including the patient responses. This exercise illuminates similarities and differences in therapy knowledge and the skills of students as they enter their clinical year.

"Typhon" Student Tracking Software

Students provide a record of the clinical sessions of the patients they see in "Typhon," an outsourced nurse practitioner student tracking system. Typhon is used by many nurse practitioner students in the US. The software provides a method for each student to enter a clinical chart for each patient they see and to update the chart each time they see the patient for follow-up. We require students to write an intake record and then write an integrated psychotherapy/medication management clinical note for each patient visit. Students with a very large clinical load enter all patients, but only need to write seven follow-up notes each week. Clinical preceptors are given access to this data for the students they supervise. University faculty supervisors can compile custom reports by student or by student group. These reports allow faculty to review clinical notes and give feedback to the student within the learning management system. The feedback is provided privately in a discussion topic that can only be accessed by the faculty supervisor and the assigned student.

Clinical Evaluation Analog Scale

This scale is used by faculty supervisors to evaluate clinical reasoning skills, self-awareness skills and student participation in online clinical supervision. Data that is analyzed to support ratings are discussion forums, moment map reflections and branching story reflections.

Faculty supervisors rate students at the middle and end of each clinical quarter and include the scale and a short summary of clinical progress as part of the mid-term and final clinical evaluations.

Mid-term and Final Clinical Evaluations

The student clinical performance evaluations include the CDS report of competency development, a summary of reporting from the Typhon system, the clinical analog scale and a separate summary of clinical psychotherapy skills as reflected in the moment map and clinical story assignments.

ETHICAL CONSIDERATIONS

We provide both formal faculty supervision and supply avenues for peer-to-peer supervision. Formal supervision requires contractual agreements. We require two contractual agreements. The first contract is an agreement between the university and the clinical site. This contract outlines requirements of both the university and the clinical site related to student professional liability insurance, confidentiality issues, and site requirements. The second contractual agreement is the course syllabus. This lays out the responsibilities of the university course to the student and what the student has to do to pass the course.

Confidentiality of patient and student information is regulated, in this instance, by the Family Educational Rights and Privacy Act of 1974 (FERPA) and the Health Insurance Portability and Accountability Act (HIPAA). FERPA is federal legislation in the US that provides protection of a student's right to privacy by specifying rules about public disclosure of student academic records and guidelines for the handling, storage and release of student data. HIPAA is federal legislation that requires health care providers to protect the privacy of patient information and to ensure the security of patient/client health data. Faculty supervisors are required to take FERPA and HIPAA training on a yearly basis and to socialize students into understanding and following the guidelines.

Because of HIPAA and FERPA guidelines, all students are required to remove any information that might identify a specific patient before submitting clinical notes, stories or moment maps. Students may use pseudonyms as long as they also state in the document that they are not using real patient names. The CDS does not collect patient information. The Typhon clinical tracking software is in compliance with HIPAA and FERPA. Patients are identified only by a number. Students assign pseudonyms for their patients and refer to them in clinical notes by the pseudonym initials.

Additional ethical considerations beyond maintaining patient confidentiality when doing psychotherapy include adequate performance evaluation and the ability to work with alternative perspectives. We have presented our extensive performance competency-based evaluation system which addresses many roles of a psychotherapist beyond psychotherapy. We also encourage our students to explore and provide evidence to support alternative perspectives. A competency that students need to demonstrate is the ability to find, evaluate and present evidence to support treatment approaches. We believe that teaching students how to apply evidence to practice and how to evaluate the quality of their practice promotes lifelong learning as progress is made in the assessments and treatments available for promoting mental health of individuals and communities.

CONCLUSION – A LOOK TO THE FUTURE IMPACT OF THE INTERVENTION

We are continuing to create partnerships with online educational development companies to build additional "Learn More" activities as vehicles to translate knowledge into action related to mental health nursing competencies. As these are created, they will be added to the CDS.

Today's online learning management systems have improved vastly over those introduced in the 1990s. Many of these programs already have features where learning activities can be mapped to competencies and an e-portfolio system where items demonstrating competency development can be stored and displayed by students. Our plan is to create a CDS which gathers student and preceptor ratings, identifies gaps in clinical psychotherapy

education, provides simulations to fill these gaps, and links seamlessly with other learning management systems that map learning activities to competencies. Such a product could be useful for the clinical supervision of mental health professionals beyond nursing because the competencies and cues can be fully customized by the clinical supervision team.

We also have plans to expand psychotherapy education into the virtual world Second Life, which is being used more and more for educational purposes by universities and companies across the world. Second Life lends itself very well to role-playing with simulated patients. It is a synchronous online activity, so we will not go into much detail. We will briefly say that we see it as a venue where faculty supervisors can model group and individual psychotherapy for students, supervise student therapy practice in a safe setting with simulated patients, and provide student practice with principles for setting up groups and methods for evaluating the efficacy of psychotherapy.

REFERENCES

Sabelli, H. (1989). *Union of opposites: A comprehensive theory of natural and human processes.* Lawrencefille, VA: Brunswick.

Sabelli, H., & Carlson-Sabelli, L. (2006). Bios, a process approach to living system theory: In honor of James and Jessie Miller. *Systems Research and Behavioral Science, 23*(3), 323–336.

Shulman, L. S. (2002). Making differences. A table of learning. *Change, 34*(6), 37–44.

Note

The technology described here was developed in part by funds from the Division of Nursing (DN), Bureau of Health Professions (BHPr), Health Resources and Services Administration (HRSA), Department of Health and Human Services (DHHS) under Project Aha! grant number 1D09HP02987 Advanced Education Nursing Grants for $478,739. It is continuing under a second BHPr DHHS grant, Filling in Competency Gaps, number D09HP09354 for $585,220. The information here, is supplied by the author and should not be construed as the official position or policy of, nor should be endorsements be inferred by the Division of Nursing, BHPr, DHHS or the U.S. Government.

Chapter 26

TRADITIONAL USES OF TECHNOLOGY IN COUNSELING EDUCATION AND SUPERVISION

Ginger Clark

INTRODUCTION

Supervision is the most highly valued element of training required for mental health providers. Close monitoring of clinical work, over a defined period, is a mandatory requirement for licensure as a mental health provider in every state in the United States and is commonly required in other countries, including the U.K. Supervision, as defined by Bernard and Goodyear (2013), consists of a relatively long-term relationship, between an experienced and novice professional, where evaluation, teaching, mentoring and guidance take place. Supervisors are expected to oversee the quality of care received by their trainees' clients and are responsible for making sure only competent and unimpaired practitioners go on to professional practice.

History of the Supervision

Traditionally, supervision was conceptualized as the trainee describing for the supervisor the critical events that occurred during the counseling session. This approach emerged out of the psychoanalytic movement, where it was expected that supervisors would pick up on areas of countertransference or omission as a results of how the trainee described the events (Salvendy,

1984). Numerous studies on the supervision process have challenged that approach as too subjective and ineffective (Goin & Kline, 1976; Muslin, Burnstein, Gredo, & Sadow, 1967; Stein, Karasu, Charles, & Buckley, 1975) and have served to stimulate the development of different approaches to supervision that provide more accurate data to the supervisor.

TYPES OF SUPERVISION

There has been very little research comparing the effectiveness of different types of supervision modalities on developing counselor competencies. Most articles that investigate the approaches to supervision focus more on describing the modalities used and the trainees' level of comfort with those methods. Almost no data is available on the differential effect of various supervision modalities on improved therapeutic outcomes (Anderson, Rigazio-DiGilio, & Kunkler, 1995), and the studies that do exist vary in the rigor of methodology used (Ellis, Ladany, Krengel, & Schult, 1996). However, many studies do find that therapist performance improved with training and supervision

(Beidas & Kendall, 2010).

There are, generally, two types of supervision that are used in counselor training programs: delayed or live supervision. Delayed supervision takes place after the counseling session has ended. The trainee is expected to either talk about the case or review an audio or video recording of the counseling session, and feedback will be given to the trainee by the supervisor and other trainees in the supervision group. Live supervision takes place during the counseling session. Observation of the session is usually done through a one-way mirror or observation room, where some form of communication between the supervisor and trainee is possible using a particular type of technology (e.g., phone, bug-in-the-ear, computer communication).

Studies assessing the types of supervision used in counselor education programs found that most reported some use of delayed supervision formats, such as: case review, audio recordings and video recordings, in addition to some live supervision approaches (Bubenzer, West, & Gold, 1991; Lee, Nichols, Nichols, & Odom, 2004; Saltzburg, S., Greene, G., & Drew, H., 2010).

Delayed Supervision
Case Review

Definition. Case review requires the trainee to bring in pertinent information about their client to their supervision meeting, where they will present this information to their supervisor and fellow trainees. Typically, a standard format of presentation about the client is provided by the supervisor for the trainee to follow, such as: (1) Demographic information, (2) Description of the problem, (3) Psycho-social history, (4) Diagnosis, (5) Theoretical conceptualization, (6) therapeutic relationship, (7) Treatment plan, (8) Progress made, (9) Areas of concern and (10) Questions.

Effects on Trainee, Client and Therapy.

Case review gives the trainee the opportunity to think more systemically about the client and how their issues developed. This encourages a more global assessment strategy on the part of the trainee. Biggs (1988) describes three essential elements to case presentation designed to increase conceptualization skills. The first is using clinical observations to support conclusions about the client, such as critical incidents in session, diagnosis and formulation of the problem. The second is incorporating the trainee's view of the therapeutic relationship and its effects on treatment. The third is laying out the treatment plan and tying it back to the client's problem, the theory being used to conceptualize the problem, the strategies being used and possible obstacles. It is assumed that the process of compiling this information will engage the trainee in the assessment, conceptualization, problem solving, and anticipatory planning that are crucial in mental health treatment.

The drawback to this approach is that it lacks the objective observation by the supervisor of how a case is progressing, and relies solely on the perspective of a novice therapist (Anderson, Rigazio-DiGilio, & Kunkler, 1995). Because of their inexperience, trainees lack the knowledge needed to know what the critical incidents in therapy are and how they as counselors may affect their client. Novice trainees do not yet have the conceptual framework to organize information from the session into the meaningful categories expected in a case review. And they often do not yet have the multicultural competency training to identify relevant cultural elements that impact the client's experience that should be discussed in supervision (Falender, Shafranske, & Falicov, 2014).

Example Scenario: A new trainee was asked to review one of her cases in supervision. The client was a 21-year-old Latino female suffering from depressive symptoms. The trainee had chosen Cognitive Therapy as her theoretical framework. She began by explaining the clients' cognitive distortions (e.g., dichotomous thinking, mind reading) and proceeded to list the client's automatic thoughts (e.g., "I am no good because I'm not helping my family while I'm in college" and "My mother resents the time and money I'm spending on school"), reflecting a basic level of understanding of the tenets of the theory and its application. When asked how she thought the clients' distortions developed, she had a difficult time tying the theory into the psychosocial assessment. She didn't categorize the information into the organizational structure of Cognitive Theory, and only tried to apply the theory to pieces of what stood out to her *after* the session, so key elements of the theoretical conceptualization were missing from her thought process. She also failed to recognize that because the client was raised in a traditionally collectivist Latino culture, these thoughts may not be seen as distortions to the client or her family and may have been well aligned with the client's value system, depending on the client's level of acculturation to the dominant (individualistic) culture vs. her culture of origin.

Ethical Considerations: In order for supervisors to adequately supervise the work their students are doing, multiple methods of assessment should be used. The supervisor should not rely solely on the trainee for information about how they are progressing in their work, but should directly observe the work they are doing to do a more objective evaluation of the trainee's clinical skills and interpersonal appropriateness for the field. Case reviews provide valuable practice in teaching students how to think about their cases and should be utilized in conjunction with other forms of supervision to help students form a more accurate view of their work and the history and progress of the client.

Relevance in Training: When clear structure is provided early in training as to what is expected in case review, it can be a valuable tool in helping students to learn how to organize the information they learn about their clients. It can give them a conceptual framework for categorizing important elements of a case so that they can learn how to determine what information is missing, and how key elements of a case may be contributing to the problem or may be able to contribute to the solution.

This structure should include a comprehensive model for integrating a client's psychosocial experience of ethnic, racial, gender, socioeconomic and sexual orientation influences, as well as other demographic characteristics that affect the client's experience and cognitive schema development. Teaching students to understand the powerful impact of external factors, such as power structures and institutionalized oppression, as well as sources of strength such as faith-based groups, culturally- and language-based affiliation and community and social media-based activism, are necessary for them to have a complete picture of the client's development and resources, as well as their presenting issue.

Audio and Video Taping

Definition: The video and audio taping of counseling sessions for supervision began in earnest in the 1960s. Capturing a full counseling session on a recording provided supervisors a way to view a trainee's work without distracting from the process by being in the room. Audio recordings provided a record of the conversation, including all of the relevant inflections, silences and side comments that reflect the therapeutic process that would not be captured in a case review. Audio recorders were less obtrusive than the large, bulky video cameras of the time, and clients were often more willing to be audio recorded than recorded on video. Most supervisors, however, prefer video recordings of sessions because it includes the non-verbal communication between the counselor and client that is so important in assessing the relationship- and power-dynamics within a session. For that reason, most supervision research has focused on video taping.

Effects on Trainee, Client and Therapy: Video and audio taping preserves the data and process of the session for the supervisor to review on their own time. Whiffen (1982) describes the benefits of using video taping in self review and supervision. It allows for stop action analysis of particular moments during a session, or patterns of behaviors across sessions. Antecedents and consequences to critical events in the session can be examined. It allows trainees to view themselves objectively, as a part of the therapy session, rather than only recalling their clients' behavior. Video permits the supervisor to observe a trainee's facial expressions, attending behaviors and reactions to resistance. The supervisor has direct access to most of the visible and audible data from the session, rather than relying on the trainee's memory, which includes biases and lack of self awareness (Haggerty & Hilsenroth, 2011).

Haggerty and Hilsenroth (2011) and Binder (1999) argue for the use of in-depth analysis of video to help trainees recognize complicated interpersonal patterns and how their reactions to these patterns affected the outcome of the session. Kagan (1980) describes a similar approach: Interpersonal Process Recall (IPR), where the trainee controls and reviews different segments of the recording during supervision. The trainee is encouraged to discuss how they were feeling at particular times in the session, and to comment on their reactions to the client. Kagan reports that IPR is especially useful in helping novice practitioners comment on underlying feelings they observed in their clients, but were afraid to address. It also gives them a chance to see things they didn't notice in the session because they were too distracted with their own performance. Trainees who used IPR as their supervision model made

more gains in developing effective counseling skills than those who received traditional types of supervision (Kagan & Krathwohl, 1967), and were able to identify when their own anxiety got the way of their use of more complex treatment approaches (Burgess, Rhodes, & Wilson, 2013).

Example Scenario: A common scenario in supervision is that students are often shocked at how they appear on video recordings. One remark that is often heard is: "I look so scared!" Students are often surprised that the emotions they felt in the session with the client were apparent in their facial expressions and body language. It is a powerful tool for showing trainees their impact on their clients. It can also be a helpful tool in showing students how they respond when they hear something from the client that does not fit with their own world view. It allows them to see the impact of cultural differences, and further motivates them to broaden their understanding of people's different experiences of the world.

Ethical Considerations: Informed consent is necessary in order for clients to feel in control of what is happening to them in therapy. If clients are uncomfortable with the recording process, trainees can be encouraged to explore clients' discomfort and to educate their them about how the recording will be used and when it will be destroyed. Ultimately, though, the decision for consent to record lies with the client (or their parents, if the client is a minor). Confidentiality is paramount when considering the use of audio or video recording. Trainees and supervisors must take all necessary precautions to ensure the security of the recording while it is in use, and its proper destruction and disposal after it is no longer needed.

Relevance in Training: Video recordings, in particular, still hold a very valuable place in the training and supervision of counselors. Technology has come a long way from large, cumbersome, expensive recording equipment. The benefits of being able to observe a trainee's work, of having them critique their own work and breaking the session down into component parts, is a crucial part of clinical training that should be retained as one of many training modalities in counseling programs (Burgess, Rhodes, & Wilson, 2013; Romans, Boswell, Carlozzi, & Ferguson, 1995). Although, immediate feedback is not possible within the session, there is value in taking time to reflect, review and analyze one's work.

LIVE SUPERVISION

Live supervision has most commonly been used in the supervision of marriage and family therapy, where teams of supervisors (and often trainees) would observe a session through a one-way mirror and would consult with the therapist through some form of communication (Frankel & Piercy, 1990). One qualitative study found that students reported that live supervision helped them to "bridge the gap" between theory and practice in applying the concepts and skills learned in their training programs (Saltzburg, Green, & Drew 2010).

In both a 2012 and 1991 survey, approximately 50% of responding counselor training programs across the United States used some form of live supervision in their training curriculum (Amerikaner & Rose, 2012; Bubenzer, West, & Gold, 1991). Many programs reported using more than one form of live supervision (e.g., 53% used cotherapy, 46% used phone-in, and 25% used bug-in-the-ear) (Bubenzer, West, & Gold, 1991). After studying student reactions to live supervision, Anderson, Rigazio-DiGilio and Kunkler (1995) suggest that the skill of the supervisor is a strong factor in the effectiveness of live supervision practices. Locke and McCollum (2001) found that clients were comfortable with the interruptions of live supervision as long as they perceived an improvement in treatment,

as a result.

Knock-at-the-Door

Definition: The lowest tech type of live supervision is the "Knock-at-the-door," where the supervisor will observe the therapy session from an observation room, and will physically enter the session to call the therapist out of the room when a change of direction in the therapeutic work is warranted. In some cases, the supervisor will join the therapist as a co-therapist, but this is not seen as desirable, as it could compromise the client's perception of the trainee's competence if the client perceives the supervisor joining the session as a "take over."

Effects on Trainee, Client and Therapy: Smith, Smith and Salts (1991) found minimal changes in the flow of the therapeutic process occurred when there was knock-at-the-door or phone-in supervision interruptions, supporting the argument that they are not distracting enough to prohibit their use. However, they point out that interruptions should be infrequent and brief. If more interruptions seem necessary, then it might be more appropriate to terminate the session. On the other hand, Scherl and Haley (2000) suggest this approach could compromise the therapist's credibility with the client, whether the supervisor joined the session as a co-therapist, or simply called the therapist out of the room to consult.

Berger and Damman (1982) argue that knock-at-the-door supervision can quicken the pace of therapy. Because the observers are not required to join in the family dynamics, they are better able to objectively observe patterns within the family, and are able to make recommendations without concern for how the family will react to them as therapists. A suggestion from the observation group can be seen by the family as an "expert prescription" that may not feel comfortable, but might be worth trying. However, the counselor's intimate knowledge of the family's culture and values and how that might inform intervention strategies should be considered.

Live supervision allows the supervisor to view the session more objectively, to observe nonverbals between the client and counselor, and to observe how the counselor implements the feedback they receive from the supervisor (this last not being possible with delayed forms of supervision). Knock-at-the-door techniques can be effective as long as clients and trainees are well prepared for these interruptions and see them as part of the therapeutic process, and not an interruption of process or indication of failure.

Example Scenario: The Knock-at-the-door technique can be particularly useful when a trainee is feeling overwhelmed with a client crisis. For example, a trainee was doing her first intake, and in the midst of the interview, the client (an adolescent Caucasian girl) disclosed that she often wished she were dead. The trainee commented on the statement, and asked the client what she meant. The client reported that she thought about suicide often, but when asked, said she did not have a plan or any means. This is where the trainee got stuck. She was not sure whether to move on with the interview since the client was apparently not an imminent threat to herself, or to process the depressive feelings surrounding the statement and inform the parents. After the trainee was asked to join the supervisor in the hall, she was instructed to do further assessment (e.g., drug and alcohol use, support system, history of prior attempts) and then to discuss with the client how her parents might be helpful to her if they knew she was feeling this bad. The parents were later brought in and a safety plan was established. The trainee said later she was very relieved to have a moment to think outside of the presence of the client, and to be able to consult with her supervisor about such a critical and potentially dangerous issue.

Relevance in Training: Knock-at-the-door supervision can be very powerful when

used sparingly. It can help trainees take a moment to gather their thoughts and consult with their supervisor, which has particular importance during the initial experience of crisis situations. Both trainee and client can feel cared for and supported when they physically see supervisors actively participating in assuring the proper standard of care, and skillfully using such occasions as teachable moments for trainees (Charlés, Ticheli-Kallikas, Tyler, & Barber-Stephens, 2005).

Phone-in Supervision

Definition: Phone-in supervision takes place in an observation room (often in the presence of other trainees) with a telephone connected to a phone in the counseling room. When the supervisor wants the trainee to change their path of inquiry or intervention, they phone the suggestion into the counseling room. The counselor, who answers the phone, is the only one who hears the suggestion, but the clients are aware that the counselor is receiving a message from the observers. This approach lessens the time between when something occurs in session that requires feedback and when the counselor gets that feedback from the supervisor, but keeps the physical presence of another person out of the room. It allows the counselor to recognize the critical moment in session, to try a particular intervention and to see the outcome of that feedback live. It also allows other trainees to observe the effects of the change (Wright, 1986).

Effects on Trainee, Client and Therapy: Frankel and Piercy (1990) reported that both supervisors and trainees found that phone-in supervision was effective in helping the counselor produce client change. When supervisors used high quality teaching and supportive statements in their calls to trainees, these counselors tended to improve their own teaching and supportive skills toward the client. The opposite was true as well. When supervisors used poor teaching skills and did not provide support in their calls, trainees' teaching and supportive behavior toward clients diminished. Support skills in supervisors made the most impact on trainees' supportive behavior toward the clients, and this behavior in turn predicted the most change in client resistance. The more support the trainee showed in the session, the more likely the family members were to be cooperative in the plan for change. These researchers point out, however, that phone-in supervision is not meant to be co-therapy, but is meant to help trainees develop their own skills. Therefore, it should be done only when the supervisor believes the trainee will not make the change on their own; when the supervisor believes the trainee *must* change directions altogether (rather than *might* try a different path), and when there is a clear, concise, supportive message that can be given to the trainee (Frankel & Piercey, 1990; Wright, 1986). Too much use of both knock-at-the-door and phone-in supervision may be disruptive for both the trainee and the client (Liddle, 1991; Scherl & Haley, 2000).

Example Scenario: In observing two MFT trainees working with a couple, a supervisor noticed that one of the trainees seemed to be exploring the option of divorce to the exclusion of assessing the strengths of the relationship and possible reasons to stay in the marriage. There appeared to be collusion between this trainee and the wife that fostered a sense of hopelessness in the session, and the second trainee and the husband were trying to approach the relationship more constructively. The supervisor made a call to the second trainee and asked her to point out this dynamic to the couple and her cotherapist. The supervisor wanted to draw attention to the covert strategies that were taking place, so that an overt assessment could be made about what everyone wanted for the relationship. The trainee that had been colluding had a chance to think about his part in taking

sides, and was able to change his approach to be more constructive. Later, he discussed how his own recent divorce was coloring his optimism about the chance this relationship had to survive.

Relevance in Training: While a ringing phone, with a phantom observer on the other end, might be more disorienting than a knock-at-the-door from a visible person, it does have its advantages. It has the effect of stopping what is happening immediately in the room, in order for the trainee to pick up the phone and listen to what is being said. This can accomplish a few things. It can first teach the trainee that it is sometimes necessary to interrupt what is happening in a session in order to stop a destructive process or focus on something important that is being missed. It can also serve as an in vivo demonstration of the process of interruption and refocus, so that the trainee can see that it can take the session down a more fruitful path.

Bug in the Ear (BITE)

Definition: Bug-in-the-ear (BITE) supervision consists of observing a session in an observation room with a direct audio connection to the trainee through discreet earpiece. The trainee's earpiece receives radio transmissions from a microphone used by the supervisor. These messages are only heard by the trainee, and not by the client. The client is unaware of any statements made to the trainee unless the trainee indicates she hearing something through her body language. The equipment is inexpensive and allows the supervisor to give real-time guidance and encouragement to the trainee during the session with the client. Other trainees can observe this process and learn from the comments being made to the counselor during the session (Boylston & Tuma, 1972; Byng-Hall, 1982; Gallant, Thyer, & Bailey, 1991; Jakob, Weck, & Bohus, 2013).

Effects on Trainee, Client and Therapy: BITE appears to be more advantageous in developing specific clinical skills (such as supportive or facilitative statements to clients) than delayed supervision (Gallant, Thyer, & Bailey, 1991; Jakob, Weck, & Bohus, 2013; Tentoni & Robb, 1977). BITE supervision also allows for the shaping of appropriate therapeutic skills through the use of immediate reinforcement, correction of ineffective behaviors, pointing out client nonverbal behavior and guidance when the counselor feels "stuck" (Gallant & Thyer, 1989; Jakob, Weck, & Bohus, 2013). This form of supervision allows the supervisor to give the trainee feedback about their work that can be implemented immediately, without interrupting the flow of the session. This prevents any loss of credibility for the therapist when the supervisor makes a suggestion, since the client is not aware of the interruption, and doesn't know the therapist may have been stuck or making an error (Byng-Hall, 1982).

In an empirical study on the effects of BITE technology on trainees, McClure and Vriend (1976) found that clients were not disturbed by the use of the BITE technology. Trainees in their study reported no development of dependence upon their supervisor, other than their reliance on it for guidance in their initial sessions. Counselors actually felt more comfortable knowing that they could utilize their supervisors' expertise to competently work with their client during the session, without having to wait for supervision for feedback.

Example Scenario: A trainee is working with an African American male client in his thirties whose mother just died of cancer. The client admits having a hard time experiencing his feelings about his mother's death. The trainee, also an African American male in is late twenties, is using language that side steps the enormity of the loss experienced by the client. The trainee seems to be treading lightly around the issue of death and the expression of emotion with this client. The supervisor gives brief, supportive, instructive

statements through the microphone, such as, "Use more direct language about the death." And later, "I can see you noticing his nonverbals as he holds back the emotion. Reflect that to him." The trainee then begins to use language like "the death of your mother," rather than "now that your mother is no longer there." He also points point out that the client seems to be holding back his tears.

Relevance in Training: BITE technology is still an effective option for a non-intrusive approach to live supervision. It is relatively simple, inexpensive technology that allows a direct connection between supervisor and trainee during the session that is not distracting to the client.

Computer-Mediated Supervision

Definition. Computer mediated supervision is a form of live supervision, where a computer monitor is placed in the counseling room, usually behind the client in clear view of the trainee. The supervisor and other observers are in an observation room, and provide written or symbolic feedback about the trainee's performance that is displayed on the computer monitor (Klitzke & Lombardo, 1991; Neukrug, 1991).

Effects on Trainee, Client and Therapy: Neukrug (1991) suggested that the visual cue of messages on a computer screen may be more easily integrated into the trainee's work than audio cues (BITE) that may interfere with the trainee's thinking process. Scherl and Haley (2000) found this approach to be less intrusive than knock-at-the-door and phone-in supervision, and effective in guiding trainee behavior. They reported that shorter messages were more likely to be implemented by the trainee, because the simple messages didn't interfere with their cognitive processing about the client.

"Direct Supervision," described by Smith, Mead, and Kinsella (1998), used a computer monitor to display symbols communicating the supervisor's perception of the client's behavior, how to respond to the client's behavior and a rating on how well the trainee did in matching those interventions. Follette and Callaghan (1995) also used symbolic communication through a "performance line," where they showed a line on a computer screen representing the trainee's performance during the session. When the trainee was on target, the line rose; when the trainee was less effective during the session, the line fell. There was no qualitative feedback given to the trainee during the session.

Rosenberg (2006) combined live supervision techniques with delayed supervision strategies in her approach called "Real-Time Training." This method provides real-time written feedback visible on a monitor to trainees *observing* a session (not the counselor), so that observing trainees are able to learn from the work of their colleague and their professor at the same time. The feedback is available to the trainee who conducted the interview after the session is over. This way the feedback does not impede the counselor's higher order clinical thinking or foster dependence on the supervisor's feedback. When they review the tape, they experience what it was like to watch themselves in real time with the supervisor's feedback.

Example Scenario: A trainee is seeing an Asian American family of four. The parents are first generation immigrants, and seeking counseling because they cannot convince their 16-year-old daughter to stay in school. Seeking counseling was their last resort and brings them shame, since the matter could not be handled within the family. In this session, the trainee is facing the client and the computer with a live text-based feed from the supervisor that is placed behind the client. The trainee begins the session by focusing on how the family is feeling, resulting in visible discomfort in the parents. A note is sent over the computer monitor to remember to focus on the parents first, as a sign of respect for

them as the head of the family. The therapist shifts focus and a supportive symbol is sent over the computer. The next message is to remind the trainee to be more directive, since the family has communicated that they came to therapy to get an expert opinion on what to do with their child. The family may decide not to return to therapy if the therapist continues to focus on feelings.

Relevance in Training: Computers can facilitate communication between supervisors and trainees, and can be programmed to provide some of the predictable/rote training that previously required a great deal of faculty resources. A distinction should be made, however, about what is best handled by computer-based platforms and what needs to be closely monitored by faculty members. Live supervision, for example, takes a very high level of resources in terms of time, vigilance, and clinical evaluation on the part of the supervisor (Rosenberg, 2006) and cannot be done without that human interaction (whether it be in-person or online). Computers can facilitate, but not replace, this process.

Ethical Considerations: Preparing both trainees and clients for the disruption caused by live supervision is paramount to its effectiveness. They should expect to be interrupted as the therapy progresses. This preparation will help trainees to maintain their focus and composure so that they don't compromise their credibility with their clients, and will help them integrate the feedback seamlessly into their work. There is an ethical obligation to clients to clearly inform them that they are being observed and that the observers may participate in their therapy. They have a right to know who is treating them, how their information is being used, and who has access to it.

Because BITE and Computer-Mediated Supervision are not immediately known to clients when it is given, it is vitally important that they be informed about its use, how it works and how it may affect the progress of their therapy. This empowers the client to make informed decisions about their own treatment. All communication should be kept on a professional level and given in the best interest of the client.

FUTURE IMPACT OF THESE FORMS OF SUPERVISION

It is not likely that any of these technologies will disappear in the near future, because they each hold value in providing different forms of information and skill building for trainees. Their implementation is what will change, and much has already changed. Computers are already being used to teach basic counseling and interviewing skills to trainees (Kenny, Parson, Gratch, & Rizzo, 2008). Video-links continue to be used for supervision, but video cameras can now be embedded in phones and laptops, and are much smaller, less distracting and in many cases less expensive. Case review is likely to remain for the value it retains in teaching students how to conceptualize their clients, but case reviews can now take place over the Internet with E-portfolios that include elements of one's clinical work (e.g., video, case notes, conceptualization and questions) (Coursol & Lewis, 2000). Live supervision can take place electronically through secure Internet-based video feeds, where supervisors and other trainees can observe sessions live and send messages through the Internet by voice (BITE), text or symbol (computer monitor or handheld device) (Casey, Bloom, & Moan, 1994; Rousmaniere & Frederickson, 2013). The delivery may change, but the key concepts being taught by these techniques appear to still be of value to the field.

REFERENCES

Amerikaner, M. , & Rose , T. (2012). Direct observation of psychology supervisees' clinical work: A snapshot of current practice. *The Clinical Supervisor, 31*, 61–80. doi: 10.1080/07325223.2012.671721.

Anderson, S. A., Rigazio-DiGilio, S. A., & Kunkler, K. P. (1995). Training and supervision in family therapy: Current issues and future directions. *Family Relations, 44*, 489–500.

Beidas, R. S., & Kendall, P. C. (2010). Training therapists in evidence-based practice: A critical review of studies from a systems-contextual perspective. *Clinical Psychology, 17*(1), 1–30. doi:10.1111/j.1468-2850.2009.01187.x

Berger, M., & Dammann, C. (1982). Live supervision as context, treatment, and training. *Family Process, 21*, 337–344.

Bernard, J., & Goodyear, R. (2013). *Fundamentals of clinical supervision* (5th ed.). Upper Saddle River, NJ: Pearson Merrill.

Biggs, D. A. (1988). The case presentation approach in clinical supervision. *Counselor Education and Supervision, 27*, 240–248.

Binder, J. L. (1999). Issues in teaching and learning time-limited psychodynamic psychotherapy. *Clinical Psychology Review, 19*, 705–719.

Boylston, W., & Tuma, J. (1972). Training mental health professionals through the use of a "bug in the ear." *American Journal of Psychiatry, 129*, 124–127.

Bubenzer, D. L., West, J. D., & Gold J. M. (1991). Use of live supervision in counselor preparation. *Counselor Education and Supervision, 30*, 301–308.

Burgess, S., Rhodes, P., & Wilson, V. (2013), Exploring the in-session reflective capacity of clinical psychology trainees: An interpersonal process recall study. *Clinical Psychologist, 17*, 122–130. doi: 10.1111/cp.12014.

Byng-Hall, J. (1982). The use of the earphone in supervision. In R. Whiffen & J. Byng-Hall (Eds.), *Family therapy supervision: Recent developments in practice* (pp. 47–56). London: Academic Press.

Casey, J. A., Bloom, J. W., & Moan, E. R. (1994). Use of technology in counselor supervision.

In L. D. Borders (Ed.), *Counseling supervision*. Greensboro: ERIC Clearinghouse on Counseling and Student Services, University of North Carolina.

Charlés, L. L., Ticheli-Kallikas, M., Tyner, K., & Barber-Stephens, B. (2005). Crisis management during "love" supervision: Clinical and instructional matters. *Journal of Marital and Family Therapy, 31*, 207–219.

Coursol, D. H., & Lewis, J. (2000). Cyber-supervision: Counselor supervision in a technological age [Online]. Alexandria, VA: American Counseling Association/ ERIC/CASS.

Ellis, M. V., Ladany, N., Krengel, M., & Schult, D. (1996). Clinical supervision research from 1981 to 1993: A methodological critique. *Journal of Counseling Psychology, 43*(1), 35–50. doi:http://dx.doi.org.libproxy2.usc.edu/10.1037/0022-0167.43.1.35.

Follette, W. C., & Callaghan, G. M. (1995). Do as I do, not as I say: A behavior-analytic approach to supervision. *Professional Psychology Research and Practice, 26*, 413–421.

Falender, C. A., Shafranske, E. P., & Falicov, C. J. (2014). *Multiculturalism and diversity in clinical supervision: A competency-based approach.* American Psychological Association.

Frankel, B. R., & Piercey, F. P. (1990). The relationship among selected supervisor, therapist, and client behaviors. *Journal of Marital and Family Therapy, 16*, 407–421.

Gallant, J. P., & Thyer, B. A. (1989). The "bug-in-the-ear" in clinical supervision: A review. *The Clinical Supervisor, 7*, 43–58.

Gallant, J. P., Thyer, B. A., & Bailey, J. S. (1991). Using bug-in-the-ear feedback in clinical supervision: Preliminary evaluations. *Research on Social Work Practice, 1*, 175–187.

Goin, M. K., & Kline, F. (1976). Countertransference: A neglected subject in supervision. *The American Journal of Psychiatry, 133*, 41–44.

Haggerty, G., & Hilsenroth, M. J. (2011). The use of video in psychotherapy supervision. *British Journal of Psychotherapy, 27*, 193–210. doi: 10.1111/j.1752-0118.2011.01232.x.

Jakob, M., Weck, F., & Bohus, M. (2013). Live supervision: From the one-way mirror to video-based online supervision. (English Version of) *Verhaltenstherapie, 23*, 170–180. doi: 10.1159/000354234.

Kagan, N. (1980). Influencing human interaction – Eighteen years with IPR. In A. K. Hess (Ed.), *Psychotherapy supervision: Theory, research and practice* (pp. 262–283). New York: Wiley.

Kagan, N., & Krathwohl, E. R. (1967). *Studies in human interaction: Interpersonal process recall stimulated by videotape.* East Lansing, MI: Michigan State University.

Kenny, P., Parsons, T. D., Gratch, J., & Rizzo, A. A. (2008, September). Evaluation of Justina: A virtual patient with PTSD. Paper presented at the 8th International Conference, Intelligent Virtual Agents, Tokyo, Japan.

Klitzke, M. J., & Lombardo, T. W. (1991). A "bug-in-the-eye" can be better than a "bug-in-the-ear": A teleprompter technique for on-line therapy skills training. *Behavior Modification, 15*, 113–117.

Lee, R. E., Nichols, D. P., Nichols, W. C., & Odom, T. (2004). Trends in family therapy supervision: The past 25 years and into the future. *Journal of Marital and Family Therapy, 30*, 61–69.

Liddle, H. A. (1991). Training and supervision in family therapy: A comprehensive and critical analysis. In A. S. Gurman & D. P. Kniskern (Eds.), *Handbook of family therapy* (Vol. 2, pp. 638–697). New York: Brunner/Mazel.

Locke, L. D., & McCollum, E. E. (2001). Clients' views of live supervision and satisfaction with therapy. *Journal of Marital and Family Therapy, 27*, 129–133.

McClure, W. J., & Vriend, J. (1976). Training counselors using absentee-cuing system. *Canadian Counselor, 10*, 120–126.

Muslin, H. L., Burnstein, A. G., Gredo, J. E., & Sadow, L. (1967). Research on the supervisory process. I. Supervisor's appraisal of the interview data. *Archives of General Psychiatry, 16,* 427–431.

Neukrug, E. S. (1991). Computer-assisted live supervision in counseling skills training. *Counselor Education and Supervision, 31,* 132–138.

Romans, J. S. C., Boswell, D. L., Carlozzi, A. F., & Ferguson, D. B. (1995). Training and supervision practices in clinical, counseling, and school psychology programs. *Professional Psychology: Research and Practice, 26,* 407–412.

Rosenberg, J. I. (2006). Real-time training: Transfer of knowledge through computer-mediated, real-time feedback. *Professional Psychology: Research and Practice, 37,* 539–546.

Rousmaniere, T. & Frederickson, J. (2013). Internet-based one-way-mirror supervision for advanced psychotherapy training. *The clinical supervisor, 32,* 40–55. doi: 10.1080/07325223.2013.778683.

Saltzburg, S., Greene, G., & Drew, H. (2010). Using live supervision in field education: Preparing social work students for clinical practice. *Families in Society: The Journal of Contemporary Social Services, 91,* 293–299. doi: http://dx.doi.org/10.1606/1044-3894.4008.

Salvendy, J. T. (1984). Improving interviewing techniques through the bug-in-the-ear.

Canadian Journal of Psychiatry, 29, 302–305.

Scherl, C. R., & Haley, J. (2000). Computer monitor supervision: A clinical note. *The American Journal of Family Therapy, 28,* 275–282.

Smith, R. C., Mead, D. E., & Kinsella, J. A. (2007). Direct supervision: Adding computer-assisted feedback and data capture to live supervision. *Journal of Marital and Family Therapy, 24,* 113–125.

Smith, C. W., Smith, T. A., & Salts, C. J., (1991). The effects of supervisory interruption on therapists and clients. *The American Journal of Family Therapy, 19,* 250–256.

Stein, S. P., Karasu, T. B., Charles, E. S., & Buckley, P. J. (1975). Supervision of the initial interview. A study of two methods. *Archives of General Psychiatry, 32,* 265–268.

Whiffen, R. (1982). The use of videotape in supervision. In R. Whiffen & J. Byng-Hall (Eds.), *Family therapy supervision: Recent development in practice* (pp. 39–56). London: Academic Press.

Tentoni, S. C., & Robb, G. P. (1977). Improving the counseling practicum through immediate radio feedback. *College Student Journal, 12,* 279–283.

Wright, L. M. (1986). An analysis of live supervision "phone-ins" in family therapy. *Journal of Marital and Family Therapy, 12,* 187–190.

Chapter 27

THE USE OF TELEPHONE TO ENRICH COUNSELOR TRAINING AND SUPERVISION

Melissa Groman

INTRODUCTION

For most of us these days, our phones are like a third arm. And although there are a variety of good options for distance work in psychotherapy training and supervision, there is still no replacement for the sound of a familiar voice over the ease, portability and reliability of the phone. The mental health community has long been using the telephone to conduct business, facilitate distance learning, contact distant personnel and provide services. However, its use remains surprisingly underreported in the realm of clinical supervision literature (Driscoll et al., 2006, pp. 1–4), and while agencies have employed the phone as a matter of course for years, the last decade has seen a swell of telephone usage among private practitioners to both offer and accept services, training, and supervision. Teleconferences for ongoing training, continuing education, practice-building coaching, and supervision and consultation remains one of the easiest, most convenient ways to access intimate, connective experiences across distance, with colleagues, experts, and consultants of choice and to pursue personal and professional development without the constraint of geographic boundaries.

But what do we miss out on by not seeing a face in front of us? What gets lost? What gets found? How do you read the room without visual clues, body language, visual transferences, eye contact? Some studies suggest that people who are limited in one sense experience a heightened experience of other senses. Those who lack sight have been known to have a heightened sense of touch or hearing. My own father, who could not hear, claimed a heightened sense of smell. In fact, when I was small child, asleep in my bed, in a different room and down the hall from my parents' bedroom, a small nightlight beside my bed caught on fire. I, sound asleep right next to the nightlight, was entirely unaware. Yet my father, also soundly asleep, claims to have smelled something burning. He awoke, followed the smell into my room and put out the fire before any real damage was done.

One facilitator of phone group supervision, Dr. Simon Feuerman, suggests that "This brings us back to the question of what is going on in the minds of supervisees while on a group phone call. Why did people seem to intuitively not talk into and against each other?" In his work on the phone, "People reported "feeling" things from other people over the phone." Feuerman then asks, "What kinds of feelings were transmitted over the phone lines? If participants were not reacting to the feelings generated by sight, what were they reacting to?"

Feuerman suggests that even though we may at some point long for a visual completion to our other senses, the removal of visual cues does allow for verbal and sensory intuition to heighten and for our mind to work, enliven, and awaken other parts of our brains. Though being without visual cues may be anxiety producing for some, the rewards may be many in the development of parts of our psyches that were previously inaccessible to us (Feuerman, 2009, p. 11).

A ROOM ON THE PHONE

In considering phone supervision, some clinicians are afraid that they will not feel truly connected to, or understood by, someone who they cannot see. As one practitioner stated, being on the phone is "like speaking into a black hole . . . talking into a void [or] . . . like sitting in a group with a blindfold on and no spatial awareness" (Driscoll et al., 2003, p. 3).

So can the relationship between consultant and therapist become established and develop over the phone and do the benefits of clinical consultation and supervision apply across the airways? Can the goals of supervision be met without visual cues and sight-induced transferences? As with face-to-face consultation, the relationship between the two parties becomes the cornerstone for good clinical work. The development of this relationship mirrors in-person supervision in several key ways. As with in-person supervision, it is recommended to have a committed and regular time to meet and an understanding of what is expected from the work. As a supervisee, possessing the willingness to voice concerns, feelings and ideas freely, not only about cases being presented, but about the supervisee's own experience of the supervision itself, is an often unstated, but essential, component of a satisfying supervisory experience.

In her work with a supervisee over the phone, counselor and Professor of Psychology at Keele University, UK, Maggie Robson "concludes that the quality of the relationship was maintained but wonders if this was only possible because of the strength of the relationship that had been established face-to-face." Professor Robson suggests that having a previously established relationship in person can contribute to the success of work over the phone. The transition can successfully be made and that, in fact, may set the stage for good phone work. Given that this is not always possible, and that many phone experiences are born out of an original distance, not a change in circumstance, is the difference of significance (Robson & Whelan, 2006, p. 202)?

An informal surveying of phone supervision participants supports the idea that, while some therapists do prefer to actually see their supervisor, or see him or her before beginning the process, the sensation of being "with" their consultant and being listened to attentively so that they may talk openly and freely, can be conveyed over the phone by the supervisor's tone, words, cadence and verbalization of visual cues as necessary. "Rather than resisting telephone supervision . . . [clinicians may find] it a more flexible (and necessary) response to life's contingencies. In some instances, telephone supervision can increase freedom of expression and may even deepen the supervisory process" (Manosevitz, 2006, p. 581).

As part of the good work of supervision, supervisors help the therapist develop an ability to step back from the reaction to the patient and talk about the experience in an emotionally relevant fashion. It may in fact be this ability to be in the moment – to step back and talk about the experience – that is the essential indication that our students and we (as supervisors and teachers) are more fully understanding the patient. So when Spotznitz described the goal of treatment as helping the patient to "say everything," he might also be describing the process of psychoanalytic education, where teachers and supervisors help students "say everything" about the patient with the goal of helping the patient do the same. (Semel, 2009, pp. 210–211)

It is the job of a good supervisor to try to make it comfortable and possible for supervisees to say everything on their mind and to be open to checking in about the consultation process and the experience of phone supervision. In using telehealth technology, supervisors must maintain a moderate level of arousal. The supervisor must be cautious to see that the supervisee is stimulated to grow without becoming overly threatened by the use of the telehealth equipment. Therefore, the supervisor, as always, must be alert to multiple levels of experience and the possibilities as well as restrictions telehealth places on both the supervisor and supervisee (Miller et al., 2003, p. 4).

In most cases where consistent regular appointments are met, the relationship between supervisor and supervisee develops on the phone as it would in person and therapists usually find that after a short period of time, they become accustomed to the 'feel' of the phone and it is not necessary to process the modality itself very often.

Frequency of meetings can also affect the way therapists experience phone supervision. Some clinicians choose weekly supervision, some biweekly and some meet monthly. Others choose to call to schedule on an "as needed" basis to process a particular case, or discuss issues as they present, instead of scheduling regular meetings where this is allowed by their relevant regulatory body. This kind of arrangement works quite well for many professionals, but does not necessarily promote the same kind of reflection and learning, or relationship development, that regular sessions

can. When evaluating the feelings, experience, and usefulness of phone supervision, meeting frequency should be taken into account.

CAVEATS AND ADAPTATIONS: WORDS AND SILENCES

When meeting on the phone, additional verbal check-ins can often be useful. Without visual cues, participants in phone supervision often find that they become much more focused on their internal experience and become accustomed to deeply concentrated listening, which many who work on the phone believe to be an added benefit of this modality. It is often customary to verbalize particular actions such as smiling, head nodding, wincing and so forth and to name the feeling behind the cue in order to express it. Participants can tend to express would-be actions, even subconscious ones, with words. Verbalizing a head nod or smile ("I am nodding vigorously right now" or "I am smiling") become more normalized over the phone in order to foster connectedness and a feeling of being present over the wire. Moreover, without the interruption of visual cues, phone participants may become internally focused and more readily aware of feelings and sensations. Voice tone, cadence and pace take on more meaning. Likewise, the ability to express feelings and say everything may become finely tuned in phone work and can benefit case presentation greatly, as well as highlighting parallel process in action. In a discussion on supervision using the telephone during the 2005 Spring meeting of Division 39 (Psychoanalysis) of the American Psychological Association, one participant likened the experience of working without visual cues to:

Freud's use of the couch to reduce the social influence and to deepen and facilitate his access to unconscious process in both participants. [She suggested] that these factors contributed to a highly enriched experience in supervision by telephone and one that was often more productive than face to face sessions. (Manosevitz, 2006, p. 580)

Phone supervision tends to facilitate mindfulness, due to the lack of social and visual distractions and the need to focus on voice and feeling only. This can often be used effectively to understand more about a case. If, for example, when discussing a particular case, phone participants (either supervisor or supervisee) can identify, in the moment, and express or explore a particular feeling or sensation, such as inadequacy, hunger, annoyance, distraction or excitement (for example), these feelings can very often be traced back to the case being presented and lead to a deeper understanding of the client's experiences. This can then be used to discuss interventions, ideas and to help supervisees build resilience and work more steadily with difficult feelings and difficult cases.

Similarly, when there is silence on the line, supervisors may ask (as they might in face-to-face supervision) if the silences are comfortable, what the function of the silence is and if it should be filled, tolerated or enjoyed. Silences over the phone can produce more anxiety than silences in a face-to-face setting. In the absence of visual cues and especially at the beginning of a phone supervisory experience, a discussion about the use of silences can help supervisor and supervisee learn about how they both prefer to employ and respond to silences and what is most helpful to the process. In phone supervision, silence may induce a more tangible fear of having been disconnected physically, not just emotionally or psychically. For this reason, participants in phone work may interrupt silences earlier than in face-to-face work. Actual phone line disconnections occur most often if one party is on a cell phone and use of cell phones is strongly discouraged for this,

as well as for security reasons.

BENEFITS AND APPEAL

Many professionals are choosing phone supervision for its convenience and ease of use. The ability to arrange access to distance learning programs, experts, colleagues or group experiences that are otherwise geographically off limits is compelling for many professionals. Many clinicians have become acquainted with the work of topic experts and specialists, authors, practice-building coaches, and others whom they believe can offer them training, new ideas, understanding, and advancement. The phone is then an obvious choice for overcoming the obstacle of distance.

Clinicians also find that consultation over the phone saves time and is efficient use of scheduling. Therapists can factor out travel time and participate from their office. Many clinicians who use the phone from their office find that they are more readily able to focus on cases, problems in cases, and ideas that they want to discuss. Though some miss the change of environment and the appeal of being in a different space physically, others believe that they are better able to concentrate and recall cases and dialogue from the familiar setting of their own office.

In rural locations and small towns, or where members of the therapy community know one another, clinicians may choose phone supervision for its anonymity and out-of-town feeling, in addition to convenience and accessibility of experts.

THE PHONE GROUP EXPERIENCE

The coming together of colleagues from far and wide is an experience like no other. Group supervision/consultation traditionally offers a rich dynamic experience, the opportunity to glean different viewpoints, study group process, get support and contribute to the work of others. As McWilliams writes in *Some Observations about Supervision and Consultation Groups:*

> The chief purpose of a supervision group is to increase the therapeutic skills of members. It offers fringe benefits in friendship, networking, comparing notes on professional issues and learning for its own sake. It provides a rare kind of sanctuary, a place where therapists – who suffer self-conscious concern about their impact on others to a greater extent than any other professionals I know – can let their hair down, kvetch, laugh, compare experiences, and find consolation. Members report that belonging to a group helps them contain their most problematic feelings when working with difficult patients because they know they can vent later to a sympathetic audience. In a group they can also build on their strengths, increase their facility in giving feedback, try out their own supervisory style and develop a realistic appreciation of their capacity to make helpful contributions. "I found my own voice here," one participant recently reflected. (McWilliams, 2004, p. 2)

Group benefits and dynamics on the phone are similar to in-person group dynamics except for the absence of visual cues. Over the course of several group meetings, members tend to become familiar with each other's voices, the use of silences and the general feeling and tone of the call.

In 2002, seeking a way to provide more accessible convenient supervision to nurses in England, Wales and Northern Ireland, the Developing Practice Network, a UK-wide network for health-care practitioners that exists to promote, support and enable developments in practice in health care settings, piloted a project to provide and study phone supervision for ten of its members.

While the overall response was positive, group members concluded that naming one another before speaking and having a round of introductions each time and checking everyone could hear each other, was evaluated positively and gave the opportunity for everyone to participate in the group. Whilst some participants reported early in the life of the group that it was easier to express feelings to others you did not know on the telephone, other self reports of meetings contradicted this, suggesting that the group appeared "cosy" and could have challenged each other more. Towards the end of the project the latter had begun, evidenced by increased levels of reflective questioning, but is suggestive that the telephone group clinical supervision method takes three to four meetings before participants can gauge others levels of comfort or discomfort and use questioning techniques and silences effectively. (Driscoll, 2006, p. 3)

Groups on the phone function best when a trained group leader runs them. It is the leader's job to make sure each participant gets their share of talking time, that participants understand the rules and guidelines for the group, and to facilitate beginning and ending on time. The leader also takes care of all administrative duties and business issues. It is also the responsibility of the group leader to protect the group and the participants from potential emotional pitfalls of group dynamics and to assure that ethical boundaries are maintained.

The nature of group phone supervision can vary greatly depending on the members, the purpose of the group and the training and theoretical orientation of the leader and the number of participants. Some groups are set up as coaching calls, mentoring sessions, continuing education or lecture-oriented learning experiences. Other groups are designed to encourage a group process, help clinicians build a support network and create an experiential learning opportunity. Certain groups may be strictly case presentation- or business-oriented, while others are more attuned to countertransference issues. As with in-person groups, phone groups, while supervisory in billing and nature, can take on the feel or experience of a therapy group. This largely depends on the leader and the participant's wishes. When choosing a phone group, professionals should have a clear understanding of the purpose of the group, how it is run, what kind of experience is being offered and what to expect.

Group leaders should be accessible to group members outside of the group for individual supervision or consultation as needed to process any feelings that come up in the group that may be outside the scope of the group. It is a widely accepted practice in many training institutes for group members to meet individually with the group leader as needed to discuss issues that seem too personal to share with the supervision group; however, issues that involve the group are usually redirected back to the group for processing.

SUPERVISION VS. CONSULTATION

While definitions of supervision vary widely depending on the applicable regulations, licensure requirements, personal needs and preferences, one example includes:

the terms supervisor and consultant are often used interchangeably. A central distinction between the two is that a supervisor has the authority to implement sanctions on a worker if there are problems with the management of a case, whereas a consultant can make recommendations but has no power . . . professional credentialing bodies have specific definitions of supervision for their purposes and it is the responsibility of both supervisor and supervisee to know what is expected from them. (NASW, 2009, p. 15)

Additionally, supervisors may, in some circumstances, be held accountable for the cases their supervisee is working with. Consultants are generally not considered responsible, nor are they ever in decision-making roles.

Where professional bodies require practitioners to have supervision with a qualified supervisor (e.g., throughout a practitioner's career in the UK, prelicenced practice in the USA, and so on), phone supervision with a supervisor out of state or country may not meet professional bodies' requirements for standards such as accreditation. Practitioners are well advised to check with their individual licensing board or professional body to learn if they may seek supervision from a distance supervisor.

A GOOD EAR

Reaching into the ethics of good practice a "good ear" can be considered a must for professional self-care, quality of service to clients and continued satisfaction and professional growth. While agency professionals are often given the opportunity to present cases and discuss work issues, private practice clinicians often work in isolation, without the routine opportunity to connect with colleagues in real time and share ideas, process feelings and unpack transferences. Schools of psychoanalysis and other training institutes tend to mandate supervision/consultation as part of the learning process; however, outside the circle of such learning programs and of agency directives, many professionals go it alone in the US, at least.

DEFINING SUPERVISION AND CONSULTATION

Semel (2004) quotes Spotnitz (1976) who presented three goals of supervision:

to increase the (supervisee's) understanding of the (client's) psycho-dynamics . . . to help the (supervisee) tolerate the feelings induced in him by the (client) . . .and to use those feelings to facilitate the progress of the case, [recognizing that the supervisee often represses those feelings rather than accept them because] feelings appear to be connected with tendencies in the [supervisee] himself . . . to help the therapist communicate in an appropriate fashion with the [client]. (Semel, 2004, p. 195)

By listening to the stories of treatment with trained and kind analytic attention, supervisors also model good practice, encourage personal, professional, and practice growth; and provide support. Having a "good ear" to listen both analytically and empathetically to the nuances of cases, the transferences, the communications and the concerns of both clinician and client is likely to yield insight, new ideas and give the therapist the feeling of being taken care of.

Other uses of supervision, and telephone supervision specifically, broadly include training, both individual and group, for specific specialist qualifications. In such instances, calls may be more structured, require advanced reading or preparation and verification of time spent.

In general, however, private consultation can really be whatever the clinician wants and needs it to be. The consultation room is the place for reflection, discovery and dialog about cases and therapeutic relationships. And just as in the work of psychotherapy, the relationship between supervisor and supervisee, consultant and consultee, can be a model for a clinician's work with clients, the key to professional resilience and an emotional safety net, especially for independently working therapists. Additional benefits and uses of consultation include having a place to discuss and plan practice building, career advancement, business decisions and practices,

ethical compliance, and applications of theory and technique. Overall, the value of being able to say whatever is on one's mind to a trusted colleague trained to guide a good supervisory relationship cannot be underestimated.

While it is true that supervision is not therapy or psychoanalysis, many therapists who seek clinical consultation find that they may appropriately use consultation to learn more about themselves. This is a natural outcome of discussing countertransference and benefits not only the therapist, but clients as well. Being understood, heard, supported, accessing new ideas and ways of thinking, not just about cases, but about the work of psychotherapy and how the therapist functions has far reaching benefits for everyone.

WHAT'S IN THE WAY?

Because the need for supervision and consultation throughout a practitioner's career is not routinely practiced in all countries or all parts of the mental health care professions, it is worth noting some of the resistances against it. Perhaps the most important function of clinical consultation is to tend to the needs of the therapist. So, with so many good reasons to engage in clinical consultation/supervision, why do some therapists hesitate to weave supervision into the fabric of their work? In an informal survey among consultation group members at the Good Practice Institute (a host of telephone supervision groups), clinicians voiced obstacles to seeking out supervision/consultation that included, but were not limited to, "lack of time or money, feelings of general competency and the idea that supervision was only necessary for new professionals or for very difficult cases" (Groman, 2009, p. 1).

These ideas were further analyzed and understood to be, in part, a defense against fear of appearing incompetent or unknowledgeable; anxiety over professional presentation (how they will be viewed by supervisor or group members); fear of rejection by peers; fear of having to share personal information; fear of conflict with other members (in group supervision), supervisor, or group leader; a wish to be seen as the expert; attachment to a fantasy that others always know how best to work; or that they as the therapist ought to know how to work without having to reflect on their cases and feelings. Though many therapists do regard consultation as a necessity for good practice and normal for therapists at all levels of experience and skill, the same resistances that sometimes surface with regard to in-person supervision may apply to phone supervision.

Ambivalence over establishing a new relationship, potentially encountering difficult feelings, skepticism about the benefits of, and necessity for, ongoing process by way of consultation, fear of market competition among colleagues and fear of investing resources into an unknown entity, also help explain why many fully licensed professionals waver about seeking organized opportunities to process their work and deny themselves the often much needed and relieving opportunity to talk and tell their own stories of treatment experiences.

Psychotherapy practice by nature may necessitate rigorous self-care in the form of a dedicated personal space to study and reflect upon our work experiences. Overcoming these resistances well enough to seek out good clinical consultation as a fundamental component of good ethical practice requires a commitment to the belief that we are all humanly in need of supportive ongoing process, self, and case study.

Given the extent of resistance among some professionals, as well as objective realities of time, money and accessibility of clinical supervisors, consultants and trained group supervision leaders, phone supervision offers a simple, resource efficient opportunity to benefit from the experience of consultation without having to work through both internal and external obstacles all at once.

SAFE AND SECURE

To ensure that supervision on the phone is private, use of a landline is recommended for person-to-person calls. Even with current technological advances, cell phones are not only considered unprotected, but they can suffer static, delay in voice delivery and disruption in service. Similarly, many cordless phones are not only static producing, but may be subject to interference and should not be considered private, although this has been changing in recent years.

Most group calls take place over teleconference lines, through teleconference companies. Most companies provide secure conferencing, but participants should be certain to discuss security with the company they are using or the group leader.

Both in individual and group phone consultation, it is rarely if ever necessary or ethical to use exact names of cases being presented. If clinicians are employing phone supervision for accountability, licensure or directive purposes, and though landlines are to be considered secure, it is advisable to use pseudonyms or first names only.

LOGISTICS

Most phone supervision is done by simple direct dialing at an appointed time, with the supervisee calling the supervisor. Some consultants prefer to use secure conference lines, but most often this is used for training, education, group supervision and consultation, and not for individual appointments. Long-distance charges may apply, so callers are advised to have a cost effective long-distance rate as part of their phone service.

Conference calling is as simple as dialing

the teleconference number and putting in the access code (arranged and given to participants by the group leader) and speaking normally into the phone. When scheduling phone sessions, all parties need to attend to differences in time zones and, if the issue applies, it is good practice to be clear about what time the call is scheduled for in everyone's home zone.

As with face-to-face supervision, fees are agreed upon between clinician and consultant. Many distance consultants have the ability to accept credit cards through online payment services. Others usually accept a check sent by regular mail.

Although not face-to-face, the supervisory call should be treated as if clinician and consultant, leader and colleagues, are in the same room. Engaging in other activities, or the temptation to do so, can be viewed as a resistance to the supervision and can, if the supervisee is willing, be studied as such and used to gain insight into the case being presented (parallel process), the therapist's own feeling state and/or the phone supervision experience itself.

CONCLUSION

In the midst of our rapidly advancing, technologically developed world, there are many proponents of the traditional face-to-face way of conducting business. There may in fact be something intangible and of real value that gets lost over the phone. Visual cues, such as eye contact and facial expressions are a powerful means of conveying connection and providing a reassuring feeling of being tended to and understood and while "communicating [verbally] effectively is a prerequisite for any clinical supervision meeting . . . [it is] magnified [when participants cannot] see each other or in some cases [do] not know each other (Driscoll, 2006, p. 3). But supporters of phone supervision suggest

that it is:

> not wise to focus exclusively on what is lost when the telephone is used, [as] . . . there is something to be gained when using the telephone because of the heightened acuity to auditory cues that can result in expanded [intersubjective] supervisory space, . . . and that [phone supervision] might provide greater opportunities for expanding and deepening the supervisory process. (Manosevitz, 2006, p. 580)

Phone supervision's appeal will likely continue to grow as technology continues to dissolve geographic limitations. The growing telehealth community only serves to increase accessibility to and familiarity with colleagues from all over the world. Professional communities are springing up in interesting and innovative forums, offering opportunities for professional, practice and personal growth; connection; peer support and continuing emotional- and idea-based education. Phone supervision in its focus and simplicity connects us easily and allows us to delve deep or just review some cases. For those who appreciate the benefits, working on the phone can be richly rewarding, satisfying and productive.

REFERENCES

Driscoll, J., Brown, B., & Buckley, A. (2006). Exploring the use of telephone group clinical supervision to support the work of practice development nurses in the Developing Practice Network (DPN). In T. Shaw & K. Sanders (Eds.), *Foundation of nursing studies dissemination series*, *3*(6), 1–4.

Feuerman, S. Y. (2009). Seeing is not believing. *The New Social Worker*. [online].[Accessed March 13, 2016]. Available from: www.socialworker.com/feature-articles/practice/seeing_is_not_believing%3A_Group_Supervision_By_Telephone/

Groman, M. (2009). Phone supervision: Un-packing resistence. *Good practice, good care for professional psychotherapists* [online]. [Accessed August 13, 2009]. Available from: http://goodpracticeinstitute.blogspot.com/2009/03/phone-supervision-unpacking-resistance.html.

Manosevitz, M. (2006). Supervision by telephone: An innovation in psychoanalytic training: A roundtable discussion. *Psychoanalytic Psychology, 23*(3), 579–582.

McWilliams, N. (2004). *Some observations about clinical supervision and consultation* [online]. [Accessed August 14, 2009]. Available from: http://www.apadiv31.org/Coop/SupervisionConsultationGroups.pdf.

Miller, T. W., Miller, J. M., Burton, D., Sprang, R., & Adams, J. (2003). Telehealth: A model for clinical supervision in allied health. *The Internet Journal of Allied Health Sciences and Practices, 1*(2) [online]. [Accessed August 14, 2009]. Available from: http://ijahsp.nova.edu/articles/1vol2/MilleretalTelehealth.html.

NASW. (2009). *Private practice resource packet.* Edison, NJ: National Association of Social Workers: New Jersey Chapter.

Robson, M., & Linda, W. (2006) Virtue out of necessity? Reflections on a telephone supervision relationship. *Counselling and Psychotherapy Research. Special Issue: Technology in Therapy. 6*(3), 202–208.

Semel, V. G. (2004). Understanding the field-work experience: How do we know when students "get it" about narcissism? *Modern Psychoanalysis, 19*(2), 193–213.

Spotnitz. (1976). Trends in modern psychoanalytic supervision. *Modern Psychoanalysis, 1*, 201–217.

Chapter 28

CYBERSUPERVISION: SUPERVISION IN A TECHNOLOGICAL AGE

Diane H. Coursol, Jacqueline Lewis, and John W. Seymour

INTRODUCTION

The evolution and increased sophistication of technology has caused it to become more frequently incorporated into the delivery of health services including the area of mental health. Today technology is used to address a variety of mental health concerns through online therapy. In fact, the military increasingly uses technology to deliver mental health services. Another use of technology in mental health is the use of videoconferencing to provide online supervision or cybersupervision.

Clinical supervision in the helping professions refers to a collaborative process in which a supervisor is responsible for promoting supervisees' professional competencies and growth while concurrently monitoring and evaluating their performance to ensure client welfare (Haynes, Corey, & Moulton, 2003). Clinical supervisors serve as providers of information, challengers of "blind spots" and consultants to supervisees. Regardless of the supervisory model or theory, the relationship between the supervisor and supervisee is paramount to successful outcome for the supervisee and the client (Corey, Corey, & Callanan, 2007; Haynes, Corey, & Moulton, 2003). Ideally, the supervision process is based upon mutual respect and technology can enhance the supervisory relationship while serving as a vehicle to review critical data addressing a range of therapeutic modalities (Rousmaniere, 2014; Wood, Miller, & Hargrove, 2005).

Historically technology has been used to enhance the supervision process through a variety of formats (Borders & Brown, 2005; Trolley & Silliker, 2005; Wood et al., 2005) such as audio and videotape, bug in the ear, bug in the eye, electronic mail, chat rooms, instant messaging, mp3 and mp4 players and videoconferencing. Technology and networked communication is now the norm and worldwide use of the Internet has become accepted practice (Lewis, Coursol, & Wahl, 2004; Lewis & Coursol, 2007; Maples & Han, 2008; Sampson, Kolodinsky, & Greeno, 1997). This suggests that as digital natives many students entering counseling programs are very comfortable using technology and have a good deal of experience with it (Lewis, Coursol, Komarenko, & Bremer, 2015).

New counselors, particularly those who are pursing licensure, increasingly want access to cybersupervision. As of 2010, in the United States, six states had regulations related to online supervision and 18 others were in the process of developing such regulations.

However, 19 states still did not allow online supervision (McAdams & Wyatt, 2010). The states that allow cybersupervision do, however, often limit the number of online hours that can be counted towards licensure (McAdams & Wyatt, 2010). However, as the demand for cybersupervision grows and as videoconferencing becomes more sophisticated, all states will likely have to address this issue.

This chapter will discuss the concept of cybersupervision in the field of mental health, describe the cybersupervision process, the requirements for implementing cybersupervision, the evolution of the cybersupervision and provide an example of the cybersupervision process using videoconferencing. It will also discuss ethical implications for the field of mental health.

CONCEPT OF CYBERSUPERVISION

Cybersupervision is the process of providing supervision over the Internet to clients at physically distant sites (Coursol & Lewis, 2000; Vaccaro & Lambie, 2007). Today, it involves the use of the Internet to provide both individual and group supervision over long distances allowing supervisors and supervisees to communicate with each other from the convenience of their computer or other forms of technology such as mobile devices (Coursol & Lewis, 2000; Rousmaniere, Abbass, Frederickson, Henning, & Tauber, 2014; Rousmaniere, Abbass, & Frederickson, 2014; Watson, 2003). When originally conceived, cybersupervision was seen as providing supervision across distances using videoconferencing instant messaging and chat with video (Coursol & Lewis, 2000). Currently, cybersupervision allows supervisors and supervisees at remote sites to interact with each other synchronously at a time that is convenient to them. Recent advances in video technology and cybersecurity now allow for the synchronous online review of video recordings via secure online streaming video websites accessible by only the supervisor and supervisee, thus enhancing the collaborative nature of cybersupervision and the development of supervisee competencies.

Cybersupervision offers several advantages that include convenience, ease of access, cost effectiveness, time efficiency, practicality, and most importantly, increases the number of available supervisors (Chapman, 2005; Sampson, Kolodinsky, & Greeno, 1997). Among all these technologies, videoconferencing offers the advantage of an audio visual format where supervisors and supervisees can see and hear each other and review supervisee sessions in real time (Rousmaniere & Frederickson, 2013).

Some of the limitations of cybersupervision include access to technology, bandwidth cost, security, user technology competence and potential technology malfunctions. (Barak, 1999; Coursol & Lewis, 2000; Jerome & Zaylor, 2000; Kanz, 2001; Panos, Cox, Roby, & Matheson, 2002; Vaccaro & Lambie, 2007). However, these limitations should be considered within the context of the pace at which technology continues to evolve. Rapid technological innovations have provided increasing access to videoconferencing technology. Today, with the availability of videoconferencing on mobile devices such as phones, iPads, tablet computers and possibly on wearable technology in the future, cybersupervision has become increasingly more cost effective and accessible thereby offering a higher quality experience than other formats. Other nontechnological challenges include the lack of technology proficiency among supervisors (Rousmaniere et al., 2014).

IMPLEMENTATION OF CYBERSUPERVISION

Among the current technologies, videoconferencing provides the most comprehensive supervision experience, therefore this section will describe the implementation of cybersupervision through videoconferencing. In order to maximize the cybersupervision experience, it is important to have the appropriate hardware and software. The minimum hardware requirements for videoconferencing include a computer, microphone and camera. Many computers today come prepackaged with built-in cameras and software. However, if the computer does not have a built-in camera, it is generally possible to find a stand-alone camera that is compatible with the user's computer.

Software requirements include appropriate videoconferencing software that is H.323 compliant. Several H.323 compliant videoconferencing software packages are available including Adobe Connect; Apple FaceTime, Cisco Jabber, Cisco TelePresence, Citrix WebEx, Google Hangout, Microsoft NetMeeting and VSee to name a few. These software programs allow one-to-one communication and also allow for multiple users to communicate simultaneously in real time. Additional software is available that allows the supervisor to record a videoconferencing session and utilize it for supervision of supervision. Adding to user convenience, today, videoconferencing software such as FaceTime, Google Hangout, Jabber and VSee have become much more readily available through apps on mobile devices. However, practitioners should be aware of the varying confidentiality and data privacy and ownership issues offered by different platforms.

Both participants are required to have an Internet connection with an Internet Provider (IP) address that will allow them to connect with each other. In order for videoconferencing to be successful, a high-speed Internet connection (e.g., cable or DSL) is recommended. Finally, it is important to request that the IP offer the appropriate security assurances for confidentiality such as encryption, authentication, and a private, secure connection.

A key element of effective cybersupervision is to ensure privacy and confidentiality of the supervisor and supervisee communication. Therefore, cybersupervision should be initiated through a private designated server housed and managed locally by a trusted IP. Complete encryption should be provided utilizing a Virtual Private Network (VPN) connection. Each individual participating in cybersupervision should have a private user account with access managed through authentication protocols at sign on. Additionally, all forms of communication should be encrypted (i.e., video, audio, and text). Furthermore, to ensure compliance with the Health Insurance Portability and Accountability Act (HIPPA), it is recommended that individuals consult with the Internet security officer of their organizations and/or their IP (Rousmaniere et al., 2014).

CYBERSUPERVISION PROCESS

Initially, both supervisors and supervisees should be trained in the use of videoconferencing technology and the protocols for connectivity (Coursol & Lewis, 2000; Panos et al., 2002; Vaccaro & Lambie, 2007). It is recommended that the supervisor and supervisee practice online supervision simulations. This will allow the participants to become comfortable with using videoconferencing, adjust to the nuances of the technology and learn how to troubleshoot potential difficulties that they may encounter.

Similar to face-to-face (F2F) supervision, cybersupervsion in the mental health context involves the discussion of confidential information about clients. Therefore, it is important to identify a secure physical location where the supervisor and supervisee can engage in the cybersupervision process. At the designated meeting time the supervisor initiates the cybersupervision process by logging on to the account with a username and password to ensure security and then proceeds to contact the supervisee through the videoconferencing software. Once the point-to-point connection has been established, the supervision session can proceed much as it does during F2F supervision. One recommendation to facilitate the supervisory relationship is to use a hybrid model. Here the supervisor and supervisee can first meet F2F prior to initiating cybersupervision and then meet F2F as needed during the supervision process (Coursol & Lewis, 2000; Vaccaro & Lambie, 2007; Wood et al., 2005).

CASE STUDY EXAMPLE

In this example the supervisor and supervisee had a pre-established supervisory relationship. They initiated the cybersupervision process by first receiving training with videoconferencing technology and in the protocols of cybersupervision. At their work locations, both participants were in secure counseling rooms to ensure confidentiality of the supervisory session. In this example, both individuals chose to use a headset for the best sound quality while a picture in picture display allowed them to simultaneously see each other during the 45-minute supervisory session.

The cybersupervision session began, like most face-to-face sessions, with a greeting and reminder that the session would be recorded consistent with the written supervision contract. The supervisee immediately began discussing impressions of a new family counseling case seen earlier that week. The family included a single parent (age 42) and daughter (age 20) who both histories of anxiety and depressive symptoms, a number of family and social stressors and a relationship characterized by conflict and closeness. After the overview, the supervisor asked about the immediacy of the family's concerns:

Supervisor: Well they've been living with a lot of this for a very, very long time.
Supervisee: Mm-hmm.
Supervisor: And they each, it sounds like, have a lot of very difficult things that they deal with. A lot of challenges. What happened recently that really got them in the door? I mean, how did they sit down and decide they need to go and talk to somebody about this specifically?
Supervisee: Well, the mom is seeing another clinician in our agency and she had contacted that clinician and said, you know I'd like to come back and do some family work. Mom reported that everybody, I guess the few social connections she has and extended family, is saying you need to let your daughter grow up, you need to have some separation, your daughter needs to start doing things more independently because her daughter, there is also some financial strain and her daughter is living at home and not working and not contributing to the family . . . (continues with details)

With the supervisee having described the more immediate pressures on the family, enmeshment was identified as a major concern within the family dynamics to be addressed in family counseling. When considering the challenges that might be faced in helping the family navigate this challenge, the supervision shifted to a consideration of how to build the therapeutic relationships with both family members. This leads to a discussion about the intervention of whether to segment (split session times) or see the family members together:

Supervisor: Ok, how would you say relationship wise, how are things going in establishing a relationship with the mom and the daughter? How do you think rapport is going for you and for them?
Supervisee: Well I think initially it's going

pretty well because they are open to something working and excited on one hand
about starting to do something, but there
is also some resistance just because this is
so ingrained and this will be a huge, any
small change is going to be a huge change
for their relationship.

Supervisor: Mm-hm

Supervisee: I felt like when I met with them
both, I don't know that I can keep working with both of them together all the time.
I feel like there is an individual thing with
both mom and daughter that needs to be
addressed as well as doing some sessions
where we are all together.

A long conversation continued on the pros
and cons of how to manage the sessions (split
or together) and how this choice had the potential to either reinforce the old patterns or
allow new patterns to develop in the family.
Several strategies were discussed for helping
family members address their ambivalent
feelings and try new ways of interacting. At
the end of the session, the supervisor and supervisee came back to the original themes of
discussing immediacy, considering judicious
use of techniques for managing enmeshment
and continuing to develop the therapeutic relationship with each family member. In the
end, the cybersupervision session was very
much like a face-to-face supervision session
in dealing with the various aspects of the supervisory process:

Supervisor: So we are going to need to wrap
up in a minute. I'm wondering if there's
anything else you'd want to throw out or
loose ends we want to tie up?

Supervisee: No, I think this discussion was
helpful. You know finding out the risks
and benefits and finding out like you said
their internal dialogue. I think that's going
to definitely be helpful for me to really
understand more about where each of
them are coming from and what each of

them are wanting and needing in this process, too.

ETHICAL IMPLICATIONS

While cybersupervision offers several benefits, it is important to recognize the ethical
issues associated with it. Some of the most
significant ethical issues are confidentiality,
informed consent, the welfare of clients and
supervisees, the response to emergency situations (Coursol & Lewis, 2000; Greenwalt,
2001; Kanz, 2001; Panos et al., 2002; Vaccaro
& Lambie, 2007; Watson, 2003) and privacy
(Baltimore, 2000). Confidentiality has unique
implications online and supervisors and supervisees must establish procedures for protecting the confidentiality and the welfare of
clients and supervisees before initiating the
cybersupervision process (Coursol & Lewis,
2000). It is also critically important to protect
the confidentiality of supervisees who, during
the supervisory process will share information about their attitudes, values, beliefs,
biases and limitations (Coursol & Lewis,
2000). Both supervisors and supervisees can
protect confidentiality by using a secure
physical location that ensures privacy and
confidentiality, sharing only information relevant to the case, avoiding the use of identifying information, using a secure server, using
appropriate authentication protocols, ensuring the encryption of all information and attending to data ownership issues (Coursol &
Lewis, 2000).

As cybersupervision is a relatively new
modality for many supervisors, supervisees,
and clients, the informed consent form should
provide a clear explanation of the cybersupervision process. Supervisors, supervisees
and clients should have an understanding of
the length of the supervision process, the duration of the supervisory sessions and the
limitations of the cybersupervision process
(Coursol & Lewis, 2000). Where relevant,

clients should be aware that their video recorded session will be reviewed by the supervisor online.

One way to ensure awareness among supervisees of the ethical issues is to train them in cybersupervision before they engage in the process. The training should address issues such as maintaining confidentiality and privacy, effective informed consent and strategies to ensure the welfare of clients and supervisees. Supervisees are likely to encounter crises, so it is imperative that there is a plan to deal with these situations prior to the beginning of cybersupervision. Therefore, supervisors should discuss the procedures for dealing with crises during the training, prior to the initiation of the cybersupervision process.

The recent attention to cybersupervision in some of the ethical codes is a positive step toward ensuring that cybersupervision will become accepted modality. Currently, some professional organizations such as the American Association of Marriage and Family Therapists (AAMFT) and the National Career Development Association (NCDA) specifically address online supervision in their code of ethics. For instance, the AAMFT code of ethics (2015) provides guidelines for supervisors and supervisees who engage in cybersupervision. It is also addressed by the National Board of Certified Counselors (NBCC) in their Policy Regarding the Provision of Distance Professional Services (2012) and the NCDA code of ethics (2015) discusses cybersupervision in the section Supervision, Training and Teaching. In addition, supervisors and supervisees should read the American Counseling Association (ACA) Code of Ethics (2014) section on distance counseling, technology, and social media. At this time, the ACA (2014) ethical guidelines are less specific and more general in their approach to addressing online supervison , in part, due to the rapidly changing nature of technology. The current ACA ethical code requires counselors to understand distance counseling and social media as they have potential to impact the profession and are directed to become more knowledgeable in providing technology-based resources to clients.

CONCLUSION

There is an increasing perception that cybersupervision is a viable modality (Barnett, 2011); Chapman, 2005; Coker, Jones, Staples, & Harbach, 2002; Coursol & Lewis, 2000, Court & Winwood, 2005; Rousmaniere et al., (2014); McAdams & Wyatt (2010); Trolley & Silliker, 2005). It appears that cybersupervision is now more accepted in the field of mental health as technology has become increasingly sophisticated and integrated into society. However, as an emerging modality, it is important to support research that provides insight into the cybersupervision process and to identify ways to make it more effective. Since many supervisors and supervisees have expanded access to technology, it is incumbent on the counseling profession that it identifies ways to enhance the cybersupervision process so that it is practiced in a manner that ensures public good.

REFERENCES

American Association of Marriage and Family Therapists. (2015). *Code of Ethics*. Retrieved from https://www.aamft.org/iMIS15/AAMFT/Content /Legal_Ethics/code_of_ethics.aspx.

American Counseling Association. (2014) *ACA code of ethics and standards of practice*. Retrieved from http://www.counseling.org/Resources/CodeOfEthics/TP/Home/CT2.aspx.

Baltimore, M. (2000). Ethical considerations in the use of technology for marriage and family counselors. *Family Journal, 8,*

390–393.

Barnett, J. E. (2011). Utilizing technological innovations to enhance psychotherapy supervision, training, and outcomes. *Psychotherapy, 48*(2), 103–108.

Barak, A. (1999). Psychological applications on the Internet: A discipline on the threshold of a new millennium. *Applied & Preventive Psychology, 8*, 231–245.

Borders, L. D., & Brown, L. L. (2005). *The new handbook of counseling supervision.* Mahwah, NJ: Lahaska Press.

Chapman, R.A. (2005.) Cybersupervision of entry level practicum supervisees: The effect on acquisition of counselor competence and confidence. *Journal of Technology in Counseling, 5* (1) Retrieved December 13, 2008 from http://jtc.colstate.edu/Vol5_1/Chapman.htm.

Coker, J. K., Jones, W. P., Staples, P. A., & Harbach, R. L. (2002). Cybersupervision in the first practicum: Implication for research and practice. *Journal of Guidance and Counseling, 18*, 33–37.

Corey, G., Corey, M. S., & Callanan, P. (2007). *Issues and ethics in the helping professions* (7th ed.). Pacific Grove, CA: Cengage Learning.

Coursol, D. H., & Lewis, J. (2000). "Cybersupervision: Close encounters in the new millennium." *Cybercounseling* [Online], 1–12. Retrieved November 12, 2005 from http://cybercounseling.uncg.edu/manuscripts/cybersupervision.htm (Available upon request from authors).

Court, J. H., & Winwood, P. (2005). Seeing the light in cyberspace: A cautionary tale of developing a practical model for cybercounseling and cybersupervision within the University of South Australia. *Journal of Technology in Counseling, 4* (1), Retrieved December 13, 2008 from http://jtc.colstate.edu/Vol4_1/Court/court.htm.

Greenwalt, B. C. (Summer 2001). Cybersupervision: Some ethical issues. [Electronic Version]. *AAMFT Supervision Bulletin,* 12–14. Retrieved January 4, 2009, at http://www.aamft.org/aspbin/FTRArticleLog.asp?article=SupBul_summer2001_12.htm&stock_number=.

Haynes, R., Corey, G., & Moulton, P. (2003). *Clinical supervision in the helping professions: A practical guide.* Pacific Grove, CA: Brooks/Cole.

Jerome, L. W., & Zaylor, C. (2000). Cyberspace: Creating a therapeutic environment for telehealth applications. *Professional Psychology: Research and Practice, 31*, 478–483.

Kanz, J. E. (2001). Clinical-supervision.com: Issues in the provision of online supervision. *Professional Psychology: Research and Practice, 32*, 415–420.

Lewis, J., Coursol, D., & Wahl, K. H. (2004). Researching the cybercounseling process: A study of the client and counselor experience. In *Cybercounseling and Cyberlearning – An Encore: Beginning and Advanced Strategies and Resources.* Washington, DC: American Counseling Association/ERIC/CASS.

Lewis, J., & Coursol, D. (2007). Addressing career issues online: The perception of counselor education professionals. *Journal of Employment Counseling, 44*, 146–154.

Lewis, J., Coursol, D., Lindstrom Bremer, K., & Kamarenko, O. (2015) Alienation Among College Students and Attitudes Toward Face-to-Face and Online Counseling: Implications for Student Learning. *Journal of Cognitive Education and Psychology, 14*(1), 28–37.

Maples, M. F., & Han, S. (2008). Cybercounseling in the United States and South Korea: Implications for counseling college students of the millennial generation and the networked generation. *Journal of Counseling and Development, 86*, 178–183.

McAdams, C. R., &Wyatt, K. (2010). The regulation of technology-assisted distance counseling and supervision in the United States: An analysis of current extent, trends, and implications. *Counselor Education and Supervision, 49*, 179–192. doi:10.1002/

j.1556–6978.2010.tb00097.x.

National Board of Certified Counselors. (2012). *Policy Regarding Practice of Distance Counseling.* Retrieved from http://www.nbcc.org/Assets/Ethics/NBCCPolicyRegardingPracticeofDistanceCounselingBoard.pdf.

National Career Development Association. (2015). *Code of Ethics.* Retrieved from http://www.ncda.org/aws/NCDA/asset_manager/get_file/3395.

Panos, P. T., Panos, A., Cox, S. E., Roby, J. L., & Matheson, K. W. (2002). Ethical issues concerning the use of videoconferencing to supervise international social work field practicum students. *Journal of Social Work Education, 38,* 421–437.

Rousmaniere, T. (2014). Using technology to enhance clinical supervision and training. In C. E. Watkins, Jr. & D. Milne (Eds.), *Handbook of clinical supervision.* Chichester: Wiley.

Rousmaniere, T., & Frederickson, J. (2013). Internet-based one-way-mirror supervision for advanced psychotherapy training. *The Clinical Supervisor, 32,* 40–55. doi: 10.1080/07325223.2013.778683

Rousmaniere, Abbass, Frederickson, Henning, & Tauber. (2014). Videoconference for psychotherapy training and supervision: Two case examples. *American Journal of Psychotherapy, 68*(2), 231–250.

Sampson, J. P., Jr., Kolodinsky, R. W., & Greeno, B. P. (1997). Counseling on the Information highway: Future possibilities and potential problems. *Journal of Counseling & Development, 75,* 203–212.

Trolley, B., & Silliker, A. (2005). The use of WebCT in the supervision of counseling interns. *Journal of Technology in Counseling, 4.* Retrieved December 13, 2008 from http://jtc.colstate.edu/Vol4_1/Trolley/Trolley.htm.

Vaccaro, N., & Lambie, G.W. (2007). Computer based counselor-in-training supervision: Ethical and practical implications for counselor educators and supervisors. *Counselor Education and Supervision, 47,* 46–57.

Watson, J. C. (2003). Computer-based Supervision: Implementing computer technology into the delivery of counseling supervision. *Journal of Technology and Counseling, 3,* http://jtc.colstate.edu/vol3_1/Watson/Watson.htm.

Wood, J. A.V., Miller, T. W., & Hargrove, D. S. (2005). Clinical supervision in rural settings: A telehealth model. *Professional Psychology, Research, and Practice, 36,* 173–179.

Chapter 29

MENTORING THERAPISTS TO WORK ONLINE EFFECTIVELY

Kate Anthony, DeeAnna Merz Nagel, Audrey Jung, and Karen Turner

INTRODUCTION

As Goss and Anthony (2004) state, familiarity with email and chat and other technologies for business and personal use does not mean a qualification in online therapy. Training in this field can exist in two ways – online via the Internet and offline via face-to-face and other more traditional teaching methods. This chapter shall consider both modalities and will discuss the importance of offering training in online therapy, some of the methods employed by trainers in teaching on the topic and what training courses tend to look like from the perspective of content.

Practitioners need to assess what levels of postgraduate training are required to be effective and ethical online. They also need to identify their responsibility in gaining, as example, Continuing Professional Development hours (CPD) and/or professional Continuing Education (CE) credits. This chapter concludes with experiential analysis from the perspective of a graduate of online training.

It is now widely becoming recognized that postgraduate training in online therapy is not only desirable, but essential. As Murphy, MacFadden, and Mitchell (2008, p. 360) state, "specific techniques are required to create a therapeutic space, join with clients and create change in a text modality that lacks nonverbal communication and tone of voice." It is strongly recommended by the main professional organization in the United Kingdom, the British Association for Counselling and Psychotherapy (BACP – www.bacp.co.uk), who shifted their position on the matter from stating it "may be required" (Goss et al., 2001), to it being "strongly recommended" in 2009 (Anthony & Goss, 2009). BACP now also provides detailed descriptions of the competencies required for online practice that may be helpful in informing curricula on the topic in any part of the world. In addition, postgraduate training courses are a stipulation of membership of the Association for Counselling and Therapy Online (http://www.acto-uk.org/).

Wilkins (2006) points out that further training is desirable because however good core training was, it is bound to have gaps and become dated, a view which is particularly pertinent to the topic of mental health and technology. While most core trainings are yet to embrace online modalities as part of their curricula (Richards & Viganó, 2013), its inclusion in Masters-level training is starting to emerge in Europe at least. Gehl, Anthony, and Nagel (2010) identify that text-based continuing education courses have existed for many years in the form of correspondence courses, and now similar courses are offered online with the advent of the Internet.

BACKGROUND

Providing online training for online therapy is a relatively young part of the profession, certainly younger than online therapy itself, and therefore literature on it is scarce. Training programmes exist in the United States, Canada and the United Kingdom, and these programmes will be discussed herein. However, a cursory review of the literature and the Internet indicates a large gap in training opportunities across the globe for online therapists (though they are available – see www.onlinetherapyinstitute.com). Derrig-Palumbo and Zeine (2005, pp.124) cite the Case Study Group of the International Society for Mental Health Online (ISMHO – www.ismho.org) as having been a useful way of training by using online forum software to discuss cases and learn from each other as peer supervisors in 2000. The American Counseling Association produced a useful textbook including chapters around "cyberlearning" (Bloom & Waltz, 2000). Hsuing (2002, p. 133) acknowledges the importance of training on the topic emerging over the following years.

Online Certificate Programs have been offered since 2004 in Canada by www.therapyonline.ca in collaboration with the University of Toronto, Faculty of Social Work and consist of three offerings beginning with an eight-week foundation course and followed by Levels I and II courses in cybercounselling. The courses focus on the delivery of therapeutic services via email (Murphy et al., 2008).

In 2007, ReadyMinds published on Distance Counseling with detailed information on the Distance Credentialed Counselor certification offered through the Center for Credentialing and Education (Malone, Miller, & Waltz,

2007). Evans (2009) notes the importance of training in relation to seeking knowledge about global variations in licensing laws (p. 161), and Jones and Stokes (2009) provide a useful checklist of questions for practitioners to ask of themselves in choosing an appropriate course for their needs (p. 138). The most up-to-date literature on the topic of training specifically for online therapy are chapters in Anthony and Nagel (2010) and Anthony, Nagel, and Goss (2010), and Anthony (2014) in the *British Journal of Guidance and Counselling.*

OFFLINE TRAINING PROGRAMMES

Typically, face-to-face (i.e., offline) training programmes take place in groups. These can be small groups of like-minded individuals who come together as individuals to learn about a specific topic at a one- or two-day workshop; groups of delegates attending conference presentations; and groups from within an organization, such as a University counselling service or charity, who employ a trainer to give bespoke training to the team, steered towards their client group.

It is often the case with conference presentations that lack of time (usually an hour) means that it is not possible to disseminate all the historical and developing information to an unfamiliar audience, let alone equip participants with the skills required, and this is particularly relevant to teaching and training around technology in mental health because of the sheer volume of new information, meaning that defining the topic (for example, what Virtual Reality environments look like and what they "are") often takes up valuable discussion time from the purpose of the technology as it relates to therapy.

When presenting on online therapy, the most basic introduction to the topic would include at least definitions of online work, some trends and statistics, reference to ethical issues, and, preferably, examples of clinical work or quotes from case study material to illustrate the topic. Other presentations can have a specific focus depending on the nature of the conference and the needs of the audience, for example: legal issues, the theory (mode – see Anthony, 2000) of the therapeutic relationship online, netiquette and written communication skills or the future of the profession in light of new technologies such as virtual reality environments. An interesting trend at the time of writing experienced by the authors is the demand for presentations on boundary keeping and the professional and personal use of social and professional networking sites, such as Facebook, Twitter and LinkedIn.

The emergence of using blended technologies for conferences is also becoming less unusual. These face-to-face presentations can also be given live online during a conference where the delegates can be present in the room, or be accessing the conference remotely from around the world, including in Second Life, chat rooms or other virtual environments. Many professional conferences are now including keynote and breakout sessions on the topics of online therapy and mental health and technology. Because of the availability of such technologies as live stream and webinar recordings, professionals may be able to participate in real-time or at a later date without an actual physical presence at the conference. This allows ethnic and cultural considerations to be made available to professionals regardless of actual geographic location. For instance, a counselor in Australia may be able to view a live feed or recorded session that took place at a conference in Africa which might include the subtleties and differences of working online in that region.

ONLINE TRAINING PROGRAMMES

The concept of taking traditional face-to-face training for such an obviously applicable subject matter into an experiential online environment is entirely appropriate and sensible. The key to an online learning environment is variety, to maintain motivation and dynamism, particularly if there is no element of live interaction. According to Lehman and Berg (2007), the use of blended technologies helps to better fulfill specific learning objectives, improve course efficiency, provide flexibility and can appeal to different situations, content and learning styles.

There are many technological tools available to the online trainer in developing a programme. Webinars are an effective way of reaching a wide international audience and, if given live, can include an element of question and answer sessions at the end. Participants can telephone in to listen or do this live through the Internet, and they can include video or PowerPoint presentations. These can also be provided to download after the event. Similarly, whole conferences can be participated in remotely via video links and chatrooms, and many online conference softwares have the capacity for delegates to "hold their hands up" remotely, agree or disagree with what the speaker is saying, or conduct a conversation on the topic both in the public chatroom and via private instant message (IM) simultaneously (Wilson & Anthony, 2015).

To present course material, pdf files can be supplied and either locked to prevent download or printing or have this enabled, depending on what is included in course materials. This has the added feature of weblinks being available directly from the text to open in a new window – useful for further reading in particular – without disturbing the flow of the main course content itself.

Assessment of students can be done in a variety of ways. The simplest of these is a take-the-test feature at the end of the course, often comprising a series of multiple choice or true/false statements but sometimes with the capability of adding more subtle response types. The trainer can set the pass mark for these as a percentage and on successfully reaching this, the trainee then gets access to a readily-filled in certificate or CPD/CE document to download and print. Practice tests can also offer immediate feedback if an answer is wrong and provide the correct answer to aid or correct learning. More intense courses accept coursework that is submitted via email for feedback direct to the trainer. Often the trainee will submit answers to questions and exercises directly to the server which the trainer can access remotely. This latter method is particularly useful to check whether a student is struggling with any elements of the course before assignments have to be formally submitted.

Trainees can also be automatically tracked to check on how much they have completed, whether tests have been passed or failed, when payments have been received and so on. Many online learning platforms can translate this data automatically into graphical form. Another useful feature is the inclusion at the end of the course of a trainee feedback questionnaire, to maintain quality and refine elements of the course that need attention.

Other useful resources that can be offered to students include features such as a bookstore of related material to the topic, an editable wiki to ensure information is up-to-date and a calendar of events of interest that the trainee may like to choose to attend. Course member Twitter feeds at the training site are also a good way of creating a vibrant training atmosphere. Creating a Facebook or other social network page dedicated to a specific conference, workshop or other training event, whether online or off, is another way to enhance the training experience, particularly pre and post-training.

With trainees who may be spread far and wide around the globe, interaction amongst them is often particularly desirable to lessen the experience of isolation they may otherwise feel – particularly on longer online courses where motivation can often decrease over

time (Bloom & Waltz, 2000). Again, there are several technological solutions to achieve this. Forums are perhaps the easiest option, where trainees can discuss course material and offer peer support asynchronously via a series of titled threads. Forums also often provide a good place for post-training communication and networking. Another benefit is for the trainer to have the ability to post and broadcast information about courses to everyone involved rather than having to email trainees individually.

Despite diverse time zones, chat rooms also have a place for synchronous communication between trainees and also for the trainer. This can be utilized as a support network and is often also a vital part of the learning when on a course about online communication, as an experiential exercise. This can be organized via forums or via a calendar system.

Finally – again with organization via forums, calendar systems or email broadcasts from the trainers, synchronous meetings can be held in virtual environments such as Second Life. The Online Therapy Institute not only has offices with pleasant virtual surroundings where trainees can meet, we also have a virtual conference centre with breakout rooms available to trainees to meet and explore. For experiential work, there can be a secure invisible "skybox" for therapeutic or supervisory use by trainers, with potential for client role-play, although see Anthony and Nagel (2010, p. 117) for discussion of appropriateness of this, or placement opportunities, subject to encryption issues meaning even more secure communication software needing to be utilized for the latter.

The aforementioned Distance Credentialed Counselor training, at one time developed and delivered by Online Therapy Institute co-founders (Nagel & Anthony, 2014; Nagel & Anthony, 2010; Nagel & Sutherland, 2007) comprised a two-day in-person workshop that was also available online. The online version was self-paced, covering the same content as the in-person training. The participant could take the course in two consecutive days or the course could be completed over time, going to the material at a later date. The asynchronous style offered blended forms of technology including pdf files with embedded hyperlinks, PowerPoint slides with audio overlay and video. The participant completed a 45-question test before exiting the course. While this course was not facilitated in real time, the participants had access to the course trainers through email contact. This is but one example of how an online therapy training course has been delivered successfully. Currently the DCC training is no longer developed or facilitated by the Online Therapy Institute co-founders as they now offer broader and more comprehensive approaches to training not only therapists, but coaches and others as well. The Online Therapy Institute's (OTI) approach to training therapists about cyberculture and telemental health is delineated below.

THE ONLINE THERAPY INSTITUTE'S (OTI) APPROACH

In formulating training programmes for training therapists in online counselling, OTI offers trainings and workshops both online and offline based on years of experience of being trainers in this topic and others, such as coaching. We have already discussed the content of offline offerings as seminars, lecture and short and long workshops above, but it is worth examining the approach to providing best-quality, flexible, online course content in more detail.

Our approach is to ensure that our online programmes meet the *needs* of individuals and organizations as well as possible. It is our experience that many practitioners wish to know more about a topic without needing a full training course. This may be simply so that they can better empathise with clients regarding communication online, or because

they wish to develop their knowledge base for accreditation or licensing purposes. However, other practitioners do wish to pursue a service provision of direct online therapy and related mental health services, and will need a higher level of tutorage and mentoring.

We also understand that teaching any material via distance technology requires adherence to the pedagogy of e-learning that currently exists (Waterhouse, 2005). Implementing sound teaching strategies is paramount to providing a solid educative experience. OTI uses blended technology to meet the needs of the audience to be trained, whether the audience is one self-paced trainee whose intrinsic motivation is to enhance clinical skills or the corporate or agency administrator whose goal is to disseminate information about online therapy to a large group of clinicians in the same work setting.

OTI students immerse themselves in an online environment to fulfill being a self-reflective practitioner, particularly when working within a text-based environment (Bolton, 2005). An essential part of this is the ongoing mentoring from course tutors who give one-to-one feedback to written assignments as the student progresses, tailored to each student's individual work and personal situation. This is supplemented in larger courses with one or two live assessments via telephone or video.

A STUDENT'S PERSPECTIVE (Karen Turner)

One of the greatest benefits of having a private practice and being a clinician for 40+ years is experience and perspective. I know (as I'm sure many readers of this book do) when clinical practices have merit and when there is more fluff than substance. It is that experience and perspective that enables me to endorse my chosen training: the Online Therapy Institute's training programme for clinicians seeking to fully understand the possibilities of the Internet along with its challenges and limitations. It is a program of substance.

When I began searching for an online course to provide further training on doing psychotherapy using Internet tools, I was looking primarily for experience and expertise. From those now offered, I chose OTI because of its online presence and what I had seen in their book, *Therapy Online* (Anthony & Nagel, 2010). The scope and depth presented in the book was impressive.

There were several other things I was looking for in an online course, such as wanting it to be self-paced and provide personal connection and feedback. I wanted to receive examples and "hands-on" training using various Internet tools like asynchronous and synchronous email work and chat rooms, and I wanted to gain confidence in using tools and communicating online. The OTI course fulfilled all of these needs.

Finally, I wanted a course that would offer a systematic approach so that I could make sense of the often confusing material I had encountered online: OTI gave me that systematic clarity and directed me to more information if I wanted it.

Like me, you may be one of the people who saw early on the power and potential of computers and the Internet as an effective tool for the mental health field. While I respected the approach, I had little training. I was sufficiently competent about using emails to make first contacts with potential clients who came to my website and wanted more information. However, I was unaware of many possibilities of computer use for clinical interventions. I had never been advised of the limitations of confidentiality in most traditional email communications. This is one of the training areas one learns through OTI.

Specifically, what I felt was needed in training for people considering expanding their skills to online work was the following:

• Addressing confidentiality issues in all relevant forms of technology from emails through video conferencing, for both clients and clinicians.
• Providing guidelines for credentials.
• Information about benefits and risks to clients of such work.
• Information and guidance on creating informed consent forms and privacy policies.
• Delineating the ethics of online work and learning about issues of where and how to practice online, geographically as well as philosophically.
• Guiding hands-on practice of online tools such as email exchanges, chat rooms and video conferencing.
• Teaching on how to do the "business" end of online work – and guidelines for how to proceed.

Online Therapy Institute has done an excellent, professional and carefully thought-out job of bringing the entire array of technologies and considerations together under one umbrella. It has been able to ascertain the skills needed for each different technology and then teach these skills very well. It also weaves them all together into a rich tapestry of blended possibilities for the eager clinician to learn.

There is a growing list of reasons why a psychotherapist (no matter the orientation) needs to take this type of training seriously, whether or not you actually decide to work in ways that use technology of any kind. Among these are:

1. First and foremost, our clients/patients are dealing with the Internet in ever-increasing numbers and are spending a great deal of time exploring it. We need to understand this involvement. There is no age or demographic restriction on using the Internet. There is an issue of the OTI online magazine *TILT* (Therapeutic Innovations in Light of

Technology) that addresses Cyberspace as Culture (Nagel & Anthony, 2012), which clearly points out how important it is for modern-day professionals to recognize cyberspace as a distinct culture in its own right, with millions upon millions of participants. As an example, I recently encountered a situation with a client who casually mentioned his online involvement with something called "Second Life" and joked about his wife being jealous of his online girlfriend. It might have been left at that had I not known that "Second Life" is an online virtual reality community [and relationships in it every bit as "real" as ones developed offline]. Because I knew this, we were able to explore his Internet interest (verging on addiction) in depth. This ended up helping not only him but also his marriage because his wife joined him in his virtual world, and her participation greatly enhanced his offline life (or so-called "first life"). The "experts" at this are sometimes our clients themselves. If we listen to what they are encountering online, we can guide them through the labyrinth of possibilities they face. If you choose to pursue this particular aspect deeply, OTI has an "Avatar Identities Certificate" program.

2. Internet addiction in all sorts of forms is increasing. Pornography, virtual realities, games, gambling, social media and the like are all fast becoming a very serious threat to our well-being when they become addictive in nature. We need to know what these addictions entail, how easy it is to become addicted and that there are few limits on what can be found and pursued on the Internet. People using and misusing these things will need help in dealing with these realities. Therefore, knowing how effective the Internet is becoming at "hooking" people into various addictive behaviors can be a great asset to therapists.

3. More people daily are seeking help through the Internet so it is becoming imperative to know how to use it for marketing and information purposes. Many of my new referrals come through my website, and are drawn to seek my assistance because they read about what I do, and believe I can help them.

4. Increasingly, people are seeking help through alternative resources such as email exchange, phone, chat rooms and virtual environments. Knowing about their options makes us informed clinicians and current with the times in which we live. Many people (perhaps most) now use Google as the first guide to resources rather than their medical doctors. This is a major shift in where people look for help. This can be very beneficial as long as the information provided is not erroneous or false. To guide ourselves and our clients, we as therapists must be aware of self-help environments such as forums and message boards and even non-credentialed people writing articles and blogs. Only then can we help guide people away from harmful, misinformed sources and towards positive, truly supportive communities.

Learning the necessary skills allows us to provide service to many people who cannot or do not want to access a therapist in person. If we choose to work with people in these new ways, expert training is mandatory and extremely useful. I've listed below a number of classifications of people interested in these new forms of therapy:

• Physically disabled people for whom coming into therapy in person is difficult. This includes people who are deaf or blind, in wheelchairs and bed-ridden. The list is vast in this category.

- People who are very busy and cannot take the time to come into therapy. This can necessitate a mixture of modalities and technologies, both in person and online.
- People who are geographically distant from the therapist and the distance is too great to come in person. I, for example, work in Colorado where weather and distance play a factor.
- People who cannot find the expertise they need within their general area and do not want to settle for less than the best clinician they can find.
- People who are phobic and/or so anxious that they are prohibited from coming into sessions. There is a good deal of controversy around these issues; some clinicians feel online work can exacerbate them. Online work, however, is better than no work or can be an entry point even for people who will be able to fully heal their phobias *only* by face-to-face work.
- People who, because of shame or abuse, find it too difficult to share their concerns in person. This category sometimes includes people who are in a domestic violence situation and need support to get out of it. Here again, there are varying points of view regarding such issues. One is that working online can make the violence worse by the spouse, partner or other abuser feeling paranoid about the online work and wondering about the content of the sessions. Many other issues involved in f2f work are also involved here online. All aspects of these controversies are comprehensively addressed in the OTI courses.
- Sometimes people are having either intense spontaneous and/or drug or meditation-induced experiences that keep them from coming in person. These

people need help in integrating their experiences into their everyday lives.
- People who prefer to express themselves in writing rather than verbally and would like chat rooms or email exchanges. Some people like to take the time to compose their responses or write in the middle of the night. This makes it possible to accommodate whatever works best for the client.
- Some people find it a great deal easier to express themselves with more candor and freedom when not facing someone in person.
- People for whom Cyberspace is a culture unto itself, and they most naturally function in their own culture. We, as clinicians, need to be able to relate to their culture, not impose our own. This is also a controversial area of exploration that is examined in the OTI courses.

The next area on which I want to comment is why you should choose Online Therapy Institute for your training. Simply put, it is the very best available and during it, you will complete it feeling that you have a good idea of how to actually go forward with what you want to do. You will be taught using a state-of-the-art curriculum in a format that is clear and very accessible. The Institute lays out a curriculum that is thorough, yet not overwhelming. They help you gain knowledge and experience in all the necessary categories to make you feel well trained to work with people seeking your services.

Importantly, you also have *personal* attention from Kate Anthony and DeeAnna Merz Nagel, the two women who have put this together. They are truly experts and have proven so in many ways. The following is a personal overview and evaluation of their "distance" mentoring/coaching style. I have written it in bullet point style for clarity:

- At first, I wasn't sure about getting

mentoring "at a distance." Then I realized that doing so would allow me to access the depth and breadth of the new technologies I wanted to learn by using them. Since one of these women was in Scotland, I most certainly would experience mentoring at a distance from Colorado! It turned out that, for me, it felt like there was no distance at all. The Internet can dissolve those barriers. Kate was my main coach and she got back to me very quickly in all instances.

- I did not miss face-to-face coaching at all. I had the greatly added advantage of going at my own pace and reading and watching the materials when I could, between clients and meetings, on my own schedule. Plus, I did not have to dress up and go to a workshop (often at some distance away), taking much valuable time and costing a good deal of money for lodging as well as the workshop.
- A really wonderful aspect to this program is that you study and implement the very tools and technologies that you are being taught and will use in the future. We learned through emails, chat rooms, forums, video examples and written academic work.
- The format of the program was very easy to follow and is laid out in a step-by-step system so that I was able to learn very logically. Since there is a great variety of information subjects, this format is most helpful.
- The format allows you to learn about subjects of interest in great depth; the coaching allowed me to get as many references to explore as I wanted. The leaders of OTI are generous with their knowledge and guidance and give you a great many references for further study.
- You can dialogue and ask questions until you are fully satisfied with the answers. This is often difficult to do in face-to-face

workshops where there are time constrictions.

- All along the way, Kate and DeeAnna explore all aspects of any given subject. Both the pros and cons are presented so that you can make up your own mind. You never feel they are "selling" you on anything. For example, a good deal of time is spent on the subject of boundaries around the geographical location of where you can legally and ethically practice your profession. Since this is a highly controversial subject, all sides are presented.
- Taking this training with OTI gives a person an experience of legitimacy, just as certification and licensing does in any endeavor. Since there is such a huge array of both ethical and unethical behavior on the Internet, having this training gives consumers some standard of care and protection. For the client, knowing your therapist has gone through this training imparts a level of trust and credibility that can help them feel more secure about the quality of care they are receiving.
- Personally, I felt a greatly heightened sense of competence when I completed this training. Plus, having the books to refer back to is a great advantage.

The suggested textbooks plus the many, many other articles, audios and videos are woven together in a format that presents a cohesive and clear overview of what can otherwise be a very overwhelming and confusing area of expertise. You are introduced to and led through subjects as diverse as how to convey emotions through emails to exploring a whole new "culture" of virtual reality. Some things we can spend the rest of our lives exploring and studying.

The following is a brief overview of the subjects that are studied in this course.

Introduction to Cyberspace (Foundation in Cyberculture)

You are taught the basics of computer and Internet use as it applies to clinical work. Kate and DeeAnna have not assumed you know these basics. They teach them to you in such a way that whether you are a newbie or an old hand at computers, you will learn a great deal about how these basic skills are applied for clinicians in mental health. You learn what's "out there," from listservs and blogging, instant messaging and chat rooms, avatars and virtual realities to podcasting and VOIP (Voice Over Internet Protocol).

Relationships in Cyberspace

You learn all about relationships in cyberspace and how they are the same and different from "regular" therapeutic relationships. Here, you'll explore the limits of confidentiality in cyberspace, and the beginnings of how to communicate here therapeutically. Just as is true with all clinical work, knowing your own reactions, fantasies and countertransference issues is vital to the work. In my own work, I came across many different areas where I needed to explore myself more deeply. For example, I was emphatically trained (as you might have been as well) that you need to have a person in your presence (f2f) to do deep clinical work. Now, I have experienced, first-hand, doing both phone and email work with people who could not come into my office for various reasons. One person, whom I talk to by phone, has said that she can concentrate far better on her own inner experience without the distraction of being in my office in person. She had very severe abuse issues necessitating that she become "hyper-vigilant" to survive the abuse. This made coming into my office very difficult. In time, we worked enough so that she was able to come in and see me in person.

Another situation involved a deaf person for whom I offered email exchanges. She reported that the emails gave her the freedom to spend a good deal of time processing the information deeply enough to be able to (in her own words) turn her life around and connect with many other resources for deaf people in her community. If I had not confronted and overcome my own biases and early training, I would have been unable to help these women and others like them.

Theoretical Considerations

The course takes us into theoretical considerations of online therapeutic relationships – both our own and others. We look at the components of what creates change online. The ideas of presence, rapport, openness and understanding how fantasy works are explored. Through exercises, we have our writing skills developed in order to convey such things as empathy, warmth, congruence and various interventions in online communication. We are generally familiar with how to do such things in person and now we begin to learn what works the same and what might be different online.

Legal and Ethical Considerations of Online Therapy

Here, we consider the legal and ethical considerations of online therapy. This is a new and emerging field and requires us to implement intelligent, creative and innovative thinking. All along the way, the teachers have been bringing up the issues of doing clinical work online both legally and ethically. In this module, we go into these issues both personally and professionally. We learn how to prepare good intake and informed consent forms and how to verbalize privacy issues. Through generous sharing of what the instructors have learned, we are encouraged to create our own forms based on their very thorough examples.

Maintaining a responsible online presence is very important and this is explored in depth, including the interface with social media and how to navigate these tricky waters. There are many ethical considerations regarding social media involvement for clinicians. Personally, I had not considered the ethical ramifications of social media until clients began asking me to "follow" or "friend" them online. After OTI, I became very aware of the confidentiality issues and boundaries involved. On a professional level, I have been able to help people deal with "bullying" issues that happen with their children on Twitter. Since there are now millions of tweets per hour, it is vitally important to understand social media issues. This subject also explores the very controversial area of legal issues involved with online jurisdiction when offering services.

Working Therapeutically Using Asynchronous Email

This module is all about using emails to deliver therapeutic information and interventions asynchronously (without people being in real time). The challenges, rewards and limitations of email exchange are explored. This includes confidentiality and the process of this modality. There are many skills, such as expressing oneself in the written word, that are needed in learning to use emails. We must understand how to use encryption in emails because of confidentiality issues. Just sending emails in the usual ways uses very little encryption, thus allowing access to our emails by anyone who has the password for our clients' accounts or knows how to bypass these. These areas are explored along with such things as how to begin such a process, how to proceed and even how to show emotional states along the way. This is a very practical, hands-on module that really helps with gaining proficiency. It also suggests a five-paragraph model for how to structure your responses.

Working Therapeutically Using Synchronous Chat

After the asynchronous email exchange, we have a module on working synchronously – both people in real time together as in a chat room. Through following the process of an actual chat session, we analyze the exchanges between a client and therapist. In this, we get to see the potential, and the challenges, of such a session. I found this subject area very helpful because I just could not see how a chat room would work. After this, I came to respect the potential power inherent in such a tool. The way it was taught was very effective, much like observing a "real" chat. This convinced me that chat is an excellent tool, and one I will definitely use.

Working Therapeutically Using Telephone and Audio

Using a phone for therapy happened to be something I have done quite a bit of work with, so felt I could understand this quite well. However, even with a good deal of experience, I learned a lot from this module. The way things are presented gave me new ways of looking at what I've been doing as well as suggesting better ways to do it in the future. Using the phone or VOIP has its own challenges and benefits and this module teaches us about those and allows us to take a look at our own skills and limitations while evaluating whether or not this tool will work for us. Over and over, this course trains us in the necessary skills and qualities to be developed while also having us see how this applies to our own life and practices.

Using Video-conferencing to Conduct Online Therapy and Omnichannelling

The whole area of video conferencing is addressed. It also has a general review of client assessment and field research. The module ends with blending technologies and how we can bring them all together in our own practices. Video conferencing is a highly controversial area, especially with using such tools as Skype with its attendant confidentiality and record ownership challenges. So, in this module, the course has us examine the practical and the ethical and legal issues involved with video. We then are given an overview of the whole area of client assessment tools and field research, both for now and in the future. Concluding all of this, we are shown ways of blending all the various technologies to see how they can fit for our individual practices – a practice Anthony (2015) calls Omnichannelled Therapy.

As you can see from this analysis, if you understand the current and coming power of doing psychological counseling and therapy via the Internet, you will want to become competent through reliable training in all of these areas. The Online Therapy Institute provided this training to me in a highly efficient, thorough, and delightful way.

CONCLUSION

We have seen in this chapter that both online and offline trainings for online therapy have their own benefits and disadvantages. Immersion in an online training as preparation for immersion in online therapeutic services seems ideal, and yet as Anthony and Merz Nagel (2010) comment: "because the training is available 24 hours a day, seven days a week, work, family and other aspects of the offline world can often be given priority over the needs of the training as and when they arise rather too easily" (p. 125).

Conversely, while offline trainings have their timetables and compulsory attendance at a certain time which engages the trainee more directly, it cannot offer the experiential element required to be an effective online practitioner. The future of training therapists to be

effective when working online seems to invite blended technologies – including face-to-face work where appropriate – to provide a suite of trainings in the use of technology for mental health that reflect the increasing blending of online and offline aspects of day-to-day living.

REFERENCES

Anthony, K. (2000). Counselling in cyberspace. *Counselling Journal, 11*(10), 625–627

Anthony, K. (2007). BACP information sheet (2nd ed.) – Online counselling. *Counselling and Psychotherapy Journal.* Retrieved 16th March 2010 from http://www.bacp.co.uk/information/information_sheets.php. Rugby: BACP.

Anthony, K. (2014). Training therapists to work effectively online and offline within digital culture. *British Journal of Guidance and Counselling.* Published online at http://www.tandfonline.com/doi/full/10.1080/03069885.2014.924617#tabModule.

Anthony, K. (2015). *Omnichannelled therapy – The future of the profession.* Published online at http://www.kateanthony.net/2015/07/omnichannelled-therapy-the-future-of-the-profession/.

Anthony, K., & Jamieson, A. (2005). *Guidelines for online counselling and psychotherapy, including Guidelines for online supervision.* (2nd ed.) Rugby: BACP.

Anthony, K., & Jones, G. (2003, May). *Training online therapists online.* Paper presented at the British Association for Counselling and Psychotherapy Research Conference, London, UK.

Anthony, K., & Goss, S. (2009). *Guidelines for online counselling and psychotherapy, including Guidelines for online supervision.* (3rd ed.) Lutterworth: BACP.

Anthony, K., & Nagel, D. M. (2010). *Therapy online (a practical guide).* London: Sage.

Bloom, J. W., & Waltz, G. R. (2000) *Cybercounselling and cyberlearning: Strategies and resources for the millenium.* Alexandria, VA: ACA/ Eric Cass.

Bolton, G. (2005). *Reflective practice: Writing and professional development.* London: Sage.

Derrig-Palumbo, K., & Zeine, F. (2005) *Online therapy: A therapist's guide to expanding your practice.* New York: Norton.

Evans, J. (2009). *Online counselling and guidance skills.* London: Sage.

Gehl, N., Anthony, K., & Nagel, D. (2010). Online training for online mental health. In K. Anthony, D. Nagel, & S. Goss (Eds.), *The use of technology in mental health: Applications, ethics and practice.* Springfield, IL: Charles C Thomas.

Goss, S., Anthony, K., Jamieson, A., & Palmer, S. (2001). *Guidelines for online counselling and psychotherapy.* Rugby: BACP.

Goss, S., & Anthony, K. (2004). Ethical and practical dimensions of online therapy. In G. Bolton, S. Howlett, C. Lago, & J. Wright (Eds.), *Writing cures* (pp. 170–178). Hove: Brunner-Routledge.

Hsuing, R. (Ed)(2002). *E-Therapy.* New York: W.W. Norton.

Jones, G., & Stokes, A. (2009). *Online counselling: A handbook for practitioners.* Basingstoke: Palgrave/Macmillan.

Lehman, R. M., & Berg, R. A.(2007). *147 tips for synchronous and blended technology teaching and learning.* WI: Atwood Publishing.

Malone, J., Miller, R., & Walz, G. (Eds.). (2007). *Distance counseling: Expanding the counselor's reach and impact.* MI: Counselling Outfitters.

Murphy, L.J., MacFadden, R.J., & Mitchell, D.L. (2008) Cybercounseling online: The development of a university-based training program for e-mail counselling. *Journal of Technology in Human Services, 26,* 447–469.

Nagel, D. M., & Anthony, K. (2009). *Ethical framework for the use of technology in mental health.* Retrieved from http://www.onlinetherapyinstitute.com/ethical-framework/. (Accessed 11th October 2010).

Nagel, D. M., & Anthony, K. (2012). Cyberspace as culture: A new paradigm for therapists and coaches. *Therapeutic Innovations in Light of Technology, 2*(4).

Nagel, D. M., & Anthony, K. (2014). Distance credentialed counselor training: Mental health concentration. Internal proprietary training document. Phoenix, AZ: ReadyMinds, a division of University of Phoenix, Apollo Group.

Nagel, D. M., & Anthony, K. (2010). Distance credentialed counselor training: Mental health concentration. Internal proprietary training document. Lyndhurst, NJ: ReadyMinds, LLC.

Nagel, D. M., Malone, J. F., & Sutherland, J. (2007). Distance credentialed counselor training: Mental health focus training handbook. Internal proprietary training document. Lyndhurst, NJ: ReadyMinds, LLC.

Richards, D., & Viganó, N. (2013). Online counseling: A narrative and critical review of the literature. *J Clin Psychol, 69:* 994–1011.

Shafer, S., & Clawson, T. (2007). The distance credentialed counselor. In J. Malone, R. Miller, & G. Walz (Eds.), *Distance counseling: Expanding the counselor's reach and impact.* MI: Counselling Outfitters.

Stofle, G. (2001). *Choosing an online therapist.* PA: White Hat Communications.

Waterhouse, S. (2005). *The power of elearning: The essential guide for teaching in the digital age.* Upper Saddle River, NJ: Pearson Education.

Wilkins, P. (2006). Professional and personal development. In C. Feltham & I. Horton (Eds.), *The SAGE handbook of counselling and psychotherapy* (2nd ed.) (pp. 546–549). London: Sage.

Wilson, J., & Anthony, K. (2015). Immersion and disinhibition: How the Internet has changed our learning. *Therapeutic Innovations in Light of Technology, 5*(2), 13–18.

Chapter 30

AN UPDATED ETHICAL FRAMEWORK FOR THE USE OF TECHNOLOGY IN SUPERVISION

LoriAnn Sykes Stretch, DeeAnna Merz Nagel, and Kate Anthony

INTRODUCTION

Distance delivery of mental health services is becoming a norm in the field of mental health (Shallcross, 2012) and the American Counseling Association (ACA, 2014), the British Association for Counselling and Psychotherapy (Anthony & Goss, 2009, 2015; Hill & Roth, 2015), the National Board of Certified Counselors (NBCC, 1997, 2009, 2012) and the Center for Credentialing and Education (CCE, 2011) have all recognized the need for ethical guidance. More and more professional bodies around the world are recognizing that distance services, including distance supervision, create unique ethical challenges. Counseling licensure and credentialing boards and organizations are also beginning to recognize the need for distance clinical supervision as a means for providing access to qualified clinical supervisors who can support practitioners providing traditional and distance mental health services.

In 2010, McAdams and Wyatt found that in the US, 14 states had regulations regarding distance counseling, six states had regulations regarding distance supervision and many others had regulations in development. As Orr (2010) noted, good supervision should be dependent on the quality of the skills of the supervisor, not upon proximity to the supervisee. Bernard and Goodyear (2014) note that supervision is a process whereby a counselor with less experience learns how to better provide services with the guidance of a counselor with more experience and skill. Supervision is distinct from teaching in that the supervisees and their clients individually determine the curriculum.

While some of the existing literature provides some guidance for distance supervision (ACA, 2014; BACP, 2009, 2015; NBCC, 1997, 2009, 2012; CCE, 2011), most of the available guidelines focus on the delivery of distance counseling. Anthony and Jamieson (2005) created a set of guidelines for supervisors for the British Association for Counselling and Psychotherapy, based on previous guidelines for online practice (Goss, Anthony, Jamieson, & Palmer, 2001) and updated by Anthony and Goss in 2009. These authors, in addition to Hill and Roth (2015), recognized that supervisors providing distance clinical supervision must account for the unique considerations related to supervisee and client consent, confidentiality and data protection/storage when offering online supervision.

The following framework is written to consolidate the best practices related to distance supervision, which "may include telecounseling (telephone), secure email communication, chat, videoconferencing or computerized stand-alone software programs" (CCE, 2011, para. 3). In addition to ACA (2014), NBCC (2012), BACP (2009, 2015) and CCE (2011), the sources reviewed included Anthony and Nagel (2009); Barnett (2011); Burrak (2008); Chapman, Baker, Nassar-McMillian, and Gerler (2011); Creaner (2013); Dawson, Harpster, Hoffman, and Phelan (2011); Dubi, Raggi, and Reynolds (2012); Durham (2001); Huggins (2015); Hurley and Hadden (2009); Lenz, Oliver, and Nelson (2011); Nelson, Nichter, and Henriksen (2010); Orr (2010); Reinhardt (2014); and Watson (2003). The goal was to combine best practices from supervision with the realities of using technology.

Guideline 1: Ethical and Statutory Considerations

Supervisors must demonstrate and promote good practice by the supervisee to ensure supervisees acquire the attitudes, skills and knowledge necessary to protect clients. Supervisors and supervisees must research and abide by all applicable legal, ethical and customary requirements of the jurisdiction in which the supervisor and supervisee practice. The supervisor and supervisee must document relevant requirements in the respective record(s). Supervisors and supervisees need to review and abide by requirements and restrictions of liability insurance and accrediting bodies as well.

Guideline 2: Informed Consent

Supervisors will review the purposes, goals, procedures, limitations, potential risks and benefits of distance services and techniques. All policies and procedures will be provided in writing and reviewed verbally before or during the supervisory relationship. Documentation of understanding by all parties (supervisor, supervisee, clients and others as warranted by the situation) will be maintained in the respective record(s).

Guideline 3: Supervisor Qualifications

Supervisors will only provide services for which the supervisor is qualified. The supervisor will provide copies of licensure, credentialing, liability insurance and training qualifications upon request. The supervisor will have a minimum of fifteen (15) hours of training in distance clinical supervision as well as an active license and authorization to provide supervision within the jurisdiction for which supervision will occur. Supervisors providing distance supervision should participate in professional organizations related to distance services and develop a network of professional colleagues for peer and supervisory support.

Guideline 4: Supervisee and Client Considerations

Supervisors will screen supervisees for appropriateness to receive supervision via distance methods. The supervisor will document objective reasons for the supervisee's appropriateness in the respective record(s). Supervisors will ensure that supervisees screen clients seeking distance services for appropriateness to receive services via distance methods. Supervisors will ensure that the supervisee utilizes objective methods for screening clients and maintains appropriate documentation in the respective record(s).

Supervisors will ensure that supervisees inform clients of the supervisory relationship and that all clients have written information on how to contact the supervisor. Written documentation of the client acknowledging the supervisory relationship and receipt of the supervisor's contact information should be maintained in the respective record(s). Supervisors will only advise the supervisee to provide services for which the supervisee is qualified to provide.

Clients and supervisees must be informed of potential hazards of distance communications, including warnings about sharing private information when using a public access or a computer that is on a shared network. Clients and supervisees should be discouraged, in writing, from saving passwords and user names when prompted by the computer. Clients and supervisees should be encouraged to review employer's policies regarding using work computers for distance services.

Guideline 5: Modes of Communication

Supervisors will review written procedures for the use of distance communication, including telephone, chat, email, social media and other distance technology. There will be a clear delineation between professional and personal accounts. Social media and methods of communication that are not encrypted end-to-end should never be used as a means of communicating confidential information. The supervisor and supervisee will document modes of communication that are acceptable, how frequent communication should be, what a reasonable response time is, when to use asynchronous versus synchronous communication and what to do in emergency/ crisis situations. Supervisors will establish and communicate procedures for how to contact an alternative on-call supervisor should the supervisor be unavailable for an extended period of time. Supervisors and supervisees are also encouraged to discuss temporal, cultural and lingual differences that may impact the supervisory process.

Supervisors will review written procedures for verifying the identity of the supervisee during each contact. The supervisor and supervisee may wish to use a code name or password to verify identities and protection of confidential information. Passwords or codes will be generated using a password protocol thereby reducing the opportunities

for being compromised. Supervisors will ensure that supervisees utilize identify verification methods with clients receiving distance services.

Supervisors and supervisees are encouraged to use asynchronous communication for logistics only and to use synchronous discussions (chats and video discussions) to negotiate professional boundaries and develop therapeutic/supervisory relationship. Emergency/crisis procedures will include a list of qualified professionals in the supervisee's location who have agreed to serve as back up local supervisors on an emergency basis.

Supervisors and supervisees are encouraged to write out thoughts and feelings and to use symbols to convey nonverbal communication to reduce opportunities for miscommunication. Likewise, supervisors and supervisees are encouraged to use common language in text communication rather than shortened online abbreviations and to ask the meaning of any abbreviations that are not understood by either party to increase clarity of communication.

Guideline 6: Technological Issues

Supervisors and supervisees need to discuss the challenges of using technology and develop an alternative means of communication should technological difficulties be experienced. Time to deal with technological difficulties should be incorporated into the overall supervision scheduling, especially during the initial sessions. Supervisors and supervisees are encouraged to schedule a session prior to the initiation of distance supervision to become familiar with the technology and work out any issues, such as firewalls, low bandwidth and Internet access.

Supervisors and supervisees need to develop and implement a written plan for reconnecting should a synchronous meeting experience technical difficulties. There should be a prearranged procedure for reconnecting or rescheduling the meeting.

Guideline 7: Contract

Supervisors and supervisees will negotiate an explicit, written contract outlining:

1. full contact information for the supervisor, including telephone numbers, fax number, email and address;
2. the listing of degrees, credentials and licenses held by the supervisor;
3. general areas of competence for which the supervisor can provide supervision (e.g., addictions, school, career, distance services);
4. a statement documenting training in supervision and experience in providing supervision;
5. a general statement addressing the model of, or approach to, supervision, including the role and responsibilities of the supervisor, objectives and goals of supervision and modalities (e.g., recordings, live observation);
6. a description of the specific evaluation criteria and the formative and summative evaluation process that will be used throughout the supervisory relationship;
7. a statement defining limits/scope of confidentiality and privileged communication within the supervisory relationship;
8. a fee schedule and payment arrangements, if applicable;
9. the emergency contact information for the supervisor and a list of back up supervisors local to the supervisee;
10. disclosure, confidentiality breaches, security and encryption policies;
11. frequency of supervision;
12. dates for review of the contract; and
13. how to address conflict and what the grievance process is for issues that cannot be resolved.

Supervisors will also discuss the benefits and limitations of using distance technology in the supervision process.

Guideline 8: Records

The supervisor, in collaboration with the supervisee, will maintain a log of clinical supervision hours that includes:

1. the date of the supervision session;
2. supervision start and stop times;
3. the modality of supervision provided, such as direct (live) observation, cotherapy, audio and video recordings and live supervision etc.;
4. documentation of all written communication during the supervisory relationship, such as chat histories, texts, instant messages, emails; and
5. notes on recommendations or interventions suggested during the supervision.

Supervisors should maintain copies of clinical supervision logs for a minimum of five years or the legally mandated time, whichever is longer, beyond termination of supervision and will provide copies to the state counseling boards and other credentialing organizations upon request.

Guideline 9: Security, Encryption and Confidentiality

Supervisors need to consider three aspects regarding data related to security laws: integrity, availability and confidentiality. Supervisors and supervisees will need to back up ePHI (electronic protected health information) incrementally, Monday through Thursday, with a full back up on Friday. Backup media should be stored offsite with a HIPAA/HITECH compliant (in US) cloud or similar encrypted technology. Supervisors and supervisees must have written policies regarding backups as well as training for anyone handling ePHI. The National Institute of Standards and

Technology (NIST) 800 series of documents provide guidance for compliance with federally mandated regulations (see http://www.nist.gov).

The supervisor and supervisee will implement procedures preventing the disclosure of confidential information. The supervisor and supervisee must be in a secure and private location while conducting supervisory sessions or consultations. Supervisors and supervisees must identify who might have access to confidential information and take precautions to prevent disclosure of confidential information, such as password protecting computers and profiles.

Identifying information about a client should not be used in any form of distance communication. Clients need to be identified by a code name or other means understood only by the supervisor and supervisee. Client information of any sort may not usually be forwarded, copied or blind copied to anyone without the explicit consent of the client. Supervisors and supervisees should agree how communications and recordings will be stored. Communications related to the supervisory relationship may not be forwarded, copied, or blind copied to anyone without the explicit consent of all parties, unless in accordance with grievance policy outlined in the supervisory contract or in cases where there is a risk of serious harm or legal requirement to disclose. Any communication disclosure must be documented in the respective record(s).

Both parties need to agree upon whether or not supervisory sessions are recorded and if so how these will be secured for confidentiality, how long recordings will be archived and how they may or may not be used. Clients must give written consent to be recorded and be informed in writing of how recordings used in supervision will be stored, archived and destroyed.

Guideline 10: Gatekeeping

Supervisors should utilize objective information about a supervisee's professional skills and performance to determine if a supervisee should be endorsed academically or professionally. Supervisors will review the specific criteria being used for evaluation during the initial session(s) and will review and document the supervisee's progress throughout the supervisory relationship through formative and summative evaluation. Supervisors will not endorse a supervisee whom they believe to be impaired professionally. The supervisor will document concerns in writing and review the concerns with the supervisee, when possible.

Guideline 11: Research

Research utilizing distance services must adhere to all relevant legal and ethical standards and must take into consideration the unique challenges of distance technology. Supervisors and supervisees seeking to use data collected through distance supervisory relationships must have the relevant training regarding the unique challenges of distance technology. Information gained through distance services may only be used in research with the explicit, written consent of all parties.

REFERENCES

American Counseling Association. (2014). *Code of ethics and standards of practice.* Alexandria, VA: Author.

Anthony, K., & Goss, S. (2009). *Guidelines for online counseling and psychotherapy including guidelines for online supervision.* (3rd ed.) Lutterworth, UK: British Association for Counselling & Psychotherapy.

Anthony, K., & Goss, S. (2015). Good practice in action 27 and 28. Lutterworth, UK: British Association for Counselling &

Psychotherapy.

Anthony, K., & Jamieson, A. (2005). *Guidelines for online counseling and psychotherapy including guidelines for online supervision.* (2nd ed.) Rugby, UK: British Association for Counselling & Psychotherapy.

Anthony, K., & Nagel, D. M. (2009). *Therapy online: A practical guide.* London: Sage.

Barnett, J. E. (2011). Utilizing technological innovations to enhance psychotherapy supervision, training, and outcomes. *Psychotherapy, 48*(2), 103–108. doi:10.1037/a0023381.

Bernard, J. M., & Goodyear, R. K. (2014). *Fundamentals of clinical supervision* (5th ed.). Boston: Pearson Education.

Burrak, F. (2008). Using videoconferencing technology to enhance supervision of student teachers. Apple Learning Interchange, Retrieved Edcommunity at apple.com.

Center for the Credentialing and Education. (2011). *Distance credentialed counselor (DCC).* Greensboro, NC: Author.

Chapman, R., Baker, S. B., Nassar-McMillian, S. C, & Gerler, E. R. (2011). Cybersupervision: Further examination of synchronous and asynchronous modalities in counseling practicum supervision. *Counselor Education & Supervision, 50*(5), 298–313.

Creaner, M. (2013). *Getting the best out of counselling & psychotherapy supervision.* London: Sage.

Dawson, L., Harpster, A., Hoffman, G., & Phelan, K. (2011). A new approach to distance counseling skill development: Applying a discrimination model of supervision. Retrieved from http://counselingoutfitters.com/vistas/vistas11/Article_46.pdf.

Dubi, M., Raggi, M., & Reynolds, J. (2012). Distance supervision: The PIDIB Model. Retrieved from http://www.counseling.org/docs/default-source/vistas/vistas_2012_article_82.pdf?sfvrsn=9.

Durham, T. G. (2001). *Clinical supervision of alcohol and drug counselors: An independent study course.* East Hartford, CT: ETP, Inc.

Goss, S. P., Anthony, K., Jamieson, A., & Palmer, S. (2001). *Guidelines for online counselling and psychotherapy.* Rugby, UK: British Association for Counselling & Psychotherapy.

Hill, A., & Roth, A. (2015). The competences required to deliver psychological therapies "at a distance." Retrieved from http://www.bacp.co.uk/admin/structure/files/pdf/13919_background_document.pdf.

Huggins, R. (2015). HIPAA risk analysis, risk management plan, and policies and procedures manual. Retrieved from https://personcenteredtech.com/security-compliance-workbook-launch-campaign/.

Hurley, G., & Hadden, K. (2009). Online video supervision: A case study. Retrieved from the National Register of Health Services Providers in Psychology.

Lenz, A. S., Oliver, M., & Nelson, K. W. (2011). In-person and computer-mediated distance group supervision: A case study. Retrieved from http://counselingoutfitters.com/vistas/vistas11/Article_67.pdf.

McAdams III, C. R., & Wyatt, K. (2010). The regulation of technology-assisted distance counseling and supervision in the United States: An analysis of current extent, trends, and implications. *Counselor Education & Supervision, 49*(3), 179–192. Retrieved from EBSCOhost.

National Board of Certified Counselors. (1997). *Standards for the ethical practice of webcounseling.* Greensboro, NC: Author.

National Board of Certified Counselors. (2009). *The practice of internet counseling.* Retrieved from http://www.nbcc.org/Assets/Ethics/internetCounseling.pdf.

National Board of Certified Counselors. (2012). NBCC policy regarding the provision of distance professional services. Retrieved from http://www.nbcc.org/Assets/Ethics/NBCC Policy Regarding the Practice of Distance Counseling – Board-Adopted Version-July 2012-PDF.

Nelson, J. A., Nichter, M., & Henriksen, R. (2010). On-line supervision and face-to-face supervision in the counseling internship: An exploratory study of similarities and differences. Retrieved from http://counselingoutfitters.com/vistas/vistas10/ Article_46.pdf.

Orr, P. P. (2010). Distance supervision: Research, findings, and considerations for art therapy. *The Arts in Psychotherapy, 37,* 106–111.

Reinhardt, R. (2014). Technology tutor: What can counselors learn from Edward Snowden? *Counseling Today.* Retrieved from http://ct.counseling.org/2014/12/technology-tutor-what-can-counselors-learn-from-edward-snowden/.

Shallcross, L. (2012). Finding technology's role in the counseling relationship. *Counseling Today, 54*(4), 26–35.

Watson, J. C. (2003). Computer-based supervision: Implementing computer technology into the delivery of counseling supervision. *Journal of Technology in Counseling, 3*(1). Retrieved from http://jtc.colstate.edu/vol3_1/Watson/Watson.htm.

Chapter 31

SUPERVISING THE DELIVERY OF ONLINE COUNSELLING SERVICES IN AN EMPLOYEE AND FAMILY ASSISTANCE PROGRAM (EFAP) SETTING

Michèle Mani and Barbara Veder

INTRODUCTION

"The twenty-first century is rapidly becoming an era of educated consumers utilizing the most up-to-date technology to assume control over their own health care" (Deleon & Folen, 2010, p. xv).

Technological advances have made it possible for online mental health services to be increasingly offered to a wide range of client populations (Mallen, Vogel, Rochlen, & Day, 2005; Richardson, Frueh, Grubaugh, Egede, & Elhai, 2009; Yuen, Goetter, Herbert & Forman, 2012). Adapting counselling to technological innovations allows practitioners to address client needs (Barak, Hen, Boniel-Nissim, & Shapire, 2008) and improve accessibility (Gros, Yoder, Tuerk, Lozano, & Acierno, 2011). Consequently, online therapeutic supervision has garnered growing attention. Anthony and Goss (2009) indicated how online counselling and supervision are evolving professional fields. This assessment remains relevant today. Certainly, there are an increasing number of resources, articles and research papers on the subject, yet online counselling remains an emerging field when compared with more traditional practices. Mallen, Vogel, Rochlen, and Day (2005) and Anthony and Merz Nagel (2010) highlighted the need for online counsellors to be informed of the special requirements involved in providing online counselling, which entails training and supervision while developing the necessary skills. Furthermore, despite the presence of significant online therapy literature and guidelines recommending specialized online training and supervision, inconsistencies remain in practice.

In their 2010 qualitative study, Finn and Barak found that, overall, e-counsellor subjects did not have formal e-counselling training. Only a minority of e-counsellors had accessed informal or formal supervision for their online practice. Moreover, there was little consensus with regard to counsellor attitudes, knowledge of current regulations or professional obligations. Even when taking study limitations into consideration, the findings strongly highlight the need for greater alignment between existing online counselling guidelines and counsellor implementation. The outcomes are particularly compelling since online counselling research often features trainees or students as sample subjects, whereas the 2010 sample was comprised of experienced counselling professionals with a relevant counselling Master's degree and an active e-counselling practice.

With technology increasingly being employed to provide clinical services, and given the discrepancies in service delivery standards, clinical supervision of online counsellors (and the use of technology to provide supervision) is gaining even more consideration. Therefore, both novice and experienced online counsellors and supervisors have the opportunity to engage in further professional development and to familiarize themselves with current ethical frameworks and guidelines.

Clinical supervision has been described as an essential aspect of ethical and effective therapy. It has also been shown to have a positive impact on significant developmental areas such as skills and self-efficacy (Wheeler & Richards, 2007). The British Association for Counselling and Psychotherapy (Anthony & Goss, 2009) emphasizes the professional obligation to receive supervisory and consultative support.

This chapter will discuss the role of clinical supervision in delivering online counselling services within an EAP setting. It will review the use of technology to provide clinical supervision (to counsellors) as well as online counselling (to clients). Recommended supervisor and counsellor (supervisee) skills and competencies will be examined. Finally, specific online modalities will be explored vis-à-vis clinical supervision. Supervisory practices, common case management challenges and urgent/nonurgent consultation processes will be discussed.

Inskipp and Proctor (as cited in Wheeler & Richards, 2007) defined clinical supervision as:

> . . . the working alliance between the supervisor and counsellor in which the counsellor offers an account (or recording) of her work, reflects on it; receives feedback and where appropriate guidance. The object of this alliance is to enable the counsellor to gain in ethical competence, confidence, compassion and creativity in order to give her best possible service to the client. (p. 54)

Regardless of the supervisor's particular role, supervision involves consultation about specific client information including background and presenting issues (Merz Nagel & Riley, 2010).

Online supervision is defined as:

> . . . the provision of supervision to e-counsellors providing online clinical service delivery. It is intended to assure the quality of online counselling and the effectiveness of therapeutic outcomes. It also promotes the knowledge skills and clinical attributes required by e-counsellors who are making the transition to text and supports their online professional development. (Yaphe & Speyer, 2010a, p 194)

For the purposes of this chapter, this definition includes online supervision for other online counselling models.

Clinical supervision can be delayed (provided after a counselling session) or live (during a counselling session). The specific online counselling modality being used often influences when supervision is offered. Online supervision is provided by various means: asynchronous exchanges (email) offer an effective way to supervise online counsellors (Yaphe & Speyer, 2010b). Cyber-supervision (including chat and videoconferencing) allows supervisors and supervisees at remote sites to interact with each other synchronously at a mutually convenient time (Coursol, Lewis, & Seymour, 2010). Furthermore, many professions, including online practitioners, choose phone support for its convenience and ease (Groman, 2010).

Employee Assistance Programs (EAP)/ Employee and Family Assistance Program (EFAP) and Clinical Supervision

Employee Assistance Programs (EAPs) are employer or group-sponsored programs that are designed to alleviate workplace issues due to a variety of issues including mental health, substance abuse, personal problems and workplace issues. These programs strive to improve employee productivity and organizational performance. EAPs are also called Employee and Family Assistance Programs (EFAPs) or Member Assistance Programs (MAPs; Employee Assistance Society of North America [EASNA], 2009, para. 1). While individual EAP/EFAPs' service models, organizational mandates and structures might share significant similarities, they can also differ. Each EAP develops its own clinical and business goals, as well as service delivery methods. Whether comparing EAPs within the same country or internationally, one may find different processes, cultures and missions.

A range of public, community and private mental health providers are at different stages of project management regarding online clinical service delivery. Some are currently examining how they might initiate services; others may be in the process of implementation, or have already integrated them. By their very nature, EAPs attend to and manage online services and clinical best practices on a different scale than individual practitioners. They are also in a unique position when it comes to meeting distance supervision and technology contingencies. Although this chapter does not reflect the supervisory practice and methodology of every EAP, the authors hope it will provide a greater understanding of EAPs' online services parameters and the supervision structure that might be offered.

For the purpose of this chapter, the specific EAP resources, structure and supervisory practices discussed will be those of Morneau Shepell, under its Shepell·fgi brand, a Canadian EFAP provider that works within a short-term counselling framework. As the Council on Accreditation (COA) has accredited Shepell·fgi, there are certain assumptions the reader can make with regard to the EAPs' practices and internal processes reviewed herein. Privacy standards, confidentiality, ethical and statutory considerations, record keeping, informed consent and clinical best practices are already established and audited. Online counselling is bound by the same professional ethics as face-to-face (F2F) counselling (Finn & Barak, 2010).

In addition, clinical supervision is an integral component of clinical service design. Supervision meets specific criteria: it is structured, accessible and provides responsive and meaningful consultation. Supervision offers consultative support for urgent and non-urgent issues that may emerge. It includes formal and informal supervision as well as peer supervision. Shepell·fgi supervisory practices also correspond with current ethical guidelines for the use of technology in supervision (Anthony & Goss, 2009; Stretch, Nagel, & Anthony, 2013). As such, the following discussion of EAP supervision will not include an examination of privacy, contracts and technological standards, as the reader may assume these (and other) requirements are in place.

Online Modalities

EAPs refer to specific requirements when developing new modalities. These include, but are not limited to: privacy standards, engaging the end users, clinical best practices, managing high-risk issues and up-front disclosure about exclusion criteria. These clinical foundations inform and essentially shape EAP clinical supervisory guidelines. This chapter will focus on three online counselling modalities: synchronized chat, e-counselling and video counselling.

Synchronous Chat

Clients are offered a single session consultation (synchronous chat) when requesting immediate online "live" contact with counsellor through the 24/7 EAP call center. This online service is referred to as "First Chat," a Shepell·fgi trademark.

Both asynchronous e-counselling and synchronous video counselling provide short-term counselling, aligned with the short-term counselling model of the more traditional EAP counselling modalities (Face-to-Face); Tele-counselling).

On a related note, many EAPs have 24/7 call centers available to their clients who need to speak with a counsellor immediately. These clients also include those in need who are already accessing short-term EAP counselling. EAP call centers often provide back-up support to clients in crisis.

Online Supervisor Core Competencies

When examining online supervision practices, supervisor qualifications are a vital factor for consideration. There is a critical need for clinical supervisors to have unique and informed understanding of the online environment as well as relevant experience. Anthony and Goss (2009) were explicit about the need for online clinical supervisors to have direct online counselling experience, along with a comprehensive understanding of the relevant issues and ethical concerns.

When discussing clinical supervision using online methods, Anthony and Merz Nagel (2010) elegantly highlighted the link between online supervisors' proficiencies and their ability to effectively supervise: "Remember that just as with online therapy, supervision via technology is not a theory or technique but a conduit to experience a professional and supportive relationship" (p.128).

EAP supervisors are in the best position to provide effective guidance, direction and consultation when they have the following core competencies:

1. Extensive counselling experience with a range of client populations.
2. Considerable years working within an EAP (familiarity with EAP clinical and organizational guidelines, systems, protocols, and procedures).
3. Experience providing direct online counselling to clients (in the modality they are supervising).
4. A robust understanding of the online modality, best practices, use of technology, troubleshooting needs, current trends and the capabilities featured in the particular online clinical service.
5. Prior supervisory or managerial experience in a clinical setting.

Online Counsellor Core Competencies

Identifying counsellor core competencies is an essential ingredient of quality online clinical service delivery. Clinical supervisors and practitioners in fields other than EAPs likely recognize the importance of recruiting counselling professionals with the unique skills appropriate for the specific service modality. Several authors articulate the specialized skills required and how a therapist may be very experienced in F2F therapy, and yet unable to effectively transfer these skills to an online environment (Mallen, Vogel, & Rochlen, 2005; Yaphe & Speyer, 2010a). Indeed, both clinical supervisors and counsellors must remain mindful of the learning curve required to master a new modality (particularly text-based counselling). Online counselling core competencies are founded on the premise that a genuine therapeutic alliance and effective counselling can be developed through online contact.

Supervising the Delivery of Online Services

Synchronous Chat

First Chat, launched in 2011, is a secure, live chat service that provides clients with immediate clinical support. Several EAPs offer their clients a single session telephone consultation through their 24/7 clinically staffed call centers. Synchronous Chat is another means for clients to access immediate, live support. It is analogous to a client telephoning a 24/7 EAP call center for support, to book adjunct services, or speak immediately with a clinical counsellor. When Chat is clinical in nature, clients experience a "one time session" with a Chat trained clinical counsellor. Similar to a single session teleconsultation, the Chat session also provides assessment, support, referrals and/or crisis intervention.

The case auditing and supervision models for Chat are incorporated as part of program development. Additional considerations include advising clients before registration of the exclusion criteria. Shepell·fgi's EFAP, for example, excludes clients in crisis and those under the age of 18. As well, clients confirm that they have read, understood and agreed to documentation relating to informed consent, privacy and confidentiality. Clients are also asked standard EAP risk questions regarding imminent risk and the use of drugs and alcohol.

Counsellor Competencies

In an EAP call center, clinical counsellors can provide both consultation and crisis management support to their clients. Due to the nature of their work, EAP clinical counsellors who cover multiple locations may have highly developed distance counselling aptitudes, with significant experience responding effectively to urgent and nonurgent presenting issues. The following core skills are essential to identifying clinical counsellors who are the best fit for online modalities:

1. The ability to convey empathy and develop rapport through text-based communication.
2. The ability to integrate traditional counselling skills with those facilitated by text-based technology.

Training and Supervision

Similar to other online modalities, the Chat supervision structure is calibrated to the counsellor's text-based experience and where they are situated on their individual learning curve. With respect to Shepell·fgi's EAP training and supervision model, Chat trainees engage in multiple live simulated chats with the supervisor. Subsequent to chatting with clients, sessions are audited and supervision takes place post-session. Supervision and training are aligned with EAP standards of care as well as clinical best practices.

Live and postsession individual supervision, offered on a scheduled and as-needed basis, has proven to be helpful in meeting training objectives and ensuring clinical quality. Session audits serve as another useful supervisory and training tool. A Chat call center environment often allows access to immediate supervision and peer support. As many EAP call centers are comprised of robust clinical teams, multiple avenues of clinical supports are available 24/7.

With Chat, supervisors have the opportunity to "listen in" to sessions and support counsellors during a chat session, in a way that is not as intrusive as various F2F live supervisory methods. Chat supervisors can log into telephone and chat cues. They can monitor live chats. Depending on the supervisory structure, supervisors can be available for live audits when counsellors request support or during risk situations. Counsellors can contact their supervisor by telephone, email or by motioning their need for assistance to their onsite colleagues or supervisors.

Examining this specific EAP Chat model, supervisors typically provide live counsellor support via phone or in person. A key rationale for not doing the support online is that counsellors report that additional text becomes distracting when they are in the midst of a chat session with a client. Calling a supervisor by phone or having a supervisor physically present to help provide direction and support is found to be more effective. Peer support and supervision are also built into the process and afford additional benefits. Chat counsellor peers provide support both live and via email. For example, a Chat counsellor might request assistance in finding external resources. Email and chat supervision is primarily used as a postsupervisory and coaching tool.

Case Management

There are a number of case management issues Chat supervisors need to keep in mind when coaching counsellors. As Chat is principally a single session counselling model, supervisory goals differ somewhat from modalities that offer short-term counselling. For example, there would not be the same pacing for subsequent client sessions or as much emphasis on cultivating the therapeutic alliance. At the same time, text-based bonding and non-local presence remain relevant supervision themes.

The following are three main themes that have emerged from repeated supervisory experience:

1. *Adapting rapport building skills to text, including using a writing style that intentionally sets the tone.*
   Similar to e-counselling, mastering the nuances of telepresence as well as client-friendly language and 'voice' are essential skills for successful text-based counselling. Rapport building depends on the counsellor's capacity to convey empathy, encouragement, compassion and understanding. As stated by Mallen, Vogel, and Rochlen (2005), unless a counsellor can communicate effectively in writing, their in-person ability to transmit empathy is "irrelevant" (p. 787). Supervisors and counsellors work collaboratively to hone the essential text-based skills.

2. *Setting and maintaining an appropriate Chat pace.*
   The Chat world is a fast-paced one. Clients expect to hear from their counsellors within a relatively short period of time. For example, if a client does not see a response for 15 seconds, this can feel like the equivalent of a minute of "dead air" on the phone. Finding the balance between replying quickly and also giving clients time to consider what is being discussed (using text-based strategies) is an important element of synchronous practice. Furthermore, depending on the client's presenting issue and use of Chat, counsellors can have difficulty containing the Chat session to less than 60 minutes, as chat sessions – at least in our particular service – are not accorded a rigid time frame and counsellors report losing track of time while chatting.

3. *Containing the Chat.*
   Clients tend to discuss and review multiple issues over the course of one chat session. Suler (2004) introduced the concept of the online "disinhibition effect" that can take place when communicating remotely. Chat counsellors have needed to adapt their approach to contain the conversation. They have extensive experience reviewing a wide range of issues with clients on the phone. Nevertheless, Chat counsellors have noticed a significant increase in the nature and extent of client disclosure compared to their teleconsultations. Chat supervisors are in an ideal position to assist counsellors with these issues. Common case challenges can be anticipated and briefings offered during supervision. Supervision supports professional development, just as it does in other modalities, while providing targeted coaching to further enhance clinical acumen and expertise.

Risk Management

EAPs must consider protocols for responding to high-risk situations, and as a result, have specific safeguards and clinical procedures in place. Even though EAPs may inform their clients that Chat is inappropriate for risk/crisis, they must be prepared for all contingencies, including those clients who are at risk and who complete the online registration. Internal back-up systems and follow-up processes are required to provide at risk clients with clinical support. How and when Chat supervisors offer support to counsellors also play an important role in ensuring that proper procedure and clinical best practices are being followed. Shepell·fgi's Chat supervision structure for risk situations includes multiple supervisory and peer support options available 24/7.

e-Counselling

Shepell·fgi's e-counselling (EC) is an asynchronous, confidential, professional counselling service available to EFAP clients directly through a secure webboard. Shepell·fgi's e-counselling service was launched in 2000. The EC platform is located on secure internal servers and uses encryption software. Both clients and counsellors are required to enter their private login credentials each time they access e-counselling, and their exchanges are posted on (and retrieved from) a private conference area. Comprehensive systems, protocols, procedures and clinical practices are in place to ensure confidentiality and privacy protection.

From the onset, clinical supervision has remained a central feature of the e-counselling team's development and expansion. One of the benefits of the asynchronous e-counselling model is that supervision can be provided at any phase of the counselling process. In effect, the consultations can be multitemporal: before, during or after sessions. Since e-counsellors respond to client exchanges asynchronously, counsellors can review case management challenges with the supervisor before composing his or her reply. This provides a unique opportunity for mid-session supervision without any disruption of the primary process. Counsellor and supervisor have time "during" the virtual session to discuss any pertinent concerns. Supervisors can review counsellor drafts and make suggestions. Collaborative discussion (by telephone or email) can take place before the counsellor's letter is posted. Mid-case consultations review possible current interventions as well as future directions.

Counsellor Competencies

EAPs need to be conscientious when recruiting and hiring counselling professionals whose skill sets match e-counselling best practices. There are several specialized skills that make a significant difference to an e-counsellor's effectiveness. In addition to the previously noted core competencies, the following represent additional professional prerequisites for online practice.

1. Above average written communication skills.
2. Confidence and competence with technology.
3. Comfort with computer-mediated counselling.
4. Ability to effectively assess clients online.
5. Facility with text-based rapport building.
6. Experience with building relationships in an online environment.

Furthermore, Mallen, Vogel, and Rochlen (2005) noted one key factor in selecting e-counsellors (trainees) is their overall desire to participate in online counselling work. Those who report a true calling to this work, with a genuine love of reading and writing, an ability to "read between the lines," and convey empathy and interventions via text, are most likely to develop text-based clinical capacities. Candidates with this range of skills are more likely to successfully transition from F2F to text-based clinical delivery. By carefully choosing candidates who best suit the medium, clinical supervisors can then focus on honing the clinician's existing aptitudes.

Training and Supervision

Different EAPs offer a wide range of supervision and training. The following represent what this EFAP considers necessary investments in supporting online staff in order to maintain and enhance consistent clinical quality. Supervisors provide extensive training, mentoring and coaching. This supervision takes place primarily by email and telephone. With more experience, counsellors transition to the more typical formal and informal clinical supervision model. Enhanced clinical accountability improves quality assurance. Moreover, counsellors can access supervision and case consultation on an ad hoc basis.

We suggest three opportunities for supervision: (a) challenging case consults for supervisory support at intake and mid-case; (b) case review post-closure to refine methods and consider different text-based approaches as needed; and (c) counsellor management support for modality specific procedures, protocols, policies and best practices.

Moreover, counsellors may also access supervision and case consultation on an as-needed basis. Group training modules and quarterly teleconferences augment individual case consults and case reviews. Creating and maintaining a group listserve where counsellors can share resources and access peer support is also helpful. As with any clinical online contact, pre-established guidelines and protocols ensure privacy and confidentiality.

Counsellors attend regularly scheduled clinical supervision meetings and trainings via videoconference/teleconference. Online synchronous tools allow the manager, supervisors and e-counsellors to review shared documents. Web conferences are a supplementary means of professional development and in-service training. Both individual and group supervision offer diverse forms of counsellor support, including but not limited to case review, counsellor/supervisor identified priorities, client feedback, debriefing and ongoing orientation to EAP/e-counselling protocols. Supervision and training integrate examples of clinical best practices.

Important factors arise when clinical supervisors consider online methods for supervision. There are multiple nuances to fully understanding text-based communication (Mallen, Vogel, & Rochlen, 2005). The lack of spontaneous clarification in email is important to consider when providing feedback and consultation to counsellors (Speyer & Zack, 2003). As Anthony and Merz Nagel (2010) articulated, "conveying empathy and emotions through email text . . . is every bit as important in a clinical relationship as they are in the therapeutic relationship" (p. 129).

This highlights the need for supervisors providing supervision via online modes to have strong written communication competencies and a thorough understanding of potential challenges. Again, when supervision takes place via email, it is critical to ensure mutual understanding and clarity.

Dunn (2012) noted how "time to think" emerges as a critical theme in asynchronous online counselling. Likewise, email consultations between supervisor and supervisee confer similar advantages to the primary process between counsellors and clients. Counsellors and supervisors can compose their letters at any time during the day or evening. They also have time to reflect on the issues before responding. When needed, either the counsellor or the supervisor can initiate synchronous phone contact.

Case Management

Predominant client issues that may lead to case consults include risk of harm to self or others, extreme life situations, impasses in the therapeutic alliance, client resistance or special needs and presenting problems that appear intractable in the scope of short-term EAP counselling. With regard to counsellor management, areas of discussion that may emerge in supervision include the need to pay close attention to the client's text, practicing client-friendly language and tone of "voice," maintaining a consistent online framework and parameters, and mastering the nuances of telepresence and feeling tone in text.

Online counselling supervision is enhanced by the supervisor's access to client and counsellor exchanges. Importantly, supervision does not depend on the counsellor's report. There is direct access to the verbatim conversation. Session dialogue is accessible via webboard transcripts. When appropriate, supervisors can read session exchanges and acquire a comprehensive understanding of what transpired. There are many benefits of accessing counsellor session exchanges to identify clinical themes and interventions for discussion (Mallen, Vogel, & Rochlen, 2005; Yaphe & Speyer, 2010b).

Risk Management

As previously discussed, EAPs must bear in mind how they will respond to clients assessed for high risk. It is critical to develop a coordinated system whereby these cases can be managed in a seamless way, both at intake and mid-session. Although the EC website clearly states exclusion criteria (including clients presenting with imminent risk or predominant addiction issues), the reader will likely not be surprised to learn that, nevertheless, there are clients at risk who continue registering for the e-counselling service. The importance of having predefined protocols in place to be operationalized for crisis intervention cannot be overestimated.

One of the advantages that EAPs have with regard to risk management is their multifaceted internal resources, systems and procedures. These confer supplementary support to supervisors, counsellors and clients. Due to the asynchronous nature of the exchanges, timely consultation and guidance can be provided to counsellors. Moreover, supervisors and counsellors have the opportunity to work closely together to ensure client safety is the highest priority. E-counselling programs have successfully managed and contained diverse client risk issues.

Given significant risk issues (outside the scope of e-counselling), EAPs can ensure that their call centre supervisors and call centre clinical counsellors are trained to triage e-service needs and respond to clients offline. An example of this process would be when call centre counsellors initiate outreach telephone calls to clients for further assessment, intervention and modality change as needed.

Video Counselling

A wide range of individual, group and health care practitioners already offer video counselling (VC) to their clients. EAPs have a unique opportunity to utilize pre-existing infrastructure and resources when expanding their service delivery. Shepell·fgi developed and launched video counselling as a core clinical service in 2011. In their model, clients require only modest technical abilities to successfully participate in video counselling, making it accessible to most. Client and counsellor communicate using a webcam, landline and encrypted custom Internet software through which both parties can see and hear each other. They can also share and create documents in real-time. In the Shepell·fgi model, given the sensitive nature of a clinical session, clients are encouraged to use their home personal computers instead of conducting sessions from their work environment.

Supervision delivery was a significant component of video counselling development and implementation. EAPs have the choice to recruit and train from within, and/or to specifically search for counsellors with previous video counselling experience.

Counsellor Competencies

Experienced Shepell·fgi EFAP face-to-face counsellors with proven clinical skills were recruited as video counsellors. The counsellors who were chosen demonstrated the following aptitudes:

1. Keen interest in delivering VC,
2. Confidence with technology,
3. Curiosity to learn new skills as they adapt to the medium, and
4. Ability to navigate the system, have tolerance for computer glitches, and troubleshoot when needed.

Training and Supervision

Matching supervisor skills with the specific mode of online delivery is an important consideration. The supervisor should be a counselling professional who understands the clinical and operational nuances of the medium and can support their team by providing counsellor training, supervision, and consultation. To facilitate the transfer of clinical skills to the video environment, the counsellors were provided with intensive individual supervision and consultation. Before meeting his or her first client, a VC counsellor has already conducted multiple practice session simulations during training. Thereafter, supervision takes place postsession to discuss:

1. Relevant clinical issues,
2. Assessment of comfort level of the client with the technology,

3. Assessment of comfort level of the counsellor with the technology, and
4. Trouble shooting any technical issues.

As with any supervision, as counsellor skills mature, the shape of supervision will adapt to the individual learning curve.

Video conferencing and telephone are often ideal modes of communication for individual training. For subsequent supervision, secure email is preferred for standard administrative or simple clinical protocol questions. Telephone is used for more urgent and serious issues, such as a duty to report or high-risk circumstances. One valuable teaching tool that promotes clinical best practice and accountability is group supervision. Video conferencing is an ideal forum for counsellors to share their knowledge, observation, and experiences. It is an additional opportunity for VC counsellors to become increasingly comfortable with the technology and to learn together as a team. Anecdotal EFAP Video counsellor feedback supports Nelson, Nichter, and Henriksen (2010) research (comparing F2F and online supervision in a counselling internship) that found online group supervision was a valued and helpful experience. The group supervision provided the necessary peer and supervisor feedback and established a safe and trusting online environment.

Case Management

In conjunction with clinical subjects, individual and group supervision often cover modality specific issues. Predictably, case management themes unique to video counselling emerged and were reviewed in supervision. Basic logistics regarding session set-up when there is more than one client was also discussed (e.g., couples/families in the same or different locations).

For example, boundary setting is paramount. Counsellors have observed that clients do not always initiate the video counselling sessions in private. Moreover, they do not necessarily mention this to their counsellor at the beginning of the session. Clients typically access video counselling from home, and another person or children might be present, yet out of the counsellor's visual field. In one scenario, 30 minutes into their session, a video counsellor realized that her client's spouse was sitting on the other side of the couch. Counsellors are encouraged during training to ask specific questions about the variables of home environment, privacy, noise, etc. There is an additional learning process that takes place when counsellors face these challenges live, rather than theoretically.

Risk Management and Supervision

Although client exclusion criteria include imminent risk, child protection issues, and current drug/alcohol addiction, clients sometimes choose to not disclose these factors at intake. These issues might emerge mid-session. The importance of developing strong risk management protocols cannot be overestimated. Similarly to other modalities, counsellors are required to notify their supervisor/manager of any imminent risk issues. Furthermore, the VC manager is available for risk and nonrisk consultations on an ad hoc basis.

There are generally two circumstances when EAP clients might benefit from a counselling modality change. The first relates to VC functionality (such as a client experiencing ongoing technical issues/discomfort or lack of privacy). Secondly, counsellors may proactively recommend F2F counselling for specific clinical issues (e.g., imminent risk, child protection issues, addiction or complex concerns). At the same time, there have been circumstances when VC counsellors were in an optimal position to provide mid-session clinical support in ways not replicable by more traditional face-to-face settings.

CONCLUSION

The combination of ongoing technical innovation and increasing comfort with nonlocal professional interventions will likely lead to a growing demand for and access to online counselling. With the growth of online counselling services comes the professional and ethical need for guidelines, protocols, and therapeutic processes to be consistently maintained and developed. Specialized supervision plays a key role in fostering clinical best practices. Both online service providers and supervisors have the responsibility and opportunity to keep informed of online service models and methods, so they can collectively hone their knowledge and skills to meet "state of the art" standards.

According to Merz Nagel and Riley (2010), "Online supervision should not be viewed as inferior. On the contrary, distance supervision via technology will allow access to skilled experts and clinical supervisors across the globe" (p. 211). The authors believe that along with other online clinical providers, EAPs have important contributions to make to the growing field of online modalities and the supervision that supports quality assurance in this rapidly evolving field.

REFERENCES

Anthony, K., & Goss, S. (2009). *Guidelines for online counselling and psychotherapy, including guidelines for online supervision* (3rd ed.). Lutterworth: British Association for Counselling and Psychotherapy.

Anthony, K., & Merz Nagel, D. (2010). *Therapy online: A practical guide*. London: Sage.

Barak, A, Hen L., Boniel-Nissim, M., & Shapire, N. (2008). A comprehensive review and a meta-analysis of the effectiveness of internet-based psychotherapeutic interventions. *Journal of Technology in Human Services, 26*(2), 109–160. doi: 10.1080/15228830802094429.

Coursol, D. H., Lewis, J., & Seymour, J. W. (2010). The use of videoconferencing to enrich counselor training and supervision. In K. Anthony, D. Nagel, & S. Goss (Eds.), *The use of technology in mental health: Applications, ethics and practice* (pp. 280–288). Springfield, IL: Charles C Thomas.

DeLeon, P., & Folen, R. (2010). Foreword. In R. Kraus, G. Stricker, & C. Speyer (Eds.), *Online counselling: A handbook for mental health professionals* (2nd ed.) (pp. ix–xvi). San Diego, CA: Elsevier Inc.

Dunn, K. (2012). A qualitative investigation into the online counselling relationship: To meet or not to meet, that is the question. *Counselling and Psychotherapy Research: Linking research with practice, 12*(4), 316–326. doi: 10.1080 /14733145.2012.669772.

EASNA. (2009). *The value of employee assistance programs.* Retrieved from http:// www.easna.org.

Finn, J., & Barak, A. (2010). A descriptive study of e-counsellor attitudes, ethics, and practice. *Counselling and Psychotherapy Research: Linking Research with Practice, 10*(4), 268-277. doi: 10.1080/14733140903380847.

Groman, M. (2010). The use of telephone to enrich counselor training and supervision. In K. Anthony, D. Nagel, & S. Goss (Eds.), *The use of technology in mental health: Applications, ethics and practice* (pp. 269–279). Springfield, IL: Charles C Thomas.

Gros, D. F., Yoder, M., Tuerk, P. W., Lozano, B. E., & Acierno, R. (2011). Exposure therapy for PTSD delivered to veterans via telehealth: Predictors of treatment completion and outcome and comparison to treatment delivered in person. *Behavior Therapy, 42*(2), 276-283. doi: 10.1016/j.beth.2010.07.005.

Mallen, M. J., Vogel, D. L., & Rochlen, A. B. (2005). The practical aspects of online counseling: Ethics, training, technology, and competency. *The Counseling Psychologist, 33*(6), 776-818. doi: 10.1177/001100000 5278625.

Mallen, M. J., Vogel, D. L., Rochlen, A. B., & Day, S. X. (2005). Online counseling: Reviewing the literature from a counseling psychology framework. *The Counseling Psychologist, 33*(6), 819-887. doi: 10.1177/00 11000005278624.

Merz Nagel, D., & Riley, S. (2010). Using chat and instant messaging (IM) to enrich counselor training and supervision. In K. Anthony, D. Nagel, & S. Goss (Eds.), *The use of technology in mental health: Applications, ethics and practice* (pp. 206–212). Springfield, IL: Charles C Thomas.

Nelson, J. A., Nichter, M., & Henriksen, R. (2010). On-line supervision and face-to-face supervision in the counseling internship: An exploratory study of similarities and differences. Retrieved from http:// counselingoutfitters.com/vistas /vistas10/ Article_46.pdf.

Richardson, L. K., Frueh, B. C., Grubaugh, A. L., Egede, L., & Elhai, J. D. (2009). Current directions in videoconferencing tele-mental health research. *Clinical Psychology: Science and Practice, 16*, 323–338.

Speyer, C., & Zack, J. (2003). Online counselling: Beyond the pros and cons. *Psychologica Magazine, 23*(2), 11–14.

Stretch, L. S., Nagel, D., & Anthony, K. (2013). Ethical framework for the use of technology in supervision. *Therapeutic Innovations in Light of Technology, 3*(2), 37–44. Retrieved from http://onlinetherapyinstitute .com/2013/01/tilt-magazine-issue-13.

Suler, J. (2004). The online disinhibition effect. *CyberPsychology & Behavior, 7*(3), 321–326.

Wheeler, S., & Richards, K. (2007). The impact of clinical supervision on counsellors and therapists, their practice and their clients. A systematic review of the literature. *Counselling and Psychotherapy Research: Linking Research with Practice, 7*(1), 54–65. doi: 10.1080/14733140601185274.

Yaphe, J., & Speyer, C. (2010a). Clinical skills for online counseling: Text-based online counseling: Email. In R. Kraus, G. Stricker, & C. Speyer (Eds.), (2010). *Online counselling: A handbook for mental health professionals* (2nd ed.), (pp. 147–167). San Diego, CA: Elsevier.

Yaphe, J., & Speyer, C. (2010b). Using email to enrich counselor training supervision. In K. Anthony, D. Nagel, & S. Goss (Eds.), *The use of technology in mental health: Applications, ethics and practice* (pp. 194–205). Springfield, IL: Charles C Thomas.

Yuen, E. K., Goetter, E. M., Herbert, J. D., & Forman, E. M. (2012). Challenges and opportunities in internet-mediated telemental health. *Profession Psychology: Research and Practice, 43*(1), 1–8. doi: 10.1037/a0025524.

Chapter 32

THE USE OF TECHNOLOGY IN CLINICAL SUPERVISION: A CASE REPORT FROM CAPE FEAR CLINIC

Jennifer Askew Buxton and John Devaney

INTRODUCTION

The Cape Fear Clinic (referred to as "CFC" or just as "the clinic" here) is a nonprofit clinic that has served low-income and uninsured patients in southeastern North Carolina for 22 years. The clinic's mission is to provide compassionate and affordable patient-centered health care to low income individuals and families in the Cape Fear region, regardless of ability to pay. Our Charity-Care qualified patients do not have any form of health insurance or government health assistance and have incomes of no more than 200% of Federal Poverty Guidelines (at the time of writing, $23,550 for a household of four people; U.S. Dept. of Health and Human Services, 2013). CFC serves all without regard to race, religion, gender, ethnicity, national origin, religion, disability or sexual orientation. Since its inception, the clinic has expanded its service offerings from the provision of basic primary care services on a first-come, first-served basis one evening per week to providing both primary care and specialty services on weekdays during both daytime and evening hours. In addition to providing medical services, the clinic provides dental services and operates an onsite pharmacy to ensure clinic patients' access to prescribed medications. The pharmacy stocks a comprehensive formulary of inexpensive medications and medications obtained for individual patients through patient assistance programs. Under an affiliation agreement between the clinic and a local health system, patients receive referral-based laboratory, radiology and other diagnostic services. The clinic's budget consists entirely of grants, donations and money collected through fundraising. In 2012, 385 volunteers worked a total of 17,215 hours at the clinic. All services and medications provided by the clinic and its affiliates are free of charge to all of the clinic's patients.

In 2004, it was determined that the clinic's patient population had an increasing need of mental health care services not available in the community. There were no services available to enable basic interventions (e.g., psychotherapy, medication therapy) for mild-to-moderate anxiety, depression and other mental health disorders among indigent, particularly Spanish-speaking, patients. Services for severe mental illness continued to be available through local crisis services, the psychiatric unit at the local health-system and the Local Management Entity (LME) and other mental health resources for the severely mentally ill.

State funding for community-based outpatient treatment of anxiety, depression and other mental health disorders in the indigent and uninsured patient population of southeastern North Carolina had been lost over the prior decade due to budget cuts, resulting in a widening of gaps in care. As a result, the clinic sought out mental health professionals to assist with patients' mental health care needs and founded the mental health clinic program in 2004 to ensure that mental health was addressed as a vital component of comprehensive health care.

The mental health care clinic was founded by a clinical psychologist. The initial stages of the clinic's operation were tedious and time-consuming, as mental health providers were required to consult with the clinic's volunteer physicians and nurse practitioners to obtain prescription medications for their patients. Due to the clinic's use of volunteer providers, the same providers were not available for consultation at each clinic session, resulting in a lack of continuity of care. In an effort to increase the efficiency and quality of care, a pharmacist volunteering in the clinic's pharmacy proposed the development of a collaborative practice model (CPM) to better meet the mental health needs of the clinic's patients.

Clinic Description

In 2006, a collaborative practice agreement was established between the volunteer pharmacist and the clinic's medical director (a practicing physician). In accordance with state laws, the pharmacist obtained a Clinical Pharmacist Practitioner (CPP) license from the state boards of pharmacy and medicine (NC Board of Pharmacy, 2013). Licensure as a CPP allowed the pharmacist to participate in patient interviews with the clinic's psychologist, provide individual patient appointments, and prescribe medications based on the physician's diagnosis and the psychologist's assessment. Under the terms of the collaborative

practice agreement (henceforth "CPP protocol"), the overseeing physician is required to review all clinic notes and endorse the pharmacist's medication recommendations. At the time of writing, there were 187 actively practicing CPPs in North Carolina, and the CPP protocol discussed here was the only such agreement in the specialty area of outpatient mental health (NC Medical Board, 2013); to our knowledge, the pharmacist at the Cape Fear Clinic Mental Health Clinic was one of only three CPPs in North Carolina practicing in the area of mental health and the other two clinicians were working in inpatient settings.

The mental health clinic, which has now been in operation for more than nine years, is run almost exclusively by volunteers. The clinic currently provides mental health services three Wednesday evenings per month. The staff includes two doctorate-level psychologists, one residency-trained doctor of pharmacy, and the psychiatrist who oversees the CPP protocol. Several non-doctorate-level counselors provide various forms of psychotherapy. The supervised and nonlicensed volunteer staff of the mental health clinic include: graduate and postgraduate psychology students, pharmacy students, pharmacy residents, and psychology practitioners in need of supervised clinical practice hours. The clinic's administrative staff is composed of undergraduate and graduate psychology students and a coordinator with previous experience as a social worker and university administrator. All services provided by the clinic are offered in both English and Spanish, as many of the practitioners and support staff are bilingual.

With the addition of a volunteer psychiatrist to the care team in January of 2012, supervision of the pharmacist was transferred from the medical director to the psychiatrist. Through the receipt of a grant in 2011, the clinical pharmacist was hired as the full-time Deputy Director, Pharmacy Services. Addition of the pharmacist to clinic staff allowed for the expansion of patient access to mental health services and support as this clinician maintains availability for patient appointments during most weekdays.

Program Description

The clinic's mental health program is structured to provide four major service types: initial evaluation, psychotherapy only, medication management only and psychotherapy plus medication management (Figure 1; Buxton, Chandler-Altendorf, & Puente, 2012). Once a referral is made and acceptance to the clinic is established, patients participate in a comprehensive initial interview conducted jointly by a doctorate-level clinical psychologist and the clinical pharmacist or by the clinic psychiatrist. Initial interviews generally last one hour and conclude with a suggested diagnosis followed by discussion and initial implementation of the most feasible treatment plan. Patients with difficult-to-diagnose conditions or disease states with unclear etiologies receive a more comprehensive evaluation, which includes psychological or neuro-psychological testing if deemed appropriate by the psychologist or psychiatrist who conducts the initial interview.

Current evidence suggests that the optimal management of many mental health conditions includes both psychotherapy and medication management (Cuijpers, van Straten, Warmerdam, & Andersson, 2009; Gorman, 2003; Solomon, Keitner, Rayn, Kelley, & Miller, 2008). Most patients referred to the mental health clinic receive psychotherapy in conjunction with pharmacotherapy. Psychotherapy is provided by licensed psychologists and counselors. The medications most commonly prescribed to clinic patients include selective serotonin-reuptake inhibitors, serotonin–norepinephrine-reuptake inhibitors, and atypical antipsychotics. Medications are selected according to American Psychiatric Association (APA) treatment guidelines and drug availability (American Psychiatric Association, 2013).

Patients receiving pharmacotherapy attend periodic visits with the pharmacist and psychologist or the psychiatrist for ongoing evaluation of the efficacy of the chosen medication

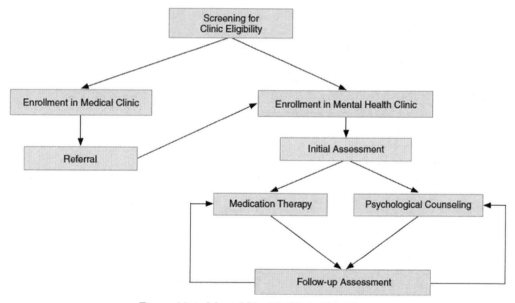

Figure 32.1. Mental Health Clinic Flowchart.

regimen (as determined via laboratory testing; patient interviews, testing, and examination; and reference to APA guidelines); these visits occur every two weeks after the initiation of medication therapy and continue through the acute phase of treatment. Once the patient has transitioned to the maintenance phase of therapy, follow-up visits occur every three to six months. Patients receiving medications that require laboratory monitoring (e.g., assessment of valproic acid levels during divalproex therapy, lipid analysis during the use of an atypical antipsychotic) are referred to a local health system for appropriate testing in accordance with treatment guidelines and medication package inserts. The results of the laboratory tests are transferred to the mental health clinic and included in the patient's medical records for interpretation by the pharmacist, psychologist, and/or supervising psychiatrist.

Patient Population

From 2010 through 2012, over 1000 mental health appointments were provided to indigent and uninsured patients by the mental health clinic staff. All patients seen in the mental health clinic must undergo the standard intake process at the medical clinic, where specialists conduct interviews and review financial documents and insurance information to verify eligibility for clinic services. Uninsured patients who meet the financial criteria described above are qualified to receive care at the clinic. In addition to the qualifications described previously, some patients must meet other criteria before receiving services at the mental health clinic. Patients with comorbid substance abuse disorders are required to actively participate in a substance abuse treatment program at one of several local agencies in order to be eligible for mental health clinic services at the clinic. Patients who are actively suicidal or psychotic are ineligible for mental health clinic

services because immediate access to the high-level services required for this patient population is unavailable at the clinic; these patients are immediately referred to crisis management services or the local health-system's inpatient psychiatric hospital or emergency department.

All patients are required to sign an informed consent agreement and contract with the mental health clinic before their first appointment. The contract discusses patient confidentiality in addition to outlining patient and provider expectations. Patients who break their contract by missing appointments without notifying clinic staff in a timely manner, refusing treatment, or engaging in inappropriate behavior are dismissed from the mental health clinic and discharged from the program and/or are sent back to the medical clinic for reevaluation, depending on the circumstances of the dismissal. All expectations are thoroughly reviewed with patients prior to their engagement in clinic services.

Psychological Testing

The purpose of the testing conducted at the mental health clinic is twofold. First, testing is used for diagnostic purposes. Psychological testing and neuropsychological testing are completed to facilitate diagnosis and to acquire standardized data for the patient's records. Testing is done by graduate psychology students or testing technicians. The tests used at the clinic include those typically used in an outpatient psychology practice, such as the Wechsler Adult Intelligence Scale (Wechsler, 1997); Trail-Making Test (Reitan & Wolfson, 1993); Mini-Mental State Examination (Folstein, Folstein, & McHugh, 1975); and Minnesota Multiphasic Personality Inventory (Butcher et al., 2001). In addition, clinic providers often administer the 12-item Short-Form Health Survey (SF-12; Ware, Kosinski, & Keller, 1996); the Alcohol Use Disorders Identification Test (AUDIT; Babor, Higgins-Biddle,

Saunders, & Monteiro, 2001); and the Patient Health Questionnaire for depression (PHQ-9; Kroenke & Spitzer, 2002). In each case, a report is generated by the student or testing technician and reviewed by a doctorate-level provider.

Secondly, testing is used as a means of monitoring and documenting treatment outcomes. Data is gathered during the initial clinic appointment to provide an overall picture of the patient's current physical and mental health status. Data is also gathered throughout the course of patients' care to enable the evaluation of the patient's response to therapy and guide future treatment. Data quantifying the estimated value of services provided and the associated staff time demands are also periodically compiled. A snapshot analysis of patient population characteristics, patient response to therapy and quantitative description of services provided has been published previously (Buxton et al., 2012).

Psychotherapy

Psychotherapy is provided by staff members fluent in English and Spanish, as well as Portuguese. There are male and female therapists, as well as doctorate- and master's-level clinicians; differing expertise areas of each clinician allows the clinic to offer a blend of specialty areas such as brain injury and dementia, pediatrics, depression, family therapy and substance abuse. In most cases, therapy is provided in 30-minute increments.

On average, each individual is seen once or twice per month. Each evening, psychotherapy services are offered, 15 to 20 patients are seen at the clinic. The typical intervention is cognitive-behavioral therapy, though some of the master's-level clinicians prefer client-centered interventions. Every effort is made to ensure that the responsible clinician's skills and personality are well suited to addressing an individual patient's problems. Each patient participating in medication management

services is seen every two to three months for evaluation of response to medication therapy. Medication management consultations are also provided on a more or less frequent basis as necessary.

Supervision

According to North Carolina statute 21 NCAC 46.3101, "the CPP written agreement shall include a plan and schedule for weekly quality control, review, and countersignature of all orders written by the CPP in a face-to-face conference between the physician and CPP" (NC Board of Pharmacy, 2013). Unlike psychology supervision, which occurs in person, much of the CPP supervision by the psychiatrist is completed in a virtual environment. As the clinic's volunteer psychiatrist attends clinic once per month, this supervision occurs in person during that week. In alternate weeks, the psychiatrist and clinical pharmacist practitioner engage in supervision via voice over Internet Protocol, or VoIP. The providers schedule a predetermined, mutually available meeting time and log into the service to meet face-to-face via Internet web conference. This process allows for the provision of supervision without requiring the volunteer psychiatrist to travel to the clinic site during weeks when direct patient care is not being provided by the psychiatrist. Patient cases are reviewed and overall clinic quality assurance processes are handled during this meeting. Both providers are available for consultation of one another via phone and text throughout the work week, adding an additional level of supervisory support.

This process has allowed the providers to carve out time during their regular work week activities for the supervision required by the CPP agreement. This arrangement also allows for increased access to prescription refills and patient assistance program medications for patients primarily managed by the psychiatrist. When a medication refill is needed or medication arrives at the clinic for a patient of the psychiatrist, the CPP can review the psychiatrist's clinical notes and care plan and provide the medication sent by the pharmaceutical company, if indicated. Patients are also instructed to contact the CPP with concerns regarding side-effects or lack of efficacy with their medication regiments. These patients' cases are also discussed in the supervisory encounters and plans of care are modified and additional patient appointments are schedule as needed. The CPP's clinical documentation is made available for countersignature in written form, with delivery to the psychiatrist's practice site via courier, or electronically. With the impending implementation of the clinic's electronic health record (EHR), documents may also be made available to the psychiatrist for countersignature via the EHR service.

Technology Implementation

In preparation for the implementation of the EHR (Allscripts Pro Suite), changes mandated by the Patient Protection and Affordable Care Act (commonly known as the Affordable Care Act (ACA or "Obamacare"), and plans to become a "hybrid" charitable clinic (accepting both charity-care patients and those with a payer source, such as Medicaid, Medicare, or private insurance), the clinic has upgraded our technological infrastructure.

Beginning with rewiring and enabling secure wireless signals between the three separate buildings on the campus, clinic administration then upgraded the server systems and established a high-speed T-1 data line that is capable of handling the traffic of the VoIP telephone system, the EHR, and future telehealth applications.

The clinic then upgraded all workstations and exam rooms with computers that are equipped with internal cameras, microphones, and speakers. These workstations are already in use to allow the face-to-face supervision in

the mental health program and are intended to be deployed in medical examination rooms to allow for real-time, face-to-face interaction of our providers and patients with interpreters and other healthcare providers in other locations as well.

Nonclinical Supervision

The Executive Director of the clinic meets with the President of the Board of Directors via video link for regular face-to-face meetings and the clinic has the ability for board members to utilize video link to join in Board Meetings when they cannot physically be present. A video link is also available to have face-to-face meetings between supervisor/supervisee and colleagues throughout our three-building campus, encouraging ease of communication between staff without physically leaving their individual workspace.

CONCLUSION

At the time of writing, the clinic has begun the initial use of the electronic record; and it is expected that, over the course of the next 12 months, remote, professional interpreters will be used on a daily basis. Currently, a limited number of Spanish-English bilingual staff and volunteers provide interpretation services, adding more work for staff and volunteers and creating barriers in access to care for patients whose primary language is not English.

The addition of remote interpretation (provided by professional, certified interpreters, in a setting where the provider, patient, and off-site interpreter can all see, hear, and interact with each other) will increase the ability of the clinic to accept and provide appropriate care to patients whose primary language can be virtually any spoken in the world.

As the clinic becomes more proficient in the utilization of technology to enhance the on-site healthcare provided, it will become possible to host students and residents requiring face-to-face supervision, where allowed by statute or professional standards. The first place this student supervision will be implemented is the mental health program where the already established supervision between the psychiatrist and CPP will be expanded to include other mental health disciplines and students seeking Licensed Professional Counselor (LPC) certification and/or other therapeutic credentials.

REFERENCES

American Psychiatric Association. (2013). Clinical practice guidelines. Retrieved from www.psychiatry.org/practice/clinical-practice-guidelines.

Babor, T. F., Higgins-Biddle, J. C., Saunders, J. B., & Monteiro, M. G. (2001). *AUDIT: The Alcohol Use Disorders Identification Test—Guidelines for use in primary care* (2nd ed.). Geneva: World Health Organization.

Butcher, J. N., Dahlstrom, W. G., Graham, J. R., Ben-Porath, Y. S., Tellegen, A., Dahlstrom, W. G., & Kaemmer, B. (2001). *MMPI-2 (Minnesota Multiphasic Personality Inventory-2): Manual for administration, scoring, and interpretation* (Rev. ed.). Minneapolis, MN: University of Minnesota Press.

Buxton, J. A., Chandler-Altendorf, A., & Puente, A. E. (2012). A novel collaborative practice model for treatment of mental illness in indigent and uninsured patients. *American Journal of Health-System Pharmacy, 69*(12), 1054–62.

Cuijpers, P., van Straten, A., Warmerdam, L., & Andersson, G. (2009). Psychotherapy versus the combination of psychotherapy and pharmacotherapy in the treatment of depression: A meta-analysis. *Depression and Anxiety, 26*(3), 279–288.

Folstein, M. F., Folstein, S. E., & McHugh, P. R. (1975). "Mini-mental state:" A practical method for grading the cognitive state of patients for the clinician. *Journal of Psychiatric Research, 12*(3), 189–198.

Gorman, J. M. (2003). A complimentary relationship: Psychotherapy and medication for anxiety and depressive disorders (Editorial). *CNS Spectrums, 8*, 326.

Kroenke, K., & Spitzer, R. L. (2002). The PHQ-9: A new depression diagnostic and severity measure. *Psychiatric Annals, 32*(9), 509–15.

North Carolina Board of Pharmacy. (2013). *North Carolina Administrative Code Pharmacy Rules.* Retrieved from http://www.ncbop.org/LawsRules/Rules.pdf.

North Carolina Board of Pharmacy. (2013).Clinical Pharmacist Practitioners. Retrieved from www.ncbop.org/pharmacists _cpp.htm.

North Carolina Medical Board. (2013). *NCMB licensee search.* Retrieved from wwwapps.ncmedboard.org/Clients/NCBOM/Public/LicenseeInformation Results.aspx.

Reitan, R. M., & Wolfson, D. (1993). *The Halstead-Reitan Neuropsychological Test Battery: Theory and clinical interpretation* (2nd ed.). Tucson, AZ: Neuropsychology Press.

Solomon, D. A., Keitner, G. I., Ryan, C. E., Kelley, J., & Miller, I. W. (2008). Preventing recurrence of bipolar I mood episodes and hospitalizations: Family psychotherapy plus pharmacotherapy versus pharmacotherapy alone. *Bipolar Disorders, 10*, 798–805. doi:10.1016/j.jad.2006.05.036.

U. S. Department of Health and Human Services, Office of the Assistant Secretary of Planning and Evaluation. (2013). *2013 Poverty Guidelines.* Retrieved from http://aspe.hhs.gov/poverty/13poverty.cfm#thresholds.

Ware, J., Jr., Kosinski, M., & Keller, S. D. (1996). A 12-item Short-Form Health Survey: Construction of scales and preliminary tests of reliability and validity. *Medical Care, 34*(3), 220–233.

Wechsler, D. (1997). *Wechsler Adult Intelligence Scale* (3rd ed.) (WAIS-3). San Antonio, TX: Harcourt Assessment.

Chapter 33

SUPERVISION IN PRIVATE PRACTICE

Anne Stokes

INTRODUCTION

Supervision throughout one's therapeutic career is a professional requirement in some countries, while others see it as solely necessary during training. Systematic reviews of supervision literature show that very little is actually known about the practice of distance supervision (Wheeler, Aveline, & Barkham, 2011) and this applies to an even greater extent to independent online supervision.

In the context of online therapy, whether or not it is demanded by regulating bodies, online supervision is essential. When working face to face, therapists usually have contact locally with fellow practitioners, to whom they can turn for support, information and advice. Working online practitioners can be or perceive themselves to be more isolated without support; therefore, online supervision becomes hugely important to ensure the well-being of both counsellor and client.

In this chapter, consideration is given to supervision in private practice, rather than of private practice – i.e., the supervisor is in private practice. It does not follow that the supervisee is also in independent practice, though they may be. Ways of conducting online supervision will be discussed including advantages and disadvantages. Initially, pros and cons of a private online supervision practice itself are noted.

Why Supervise Online in Private Practice?

There are two aspects to this question: (a) why supervise online and (b) why do this in independent practice? While not ignoring the first question, the emphasis here is on working independently. Elsewhere in this book, therapeutic advantages of supervising online have been demonstrated, including the ability to parallel the context of client work. As early as 1997, there were experiments in online supervision for social workers in the U.S. (Stofle & Hamilton, 1998).

The advantages of online supervision in private practice can be seen in relationship to both supervisor and supervisee. The supervisee is able to choose from a wider range of supervisors and is not restricted to a geographic area. This is particularly useful if the supervisee works with a specific client group (Jones & Stokes, 2009). For online supervisees, there is a practical advantage in being able to enhance skills and technology awareness through receiving expert supervision online that may not be available in person locally (Evans, 2009).

For the supervisor, there is considerable freedom in working independently. Choices can be made in arranging one's schedule – how many supervisees to take, which days or hours to work and the greater ability to manage a flexible schedule to accommodate both the supervisor and the supervisee. The disadvantage of this freedom to can be that the supervisor becomes overaccommodating and allows the schedule to control the supervisor rather than the other way around.

There are also choices in fee structures. Instead of being salaried with no flexibility, supervisors may offer different fees to different supervisees – trainees, beginning counsellors, mature therapists, counsellors working as volunteers, etc. This is not to suggest that there ought to be different structure, but simply to demonstrate the greater freedom to do so.

There is also freedom to choose one's supervisees and play to one's strengths, develop new areas of interest, and supervise a mixture of 'ages and stages' of online practitioners. Another freedom is the ability to offer group or individual online supervision, and keep to a preferred way of working (synchronously or asynchronously) or offer a mixture.

Having outlined these advantages, there are also disadvantages. As mentioned, supervising in private practice can be isolating. Practitioners need to develop online communities and engage in online supervision of supervision when possible. Often supervisors in private practice are poor at pacing themselves, certainly in initial stages of establishing themselves. They find that they work with supervisees early in the morning and late into the evening, particularly if working across time zones. This may suit some practitioners, leaving them blocks of time during the day to be away from the computer.

However, the temptation is to fill those hours in between and burn out. One of the reasons that this can be a temptation is that online supervision is still a comparatively new discipline. Independent practitioners can find themselves accepting all requests for supervision, just in case the market dries up and their income dwindles. This is a genuine concern, but can lead to unethical practice.

Finally, while many practitioners enjoy avoiding the shackles and restrictions of working within an organisation, independent practice does not suit everyone. There is no 'organisational buffer.' The supervisor does not have the weight of the organisation in terms of back-up in professional, ethical, and legal dilemmas. The supervisor make the decisions and carries the responsibility for the decisions.

As a practitioner in private practice, supervisors have the responsibility for the storage of data on the individual's computer. Once supervisor has developed protocols to ensure data confidentiality, the protocols must be followed, since as Cavanagh, Shapiro, and Zack (2003) suggest, protocols are only as good as their implementation. Supervisors do not have an IT or legal department to ensure both good practice and compliance to legal requirements. There needs to be an awareness of the regulatory bodies that govern the supervisory work. For example in England, as an online supervisor, supervisors would almost certainly need to be registered with the Information Commissioner. Therefore, supervisors need to check out what is needed in the country in which supervision is provided.

Ways of Conducting Online Supervision

There are parallels between the conduct of online therapy and online supervision, even though they have a different emphasis. There is synchronous and asynchronous supervision, and within the former, there are the possibilities of text, voice or video. Before looking at these different possibilities, supervisors and supervises need to work in as technologically safe a way as is possible. So whatever version of online supervision is undertaken, individual computers and folders should be securely password protected, as well as utilise encrypted means of communicating (Stretch, Nagel, & Anthony, 2013).

Some online supervisors and supervisees use the same mode of communication in supervision as in the supervisee's client work. So if the supervisee works by text, the supervision would take place via text. If the clinical work is by video link, then the supervision would happen via video as well. Of course, many supervisees do use several online methods of working with clients, so the mode of communication may be multimodal.

Supervisee should send a list of clients and a brief update on the number of sessions, and clinical issues on a regular basis to the supervisor, as not all clients are likely to be discussed in each session whether by email or in real time. This enables the supervisor to have a better understanding of the clinical work and can help the supervisor spot any issues that are being missed and need to be brought into supervision. In some countries or states, the supervisor may have a legal accountability for her supervisee's work, rather than just a professional responsibility towards the supervisee and clients. In such a context, it is not just good practice to have this overview, but imperative.

An example of how this might be laid out is below. The supervisee sent the follow, "I've had 13 sessions since last supervision and have listed these here [Figure 33.1]. It's low because of Christmas and New Year holidays. Lots of clients decided to not come during that period."

Some supervisees might also choose to say something about what is going on in a more general way, particularly if the supervision is by text, where unlike voice/video supervision, there may be less opportunity for relationship building and context setting. Additional pieces of information that may be useful for the supervisee to report to the supervisor in writing are

1. Where I am professionally,
2. My health, and/or
3. Things from my nonprofessional life that may affect my work.

Asynchronous Online Supervision

Asynchronous supervision can happen in a variety of ways and exactly how the independent supervisor contracts with supervisee will depend on the preferences of both parties. There should be a statement in the initial contract outlining the agreed method, which should be reviewed from time to time and adaptions made.

The most common supervisory exchange is through email. One method is through the straightforward exchange of one email from the supervisee and a response from the supervisor. This would constitute one online supervision session. In other contracts, there might be two or more exchanges in a given period, together forming one supervision session. While this imparts a more dynamic sense to the work, it is much harder to cost, as the amount of time needed will vary from session to session. It is also less easy for the supervisor to plan how much time is needed each week or a month for this form of supervision. However, both supervisor and supervisee adopting this style usually find a compromise whereby sometimes more time is spent for the same fee and other times less than might have been envisaged. There does need to be trust and goodwill on both sides if this arrangement is to work effectively.

There also needs to be an agreement about any between emails contact. The supervisor has to be clear whether this is solely for emergencies or whether it can be used for less pressing issues. The supervisee needs to know whether there are days when the supervisor will not be online, so the supervisee is not left in a state of anxiety regarding timing of a response.

A short extract of an email exchange is shown below (Figure 33.2). In the exchange, the supervisor responds within the supervisee's text. It might also be written in a different colour as well as a different font. This type of exchange works for some practitioners and

Date	Client code	Time where synchronous	Contact code/ venue	Issues dealt with
17.12.12	Peter		Email exchange	Session 11 Evaluations and endings
17.12.12	Jo		Email exchange	Introductory session Boundaries, Background
17.12.12	Belinda	1hour	Video	Session 1 Contracting and clarifying goals
17.12.12	Tom	1hour	Video	Session 3 Personal development issues related to work issues
18.12.12	Sam		Email exchange	Session 13 How will he know when he wants to end.
18.12.12	Mary	1 hour	Text	Session 2 Personal boundaries – wonder how this relates to our work?
7.1.13	Babs		Email exchange	Session 1 Present and preferred scenario of life
7.1.13	Lisa	1hour	Voice	One off session Serious child illness – I want to bring this client to supervision
7.1.13	Tom	1hour	Video	Session 4 Review and commitment to new contract
8.1.13	John	1hour	Video	Session 3 Anger issues – anger with me?
8.1.13	Sally	DNA	Email client	Non-contact issues: possibly bring to supervision
8.1.13	Sam		Email exchange	Session 14 Useful exchange on endings
8.1.13	Mary	1hour	Text	Session 3 Relationship and abandonment issues
Sessions this time		(Including 1DNA) 13		
Total sessions so far		111.30		

Figure 33.1.

Hi Lizzie,

I've attached my usual overview of my client work with this email. ***Thanks, Chris; I always appreciate having this.*** I think things are going well in most cases, ***Good – it feels as if you are becoming more confident about your online work now. Is that how you see it?*** but I want to bring a couple of clients here to look at what might be going on. I'll also just respond to a couple of things you brought up in our last exchange, if that's OK. ***Yes that's fine – these on-going exchanges can often shed light on what's going on in the counselling process.***

Chris has had a bit of a setback. You'll remember that his father's funeral was early December. That went reasonably OK – he felt that he was able to hold back his own feelings about his father appropriately, so that it didn't interfere with what his mother and siblings needed to do on that occasion. ***I recall your work with him about reasons for doing this, and if he felt it was the right thing to do, strategies for managing. Did he use these?*** However afterwards he really got into his anger with his dad – I guess he'd been holding back till after the funeral. ***Yes that feels likely.*** His last email was so angry and almost irrational that I was a bit concerned about his well-being. ***Do you mean physical or mental well-being – or both? What are your fears here? I'm aware from reading the extract that I wasn't sure if there was implied threat of violence – or am I reading too much into his words?*** And also his ability to hold it together at work, as there seemed to be some leakage there. ***Yes – I can see that his comments about that interaction with his manager might well have been triggered by issues with his father. On the other hand, if Chris is reporting the exchange as it happened, the manager was somewhat attacking.*** I'll attach an extract from his email so you can see what I mean. ***Thanks. May I just check what your contract is with Chris, with regards to me seeing extracts from his emails? Does he know this could happen, or do you feel that having told him that you are in online supervision, you have covered this sufficiently? Just thinking how this could link with that other issue he brought to you about never having any privacy as a young person, because his mother took his diary to his father to read.*** I'm not due to reply till next Tuesday, so I'll have had time to read your thoughts before then. ***OK – this has given you a little time to further reflect.*** I think I don't want to go in too challengingly. ***Hmm – I'm curious about this. Can you say a bit about the reasons for not wanting to go in too challengingly – I'm not suggesting you ought to do so, simply exploring this with you. Is there a parallel here with his old fear of challenging his dad? Or is it about his welfare? Or what's your own reaction to anger from another person – might he be angry with you? A lot of questions! Ignore those that aren't relevant for you!***

The other client I want to look at in greater depth is Bessie. We've now had 10 sessions and I think we are both stuck! ***OK – so an odd question to you! What would you both be doing if you weren't stuck? And when you have come up with an answer to that, where in your work that this is already happening (or did happen) a bit?***

Figure 33.2. Excerpt of Asynchronous Email Supervision.

not for others. Some supervisors (or supervisees) prefer the reply to be a separate, stand-alone email. There is no right or wrong; practitioners have to establish what works best for them.

Another way asynchronous supervision can take place is through the use of a forum on a website. In contracted, on-going online supervision, the independent supervisor sets up her own secure forum/noticeboard to which supervisees have access. The supervision document is posted there, followed by the supervisor's reply in much the same way as outlined above.

Alternatively, supervision or consultation can be a non-contractual arrangement. In a noncontractual arrangement, the supervisor sets up a forum on a website, to which any counsellor can bring supervision queries or dilemmas. Obviously, there needs to be a mechanism for paying for a response, using a secure check-out such as Google or Paypal. This can be particularly useful for the supervisor in private practice with a particular speciality, such as working with pornography, trauma or particular illnesses. It is also very useful for supervisees if their regular online supervisor has limited experience in a specific field when ethical, professional, or legal issues arise.

An advantage of asynchronous supervision is that the generated text enables the independent online supervisor to reflect on and evaluate on his or her supervision practice, perhaps using Interpersonal Process Recall (IPR). Dobson (2006) considers the use of videos in F2F supervision for evaluating the work of counsellor and supervisor, and much of what she explores also applies to asynchronous online supervision.

Synchronous Online Supervision

In many ways, synchronous supervision can feel more like F2F supervision, which is why some supervisors and supervisees in private practice prefer this mode of supervision. However, supervisors and supervisees must be careful not to make assumptions about overlaps as in reality there are probably more differences than similarities between F2F and synchronous supervision. The three ways of doing this are by using text, by using voice or by using voice and webcam.

Synchronous Text

A common way of conducting supervision by live text in private practice is to use one of the existing platforms or instant messaging programs. Some supervisors have even set up live text through their own website, and this may have some advantages in terms of professionalism and security. However, in reality, this option may be a costly option for less technically literate or competent practitioners and could require the on-going services of a webmaster/IT specialist.

Sessions are arranged in exactly the same way as in F2F supervision with regard to date and time. As with all online practice, arrangements for breakdown of technology are stated within the contract. One of the advantages of live text supervision is the balance of a spontaneity that is much less possible asynchronously, as well as the benefit of having a record of the supervision.

A disadvantage of this way of working may be the typing speed – or a lack of – by participants. One supervisee reported that in a group, she felt limited by having to look at the keys to type and by the time she looked back at the screen "so much seemed to have happened" (Cummings, 2002). Supervisees may feel that they "get less done" in the time. Either party might drift off rather than staying focussed while the other is typing. Conversely, it does give some reflection time. As in all supervision, quick reviews at the end of sessions, and more formal periodic reviews, should highlight what is working and what is not.

Below is an excerpt of how a very small part of the conversation might happen (see Figure 33.3). To give some authenticity, there are "typos" within the text, as it is important for neither party to become over conscious of their typing, distracting them from the work taking place. This supervisee uses the technique of putting several small sections of writing in turn on to the screen, which gives the supervisor a chance to take in what is being said more quickly. The supervisee shows that he has not finished "speaking" by using ellipses (. . .) to indicate he will continue.

[10:04:56] Anne: So where do you want to begin?

[10:05:34] Mike: I think for once can do clients straight away and not problems of technology!

[10:05:49] Anne: Excellent! Go ahead.

[10:06:52] Mike: This is one I think I mentioned a while ago – first started counselling her a couple of months ago – had had previous contract about 3 years ago

[10:07:15] Anne: Yes I think I have the right one in my head.

[10:08:02] Mike: Basically there a small part of me that questions whether one young person (22) can have so much happen to them in their live. . . .

[10:08:05] Mike: life. . . .

[10:10:24] Mike: Since childhood they have been subjected to sexual abuse from grandfather, 'hired' out by father for sexual favours, found out brother was conceived through a rape attack, mother died of a tumour, father died, aunt hung herself and now brother is on critical list in intensive care. Add to that they are transgender.

[10:10:52] Anne: Wow. A lot for you both?

[10:11:12] Mike: It feels genuine in at least what they are telling me and how much its affecting them mentally

[10:12:41] Anne: So I guess it may or may not be all factually true, but they perceive their life in these terms and have been very affected by whatever has happened to them? And there is a part of you that feels that it could be factually true? Or are you actually saying that small questioning part is actually very large?

[10:14:20] Mike: That's one of the hardest parts of working on line – it's only the written word that we can go by – I've nothing else to base this on. But having worked with her before as well it's hard not to believe it's true apart from there's so much of it. If that makes sense?

Figure 33.3. Excerpt of Synchronous Text Supervision.

Voice Alone

Voice supervision is a way of offering supervision in independent practice that includes the most traditional and the newer forms of technology. Voice supervision can include the use of the telephone as well as VoIP (Voice over Internet Protocol). The use of the telephone for therapy and supervision has long been widely accepted, and readers will be familiar with its advantages and disadvantages (Sanders, 2007). The main difference in choosing between a telephone and VoIP is in regard to technology and not the use of supervision by voice per se. Since its introduction in 2004, increasing numbers of practitioners use VoIP.

There are several advantages to using VoIP. The biggest single one over standard telephone systems is cost – calls between VoIP users are usually free. In most cases, by paying a small sum, supervisors can also call landline and mobile phones, with international calls being much less expensive than through a public telephone network. Supervisors can pay as the service is used or buy a subscription. Another advantage of this form of supervision is the ability to record sessions – once again, consider the security of your system.

A disadvantage is that communication on

the IP network is generally less reliable than a public telephone network. These systems depend on having fast, consistent broadband connections. Therefore, supervisors may experience occasional problems of delayed speech and/or echoes. Readers who can remember glitches in international phone calls some 30 years ago will recall the stilted communication resulting from these snags! Also, not all consumer VoIP solutions support encryption, although having a secure call is much easier to implement with VoIP than with traditional phone lines. So, while recognising that supervision has been offered by phone for years without enormous concern about people listening in, if you decide to use VoIP for supervision, consider a provider that automatically encrypts communications.

Voice with Webcam

Voice with webcam has perhaps the most advantages and disadvantages for supervision in terms of the use of technology. It is exciting and useful to work in such a way that a supervisee and the supervisor can see and hear each other. In this mode, the participants have all the clues that would be present in F2F supervision – voice, body language, and a sense of intimacy. Seeing the supervisee can help with focus and intimacy. Likewise, spontaneity and creativity can flow. The supervisor and supervisee can work together with drawings, pebbles, puppets, etc. With some videoconferencing programs, video clips and slide presentations are also possible. This can be particularly useful to independent practitioners working with trainees or newly qualified counsellors, where there may be a greater "teaching" element in the supervision. As Bellafiore, Colòn, and Rosenberg (2004) suggest, multimedia presentations can serve to enrich the experience in group supervision as well.

However, supervisors in independent practice may not have access to the best and quickest broadband connections, as they are often not within city centres or business parks with fast ADSL connections. This will also applies to the supervisees. If images constantly pixelate, voices become distorted or delayed, or connections are frequently lost, then this is not the supervision vehicle of choice. Aside from anything else, technological difficulties are highly distracting, and the focus is on the technology instead of the supervision. Having said that, if a good relationship has been built up between supervisor and supervisee, trying videoconferencing is worthwhile. The session can always resort to text communication on occasions when connections will not support the video link.

CONCLUSION

One final area for the online supervisor to consider is the value of undertaking a specific training in online supervision. In the same way as it is now considered sound ethical practice to undertake post initial F2F training to work as an online counsellor, there is a growing recognition of importance of online supervision training to adapt to the particulars of online supervision (Stretch, Nagel, & Anthony, 2013). Anthony and Nagel (2012) assert that even well-intentioned practitioners often do not know what they do not know until it is too late; online supervision training may well help to highlight the unknown.

This chapter has considered some of the advantages and disadvantages of working as an independent online supervisor, and also ways in which supervision sessions can be conducted. There are other issues for independent supervisors to consider, including managing time and risk, financial planning, business plans, marketing, and support networks. However, as these are generic issues for all independent practitioners, and not specifically online practitioners, they have not been explored here. Practitioners could consider these issues through further reading and research (Bor & Stokes 2011; Hemmings & Field 2007; McMahon, Palmer, & Wilding, 2005). And as Joinson (2003) states, people choose the tools they wish to use and those suiting their psychological requirements, and this must surely apply to the online supervisor in independent practice.

REFERENCES

Anthony, K., & Nagel, D. (2012). A brave new world: Coaching online. *Coaching Today, 1*(1), 33–37.

Bor, R., & Stokes, A. (2011). *Setting up in independent practice: A handbook for counsellors, therapists and psychologists.* Basingstoke: Palgrave/MacMillan.

Bellafiore, D. R., Colòn, Y., & Rosenberg, P. (2004). Online counseling groups. In R. Kraus, J. Zack, & G. Stricker (Eds.), *Online counseling: A handbook for mental health professionals* (pp. 197–216). San Diego, CA: Elsevier Academic Press.

Cavanagh, K., Shapiro, D., & Zack, J. (2003). The computer plays therapist: The challenges and opportunities of psychotherapeutic software. In S. Goss & K. Anthony (Eds.), *Technology in counselling and psychotherapy practice: A practitioner's guide* (pp. 143–164). Basingstoke: Palgrave/Macmillan.

Cummings, P. (2002). Cybervision: Virtual peer group counselling supervision – hindrance or help? *Counselling and Psychotherapy Research, 2*(4), 223–229.

Dodson, M. A. (2006, Winter). Counselling in the spotlight. *Counselling at Work,* 11–15.

Evans, J. (2009). *Online counselling and guidance skills: A resource for trainees and practitioners.* London: Sage. http://dx.doi.org/ 10.41359781446216705.

Hemmings, A., & Field, R. (2007). *Counselling and psychotherapy in contemporary private practice.* Hove: Routledge.

Joinson, A. (2003). *Understanding the psychology of internet behaviour: Virtual worlds, real lives.* Basingstoke: Palgrave/Macmillan.

Jones, G., & Stokes, A. (2009). *Online counselling: A handbook for practitioners.* Basingstoke: Palgrave/Macmillan.

McMahon, G., Palmer, S., & Wilding, C. (2005). *The essential skills for setting up a counselling and psychotherapy practice.* London: Routledge.

Sanders, P. (2007). *Using counselling skills on the telephone and in computer-mediated communication* (3rd ed.). Ross-on-Wye: PCCS Books.

Stofle, G., & Hamilton, S. (1998). Online supervision for social workers. *The New Social Worker, 5*(4) Retrieved from http://bugfix. metropublisher.net/feature-articles/field-placement/Online_Supervision _for_Social_Workers/.

Stretch, L. S., Nagel, D., & Anthony, K. (2013). Ethical framework for the use of technology in supervision. *Therapeutic Innovations in Light of Technology, 3*(2), 37–44. Retrieved from http://onlinetherapyinstitute. com/2013/01/tilt-magazine-issue-13.

Wheeler, S., Aveline. M., & Barkham, M. (2011). Practice-based supervision research: A network of researchers using a common toolkit. *Counselling and Psychotherapy Research, 11*(2), 88–96. doi 10.1080/14733145.2011.562982.

Chapter 34

DISTANCE GROUP SUPERVISION FOR PLAY THERAPY

LoriAnn Sykes Stretch and Kristin Ann Vincenzes

INTRODUCTION

Clinical supervision is an essential process that ultimately helps the client by developing the skills of a less experienced professional (Bernard & Goodyear, 2009). Supervisors have the responsibility to ensure the competency of the supervisee so that he or she can effectively apply fundamental skills to the field (Kaufman & Schwartz, 2003). In order to achieve this goal, the supervisor is often a facilitator in increasing the supervisee's professional growth. This is done by offering support, directly teaching specific skills and by helping the supervisee amplify his or her own self-awareness (Bernard & Goodyear, 2009). Supervision is an essential requirement for new mental health professionals attempting to get state licensure; however, it is also a fundamental process when working with new client populations, integrating innovative intervention techniques and continuing professional development.

One client population that requires a unique skillset is children. In addition to understanding the cognitive and developmental nature of a child, certain counseling models of intervention need to be studied so that children's needs are effectively met. Children lack the verbal ability to efficiently communicate regarding their experiences and/or feelings; therefore, creative intervention models are pertinent when working with this population (Landreth, 2012). One such model is called play therapy, which is used most often with children ages three to 11 years, but specific techniques can also benefit adolescents and adults (Carmichael, 2006).

The interest in play therapy is growing exponentially because the approach builds on a child's natural way of learning about his or her environment (Landreth, 2012). Furthermore, play is a universal language for children around the world; thus, the intervention has been proven to be globally successful with a wide variety of social, emotional, behavioral and academic concerns (Bratton, Ray, & Rhine, 2005; Landreth, 2012). Due to the uniqueness of the play therapy model, providing play therapy requires extensive education, training, experience and supervision in order to be effectively implemented.

Supervision is necessary for mental health professionals seeking to both learn play therapy and acquire the credentials of a registered play therapist (RPT). Supervisors, specifically in play therapy, serve as role models (Moustakas, 1959) in helping the supervisee gain a stronger sense of self-awareness as well as knowledge for the basic and advanced skills used in play therapy (Dee, 2004). In accordance with these skills, play therapy heavily relies on the nonverbal component of play. Thus the supervisor's role is to also help the supervisee understand the theory behind play therapy (Homeyer & Morrison, 2008). As the supervisor models the importance of genuineness and acceptance with the supervisee, this experiential process can be transferred to the counselor-child relationship (Krantz & Lund, 1994).

For professionals interested in becoming a registered play therapist (RPT), there are explicit requirements that need to be met, particularly in relation to supervision, that are above and beyond the compulsory education and state licensure mandates. Specifically, professionals desiring to be a registered play therapist are required to have 500 hours of supervised play therapy experience (Association of Play Therapy, 2013a).

Due to the specialization of this intervention model, the Association of Play Therapy (APT, 2013a) recommends applicants complete the required supervision with a Registered Play Therapist-Supervisor (RPT-S) who has specialized training in play therapy. A non-RPT-S may provide the concurrent play therapy supervision; however, an applicant will have to acquire 50 hours of supervision with a non-RPT-S versus 35 hours of supervision with a RPT-S (APT, 2013a).

Although the interest in play therapy is growing, interested practitioners may be challenged to find a RPT-S who is willing to provide the supervision necessary to successfully complete the credential's requirements. APT (2013a) has rigorous stipulations and requirements for professionals who want to serve as registered play therapist supervisors. These credentials serve as the driving force to ensure both client welfare and to preserve the professionalism of play therapy (Homeyer & Morrison, 2008). In 2012, just over 1,000 registered play therapist-supervisors

offered supervision according to APT (2013b). The extreme shortage of registered play therapist supervisors, especially globally, significantly impacts the growth opportunities for professionals to effectively integrate this model worldwide.

The paucity of registered play therapist supervisors also impacts the continued critical development of those currently credentialed as supervisors. Professional play therapists supervisors are expected to consult with other registered play therapist supervisors to further develop one's skills, safeguard against potential legal issues and provide substantive care to their supervisees and clients (Hagg Granello, Kindsvatter, Granello, Underfer-Babalis, & Hartwig Moorhead, 2008). Peer supervision is a fundamental process that aides in the critical analysis of one's own practice (Hagg Granello et al., 2008); therefore, there is a substantial need to increase the growth of registered play therapist supervisors to serve as both clinical supervisors as well as peer supervisors. This will further catapult the professionalism in play therapy by developing competent knowledgeable practitioners and supervisors.

Peer Supervision Model

A small private practice in a rural portion of North Carolina had four mental health practitioners seeking supervision for play therapy. All of the practitioners wanted to pursue the RPT credential. The group decided to recruit a RPT-S to provide supervision on-site at the facility. At the time of recruitment, the practice was serving approximately 100 clients per week with a staff of 21 practitioners and three administrative staff members. Approximately 50 percent of the client population were children, teens and their families. In addition, the Clinical Director of the practice was serving as a therapeutic consultant to a local alternative school (K–12) and three Level IV group homes.

Initially, the group searched the APT's

"Find Play Therapists" site (2013c) seeking a RPT-S in the local area. One RPT-S was found; however, upon contact, she indicated she was not in a position to provide on-site supervision due to the distance (> 25 miles each way) and the travel time, nor was she comfortable with providing distance supervision using technology. Next, the initial group of therapists began networking with colleagues trying to identify a RPT-S that would be willing to either travel to the site or provide distance supervision. At the time, APT did not have specific guidelines regarding when or how distance supervision could be done. Now, APT (2013a) defines "non-contact or distance supervision" (p. 5) as supervision that occurs "via telephone or online to discuss . . . play therapy notes, reports, or session video" (p. 5).

Eventually, the group located one RPT-S in South Carolina who was dually licensed in South Carolina and North Carolina and who was willing to experiment with distance supervision. At the time, no other RPT-S in North Carolina was willing to travel to the site or provide distance supervision. Now, nine supervisors listed in the "Find Play Therapists" database (APT, 2013c) indicate they will provide distance supervision (one of which is the RPT-S who participated in this model). The RPT-S contacted APT directly and learned that she could in fact provide distance supervision. The RPT-S agreed to meet with the group, as well as other professionals in the community who were interested in pursuing the RPT credential, once a month for two to three hours via videoconferencing and once a quarter the group would cover her expenses to travel to the site for a face-to-face group supervision session. Finally, the first distance supervision session was scheduled for the following month.

In total, the group met for ten distance supervision sessions and two face-to-face supervision sessions. During the initial face-to-face supervision session, the supervisor familiarized herself with the group members and reviewed

confidentiality guidelines and precautions. The group agreed to utilize pseudonyms for all clients and to provide only enough clinical information for the case to be discussed objectively. In addition, the supervisor had each participant identify a local professional mental health provider who could serve as a peer support in times of clinical crisis in the event the supervisor was not immediately accessible. The group had a lengthy discussion of ethics, particularly regarding the importance of informing clients that the clinician would be participating in distance supervision. The group agreed to seek written informed consent for all cases that would be presented.

During the distance supervision sessions, the RPT-S and one group member met online 30 minutes prior to the initial session to test the technology. Initially, the group utilized a video platform and a wireless Internet connection. Quickly, the facilitators realized that a hard line connection to the Internet would be necessary for a steady connection. Once the technical issues were resolved, each group member (four at the initial meeting) presented a case for discussion and consultation. The RPT-S provided support through Socratic questioning, reviewing experiential materials from sessions (such as art work, sandtray pictures, and crafts), reviewing recorded sessions and facilitating peer-to-peer discussions. The RPT-S grounded her feedback in play therapy theory, best practices, developmental theories and peer reviewed articles. In addition, despite being almost 300 hundred miles away and over four hours away, the supervisor was knowledgeable of community resources in the area surrounding the site.

Over the course of ten sessions and two face-to-face sessions, the group reviewed cases from a variety of settings including, therapeutic foster care, public schools, an alternative school (K–12), group homes and private practice. The group members were a combination of counselors, marriage and family therapists and social workers. The group members reported the cross disciplinary nature of the supervision sessions strengthened networking and knowledge of the group members. Most importantly, being able to access an expert in play therapy was invaluable and could have not been as achieved without the use of technology.

The distance group supervision model worked very well under the circumstances. The site was able to provide expert support to the staff and support the professional staff members' desire to pursue the RPT credential. Some of the challenges faced were connectivity issues, scheduling and attendance. One of the other challenges was reviewing recorded clinical data (e.g., session recordings) as a group. The group had to watch the content separate from the supervisor and simply cued the supervisor to what section to watch and then came back together to discuss. Suitable solutions were developed with the level of technology that was available at the time and now newer technology is available that can do so much more. The group learned to be flexible and creative with the use of technology and the accompanying challenges.

In future distance group supervision models, facilitators are encouraged to utilize more secure videoconferencing software. In addition, facilitators need to thoroughly review legal and ethical guidelines. Professional associations, such as ACA (2013), NBCC (2012), and APT (2013a), are providing more guidance regarding the use of distance technologies in both clinical practice and supervision. Finally, more research needs to be conducted to better understand best practices for distance supervision.

REFERENCES

American Counseling Association. (2013). *Ethics and professional standards.* Alexandria, VA: Author. Retrieved http://www.counseling.org/knowledge-center/ethics.

Association for Play Therapy. (2013a). *Play therapy makes a difference!* Retrieved from http://www.a4pt.org/ps.index.cfm?ID=1653

Association for Play Therapy. (2013b). *2012 growth report.* Clovis, CS: Author.

Association for Play Therapy. (2013c). *Find play therapists.* Retrieved from http://www.a4pt.org/directory.cfm?task=results.

Bernard, J. M., & Goodyear, R. K. (2009). *Fundamentals of clinical supervision* (4th ed.). Upper Saddle River, NJ: Pearson Education.

Bratton, S., Ray, D., & Rhine, T. (2005). The efficacy of play therapy with children: A meta-analytic review of treatment outcomes. *Journal of Professional Psychology Research and Practice, 36*(4), 376–390.

Carmichael, K. D. (2006). *Play therapy: An introduction.* Glenview, IL: Prentice-Hall.

Dee, R. (2004). Supervision of basic and advanced skills in play therapy. *Journal of Professional Counseling: Practice, Theory, & Research, 32*(2), 28–41.

Haag Granello, D., Kindsvatter, A., Granello, P. F., Underfer-Babalis, J., & Hartwig Moorhead, H. J. (2008). Multiple perspectives in supervision: Using a peer consultation model to enhance supervisor development. *Counselor Education and Supervision, 48*, 32–47.

Homeyer, L. E., & Morrison, M. O. (2008). Play therapy: Practice, issues, and trends. *American Journal of Play, 1*(2), 210–228.

Kaufman, J., & Schwartz, T. (2003). Models of supervision: Shaping professional identity. *Clinical Supervisor, 22*(1), 143–158.

Kranz, P., & Lund, N. L. (1994). Recommendations for supervising play therapists. *International Journal of Play Therapy, 3*(2), 45–52.

Landreth, G. (2012). *The art of the relationship* (3rd ed.). New York: Taylor & Francis.

Moustakas, C. (1959). *Psychotherapy with children.* New York: Harper and Row.

NBCC. (2012). *NBCC policy regarding the provision of distance professional services.* Greensboro, NC: Author.

Chapter 35

PRACTICA AND INTERNSHIP FIELD PLACEMENTS USING CYBERSUPERVISION

Jonathan Lent, Andrew Burck and LoriAnn Sykes Stretch

INTRODUCTION

Technology in counseling and supervision is a growing trend and counselor educators and supervisors need to be informed and competent in the effective use of technology (Baker, 2011; Coker & Schooley, 2012; Finn & Barak, 2010; Kraus, Sticker, & Speyer, 2010; Oravec, 2000). Technology has played a role in counseling and supervision since the 1940s when Carl Rogers demonstrated the utility of audiotape recordings of clinical sessions (Jencius, Baltimore, & Getz, 2009). Even today, audio recording has remained a primary use of technology in supervision in practica and internship.

Watson (2003) first used the term "cybersupervision" to describe supervision interactions which occur via the World Wide Web. Watson investigated the potential of applying technologically-based methods to counseling practicum interactions between supervisors and supervisees. Since the introduction of these methods of supervision, technology has grown and provided the ability to utilize more advanced methods to conduct supervision. Some previous methods of technology used in counseling and supervision include video recordings, "bug-in-the-ear" and "bug-in-the-eye" (Bernard & Goodyear, 2009; Powell & Brodsky, 2004). Beyond these technological

advances, technology has progressed and provided a variety of other methods to conduct supervision. The advent of this new technology has been referred to as cybersupervision (Chapman, Baker, Nassar-McMilliam, & Gerler, 2011), psychotechnology (Maheu, 2003), e-supervision (Dudding & Justice, 2004), technology-assisted distance supervision (TADS; McAdams & Wyatt, 2010) and technology-assisted distance counseling supervision (TADCS; Dawson, Harpster, Hoffman, & Phelan (2011).

According to Watson (2003) and Byrne and Hartley (2010), technology will play a significant role in the counseling profession as well as the supervisory process. Due to the various technological resources available for educators and counseling supervisors, these individuals need to become more familiar with the use of technology in supervision. Examples of currently available technological resources include electronic mail (e-mail), synchronous and asynchronous chat, voice over Internet (VOIP) and video conferencing. Although each of these communication modalities may be readily available to supervisors, competence in using such technology when providing supervision to counselor trainees can be a daunting task. In addition, the actual preparation and facilitation of cybersupervision can be challenging. This could especially be true for individuals who do not have a strong understanding or previous experiences with the use of technology. Along with comfort and familiarity with technology, supervisors are also faced with a number of ethical concerns that relate to the use of technology in supervision (ACA, 2013; Anthony, Nagel, & Stretch, 2013; NBCC, 2012). Two of the most alarming concerns faced by supervisors when attempting to implement technology into supervision are confidentiality and informed consent (McAdams & Wyatt, 2010; Vaccaro & Lambie, 2007). When taking into account the difficulties individuals may have with the actual implementation of technology, along with the ethical concerns that are present, supervisors may be reluctant to incorporate technology into their role as supervisors.

There are two major types of communication when using technology: synchronous and asynchronous communication. Research supports both synchronous and asynchronous methods of communication and can be effective tools for teaching and learning (Abbass et al., 2011; Chapman et al., 2011; Coker & Schooley, 2012; Conn, Roberts, & Powell, 2009; Garrison & Kanuka, 2004; Hampel, 2006; Lenz, Oliver, & Nelson, 2011; Stebnicki & Glover, 2001). Conn et al. (2009) identified the experience of students with technology-assisted supervision has been positive and there was no effect on the perceived quality of supervision when compared with face-to-face supervision. While cybersupervision may be most convenient for supervisors and students alike, determining if this is the most appropriate method to conduct supervision is important to consider (McCracken, 2004; Nelson, Nichter, & Henriksen, 2010).

The Process of Supervision

Bernard and Goodyear (2009) defined supervision as "an intervention provided by a more senior member of the profession to a more junior member of the same profession. This relationship is evaluative, extends over time and has the simultaneous purposes of enhancing professional functioning of the more junior person(s), monitoring the quality of professional services offered to clients" (p. 8). Traditionally, counseling supervision consisted of live, face-to-face meetings and has progressed to include a variety of technical modalities: electronic mail (e-mail), threaded discussions, synchronous chat, voice over internet (VOIP) and video conferencing. Successful use of distance supervision in clinical training programs is well-documented (Abbass et al., 2011; Barnett, 2011; Chapman, 2006; Coker & Schooley, 2012; Conn et al., 2009; Lenz et al., 2011; Watson, 2003; Wilson, 2001). Regardless of the format through which supervision is provided, Bernard and Goodyear's (2009) definition of supervision describes the supervisory relationship between the counselor educator and counselor trainee.

Special Considerations for Students in Rural Areas

Both authors work in a very rural area of the country and have noted that students often travel two or more hours to attend the fieldwork courses, which are land-based courses versus the content courses which are offered in an online format. In addition, the rural environment provided some unique challenges. While there is a perception that rural environment can be accurately defined, there are many unique aspects of a rural environment (Helbok, 2003). Rural environments have been defined based on the number of individuals in a population that is less than an urban areas (United States Bureau of Census, 2013) and having a population less than 5,000 individuals (Helbok, 2003). Rural environments are, by nature, isolated geographically, have a small population, and a greater distance to resources, and other mental health professionals (Barnett & Henshaw, 2002). While there is no consistent definition of rural environments, there are some traits of the population that are pertinent to supervisor and the supervisee.

Rural environments tend to be heterogeneous in nature, not accepting of diverse populations, have a greater number of individuals with disabilities and elderly, have higher rates of illiteracy and lack of formal education (Wagenfeld, 2003). In addition, there is a greater increase of poverty in rural settings especially with diverse populations and children (Strange, Johnson, Showalter, & Klein, 2012). There is increased need for medical services because of the higher rate of illness; however, the medical services are often below standards (Werth, Hastings, & Riding-Malon, 2010). Individuals in rural environments have unique characteristics of which supervisees and supervisors must be aware.

One of the challenges facing these counselor educators supervising practica and internship students in rural areas is finding an appropriate site placement and having access to supervision time with the University supervisor. The traditional, land-based approach to counseling practica and internship lends itself easily to face-to-face (F2F) interaction between supervisors and supervisees; however, with demand growing for online courses, issues with commuting, and the increasing popularity of distance education programs in counselor education, cybersupervision is a beneficial means of providing supervision for changing student populations (Chapman et al., 2011; Reese, Aldarondo, Lee, Miller, & Burton, 2009; Nelson et al., 2010). With technology advancing at a rapid rate, utilizing the Web and technological resources to meet the flexible and diverse needs of supervisees is important to consider and explore (Clingerman & Bernard, 2004). Counselor educators may be interested in, or required to provide, supervision to counselor trainees who are completing practica or internship at a distance in cases where regular face-to-face meetings are not possible.

Preparation and Implementation of Cybersupervision for Distance Supervision

Lent, the first author, utilized cybersupervision when first teaching the School Counseling Internship course at Marshall University. The graduate program in counseling at Marshall University services students across the tri-state area (Kentucky, Ohio, and West Virginia). A number of students completed a large portion of the program online; however, the Internship experience required class meetings in order for students to complete the course. Many of these students resided in locations several hours away from the main campus in Huntington, West Virginia. This resulted, in the past, in students driving several hours to attend the internship seminars. With the advent of computer technology, high-speed Internet connections, and Blackboard as a course delivery format, this opened the door for using cybersupervision to assist these students.

For counselor educators who do not have a strong knowledge or understanding of technology, developing and implementing cybersupervision can be a daunting task. Along with the difficulties associated with securing a proper site, there were a myriad of concerns related to technology use for supervision. Chapman (2008) describes the two methods of electronically mediated supervision: live or real time (synchronous) and delayed time (asynchronous). Supervisors will need to determine which modality is most beneficial and feasible for their situation. Although limited, research has supported the use of both synchronous and asynchronous communication for counselor supervision (Clingerman & Bernard, 2004).

To establish their respective cybersupervision programs, the authors had to ensure everyone involved had the basic hardware necessary, including a computer with at least a Pentium 4 or higher CPU, two GB of RAM, a 100 megabit network card and a broadband connection of at least 512 kbps. All participants needed an Internet connection in order to connect to the Internet to utilize videoconferencing software, discussion boards, instant messaging services and email. The participants were required to have a webcam with either a built in microphone an external microphone.

In developing a cybersupervision program for one specific student, Lent, the first author, had to determine the level of technological comfort and competency of a supervisee from a distance. Lent determined the student's competency and comfort via telephone and email. Supervisors have to address is the issue of technology competence. Supervisors' have to ensure that supervisees have the knowledge and skill to use technology in order to engage in online supervision (ACES Technology Interest Network, 2007; Anthony, Nagel, & Stretch, 2013; Mallen, Vogel, & Rochlen, 2005; Vaccaro & Lambie, 2007). The supervisee may need training in order to engage in online supervision. The quality of technology as well as the technical training of supervisors and supervisees can contribute to the quality of the distance supervision experience (McCracken, 2004; Nelson et al., 2010; Shallcross, 2012).

Once all the logistical concerns were addressed and the supervisee shared that she was comfortable with the process, Lent consulted with university support staff to determine which technology to use to conduct the cybersupervision. The most reasonable option in this case was to use Wimba, which was included within Blackboard at the university. Wimba allowed Lent to communicate both verbally and nonverbally using videoconferencing for cybersupervision with the student. Wimba allowed the supervisee to engage in both the group and individual supervision sessions throughout the Internship semester.

Upon completion of the semester, feedback was sought from the supervisee on her experience. The supervisee reported that, although different, this method of cybersupervision was convenient and allowed for participation from the remote location. Similarly, research on cybersupervision has demonstrated lower supervision costs, increased accessibility, reduction in travel restrictions, immediate access to supervisor, reduction in isolation, access to expert consultation and increased interaction (Burrak, 2008; McAdams & Wyatt, 2010; Orr, 2010).

Some important lessons to consider when implementing a cybersupervision program include the following: factor in time to work out technical glitches, provide training for new technologies, assess readiness for technology-assisted supervision, understand legal and ethical requirements, review raw clinical data, provide ongoing evaluation of supervisee skills, ensure a secure transmission of information and engage in a continuous program evaluation process (Hurley & Hadden, 2009; McAdams & Wyatt, 2010).

REFERENCES

Abbass, A., Arthey, S., Elliott, J., Fedak, T., Nowoweiski, D., Markovski, J., & Nowoweiski, S. (2011). Web-conference supervision for advanced psychotherapy training: A practical guide. *Psychotherapy, 48,* 109–118. doi: 10.1037/a0022427.

American Counseling Association. (2013). *Ethics & professional standards.* Alexandria, VA: Author. Retrieved from http://www.counseling.org/knowledge-center/ethics.

ACES Technology Interest Network. (2007). *Technology competencies for counselor education: Recommended guidelines for program development.* Retrieved from files .acesonline. net/doc/2007_aces_technology _competencies.pdf.

Anthony, K., Nagel, D. M., & Stretch, L. S.

(2013). *The use of technology in clinical supervision and training: Mental health applications.* Springfield, IL: Charles C Thomas.

Baker, K. (2011). Online counseling: The good, the bad, and the possibilities. *Counseling Psychology Quarterly, 24,* 341–346. doi: 10.1080/09515070.2011.632875.

Barnett, J. E. (2011). Utilizing technological innovations to enhance psychotherapy supervision, training, and outcomes. *Psychotherapy, 48*(2), 103–108. doi:10.1037/a0023381.

Barnett, J. E., & Henshaw, E. A. (2002). Ethical, clinical and risk management issues in rural practice. In L. VandeCreek & T. L. Jackson (Eds.), *Innovations in clinical practice: A source book* (Vol. 20, pp. 411–422). Sarasota, FL: Professional Resources Press/Professional Resources Exchange.

Bernard, J. M., & Goodyear, R. K. (2009). *Fundamentals of clinical supervision.* Upper Saddle River, NJ: Pearson.

Burrak, F. (2008). *Using videoconferencing: Technology to enhance supervision of student teachers.* Apple Learning Interchange. Retrieved Edcommunity at apple.com.

Byrne, A., & Harltey, M. T. (2010). Digital technology in the 21st century: Considerations for clinical supervision in rehabilitation education. *Rehabilitation Education, 24*(1 & 2), 57–68.

Chapman, R. A. (2008). Cybersupervision of entry level practicum supervisees: The effect on acquisition of counselor competence and confidence. *Journal of Technology in Counseling, 5*(1). Retrieved from http://jtc.columbusstate.edu/Vol5_1/Chapman.htm.

Chapman, R. A., Baker, S. B., Nassar-McMillan, S. C., & Gerler, Jr., E. R. (2011). Cybersupervision: Further examination of synchronous and asynchronous modalities of counseling practicum supervision. *Counselor Education & Supervision, 50,* 298–313.

Clingerman, T. L., & Bernard, J. M. (2004). An investigation of the use of e-mail as a supplemental modality for clinical supervision. *Counselor Education and Supervision, 44,* 82–95.

Coker, J. K., & Schooley, A. (2012). Investigating the effectiveness of clinical supervision in a CACREP accredited counseling program. In G. R. Walz, J. C. Bleuer, & R. K. Yep (Eds.), *Ideas and research you can use: VISTAS 2012* (pp. 1–10). Retrieved from http://www.counseling.org/Resources.

Conn, S. R., Roberts, R. L., & Powell, B. M. (2009). Attitudes and satisfaction with a hybrid model of counseling supervision. *Educational Technology & Society, 12,* 298–306.

Dawson, L., Harpster, A., Hoffman, G., & Phelan, K. (2011). A new approach to distance counseling skill development: Applying a discrimination model of supervision. Retrieved from http://counselingoutfitters.com/vistas/vistas11/Article_46.pdf.

Dudding, C. C., & Justice, L. M. (2004). An e-supervision model: Videoconferencing as a clinical training tool. *Communication Disorders Quarterly, 25,* 145–151.

Finn, J., & Barak, A. (2010). A descriptive study of 3-counsellor attitudes, ethics, and practice. *Counselling and Psychotherapy Research, 10,* 268–277.

Garrison, D. R., & Kanuka, H. (2004). Blended learning: Uncovering its transformative potential in higher education. *Internet and Higher Education, 7,* 95-105.

Hampel, R. (2006). Rethinking task design for the digital age: A framework for language teaching and learning in a synchronous online environment. *ReCALL, 18,* 105–121.

Helbok, C. M. (2003). The practice of psychology in rural communities: Potential ethical dilemmas. *Ethics & Behavior, 13*(4), 367–384.

Hurley, G., & Hadden, K. (2009). Online video supervision: A case study. Retrieved from the National Registry of Health Service Providers in Psychology.

Jencius, M., Baltimore, M. L., & Getz, H. G.

(2009). Innovative uses of technology in clinical supervision. In Culbreth & Brown (Eds.), *State of the art in clinical supervision.* New York: Taylor Francis/Routeledge.

Kraus, R., Stricker, G., & Speyer, C. (2010). *Online counseling: A handbook for mental health professionals.* Waltham, MA: Academic Press.

Lenz, A. S., Oliver, M., & Nelson, K W. (2011). In-person and computer-mediated distance group supervision: A case study. Retrieved from http://counselingoutfitters .com/vistas/vistas11/Article_67.pdf.

Maheu, M. M. (2003). The online clinical practice management model. *Psychotherapy: Theory, Research, Practice, Training, 40*(1), 20–32. doi:10.1037/0033-3204.40.1-2.20.

Mallen, M. J., Vogel, D. L., & Rochlen, A. B. (2005). The practical aspects of online counseling: Ethics, training, technology, and competency. *The Counseling Psychologist, 33,* 776–818.

McAdams III, C. R., & Wyatt, K. L. (2010). The regulation of technology-assisted distance counseling and supervision in the United States: An analysis of current extent, trends and implications. *Counselor Education & Supervision, 49,* 179–192.

McCracken, J. A. (2004). An intensive single subject investigation of clinical supervision: In-person and distance formats. Oklahoma State University. ProQuest Dissertations and Theses. Retrieved from Proquest.

NBCC. (2012). *NBCC policy regarding the provision of distance professional services.* Greensboro, NC: Author.

Nelson, J. A., Nichter, M., & Henriksen, R. (2010). On-line supervision and face-to-face supervision in the counseling internship: An exploratory study of similarities and differences. Retrieved from http:// counselingoutfitters.com/vistas /vistas10/ Article _46.pdf.

Oravec, J. (2000). Online counseling and the Internet: Perspectives for mental health care supervision and education. *Journal of Mental Health, 9,* 121–135.

Orr, P. P. (2010). Distance supervision: Research, findings, and considerations for art therapy. *The Arts in Psychotherapy, 37,* 106–111. doi:10.1016/j.aip.2010.02.002.

Powell, D. J., & Brodsky, A. (2004). *Clinical supervision in alcohol and drug abuse counseling: Principles, models, methods* (Rev. ed.). San Francisco: Jossey-Bass.

Reese, R. J., Aldarondo, F., Anderson, C. R., Lee, S. J., Miller, T. W., & Burton, D. (2009). Telehealth in clinical supervision: A comparison of supervision formats. *Journal of Telemedicine and Telecare, 15,* 356–361.

Shallcross, L. (2012). Finding technology's role in the counseling relationship. *Counseling Today, 54*(4), 26–35.

Stebnicki, M. A., & Glover, N. M. (2001). E-supervision as a complementary approach to traditional face-to-face clinical supervision in rehabilitation counseling: Problems and solutions. *Rehabilitation Education, 15,* 283–293.

Strange, M., Johnson, J., Showalter, D., & Klein, R. (2012). Why rural matters 2011-12: The condition of rural education in the 50 states. A report of the Rural School and Community Trust Program. Washington, DC: Rural School and Community Trust.

United States Census Bureau. (2013). *Urban and rural classification.* Retrieved from http://www.census.gov/geo/reference/ urban-rural.html.

Vaccaro, N., & Lambie, G. W. (2007). Computer-based counselor-in-training supervision: Ethical and practical implications for counselor educators and supervisors. *Counselor Education and Supervision, 47,* 46–57.

Wagenfeld, M. O. (2003). A snapshot of rural and frontier America. In B. Stamm (Ed.), *Rural behavioral health care: An interdisciplinary guide* (pp. 33–40). Washington, DC: American Psychological Association.

Watson, J. C. (2003). Computer-based

supervision: Implementing computer technology into the delivery of counseling supervision. *Journal of Technology and Counseling*, 3. Retrieved from http://jtc.columbus state.edu/Vol4_1/Watson/Watson.htm.

Werth, J. L. Jr., Hastings, S. L., & Riding-Malon, R. (2010). Ethical challenges of practicing in rural areas. *Journal of Clinical Psychology in Session*, *66*(5), 537–548.

Wilson, S. E. (2001). The application of technology to counselor education: Video conferencing in distance supervision. St. Mary's University of San Antonio. ProQuest Dissertations and Theses. Retrieved from Proquest.

Chapter 36

TEACHING COUNSELING TECHNIQUES USING TECHNOLOGY

KaRae' N. Carey and LoriAnn Sykes Stretch

INTRODUCTION

Edwards (2013) and Goss and Hooley (2015) note the long history of clinical supervisors using distance technology for training and supervision. In fact, Rogers (1942) discussed the use of audio recordings, which has remained a primary use of technology in counselor education for teaching and supervising counseling technique development. Specifically, students are often required to demonstrate their proficiency of micro-skills in the field of counseling by conducting mock counseling sessions, which are recorded and submitted to the instructor for critique and review. Through the review of the recording submitted, instructors are able to provide appropriate feedback to students regarding their proficiency of counseling skills and challenge them to continue to improve their counseling techniques.

Students are being taught professional counseling techniques in both land-based and hybrid (combined online/land based) classroom environments. Research supports both land-based and online methods of learning as effective tools for teaching and learning counseling techniques (Barnett, 2011; Coker & Schooley, 2012; Dubi, Ragg, & Reynolds, 2012; Karam, Clymer, Elias, & Calahan, 2014; Wilson, Brown, Wood, & Farkas, 2013). The use of technology in counselor training is becoming increasingly popular (Allen & Seaman, 2103; Lyke & Frank, 2012; Rapacki & McBride, 2014; U.S. Department of Education, 2014).

Rousmaniere, Abbass, and Frederickson (2014) noted that much of the research on skills development and supervision utilizing distance technology has attempted to prove that online methods of teaching and supervision are as good as traditional methods, yet many of the traditional methods have mixed reviews in the literature. Rousmaniere et al. (2014) instead challenge the field to view online methods of training as a new, standalone technique that is valid and the preferred method for the younger generation of counselors and counselor educators who are accustomed to technology being integrated into all aspects of their world. Clearly, technology will continue to play an ever-evolving role in how counselors are trained (Anthony, 2015).

Counseling Techniques Expected Outcomes

There are many expectations for those studying counseling techniques. In the US, under the 2016 Council for Accreditation of Counseling and Related Educational Programs

(CACREP) Standards, for example, counseling students are expected to be able to identify "counselor characteristics and behaviors that influence the helping process" (Section II.F.5.f.). In addition, students should be able to demonstrate "essential interviewing, counseling, and case conceptualization skills; developmentally relevant counseling treatment or intervention plans; development of measurable outcomes for clients; and empirically-based counseling strategies and techniques for prevention, intervention, and advocacy" (Section II.F.5.g.-j.).

At the completion of a counseling techniques course, students should be able to evaluate the influence of their own personal attitudes, values and beliefs on the delivery of counseling skills and techniques. Student should be able to demonstrate beginning and intermediate counseling techniques and skills as well as assess personal insights, strengths, limitations and challenges related to demonstrating counseling techniques and skills. In this chapter, we will describe two online counseling techniques courses, which strive to meet these standards through the use of distance technology.

Counseling Techniques Course Process

Course 1

During the eleven weeks of this counseling techniques course, students incorporate theory and use appropriate counseling techniques, which is essential to counseling practice. The course utilizes Blackboard, an asynchronous learning management system (LMS; Blackboard, 2015). Blackboard incorporates tools for course creation, delivery and management; course assessments; grading; and plagiarism prevention through TurnItIn.

Each week, students are expected to post in an asynchronous learning platform (Blackboard) their understandings and, across the term, demonstrate mastery of the following concepts: (a) integrating theoretical orientation into counseling techniques and how this orientation might impact their future clinical practice, (b) how their personal values impact the counselor role, (c) how to begin an initial counseling session and identify appropriate counseling skills used in an initial counseling session, (d) identification of the difference between and proper uses of open- and closed-ended questions, (e) understanding culture and ethnicity and how appropriate implementation of proxemics and haptics, (f) understanding culture and nonverbal communication, (g) appropriate confrontation in counseling, (h) properly closing a series of sessions (course of therapy) and a single session of counseling, (i) proper use of multisensory techniques, and (j) application of creative counseling techniques.

Students are expected to submit through Blackboard a weekly journal, which reflects their individual experiences with learning objectives throughout the course. Specifically, students are to contemplate and reflect on (a) demonstrating their skills on video for the instructor; (b) their own world view, attitudes, and beliefs; (c) using micro-skills learned in the course; (d) self-assessment and evaluation; (e) use of logical consequences; (f) maintaining focus in the counseling session; (g) providing information and psychoeducation; (i) appropriate use of self-disclosure; and (j) working with challenging clients.

As a component of the counseling techniques course, students are also expected to record a total of five videos. The videos consist of four 10-minute videos and one 20-minute capstone video project. The videos are intended to demonstrate student counselor competence in the applied clinical skills of providing informed consent, attending behaviors, encouraging the client, paraphrasing with checkout, reflection of feeling, proxemics/haptics, nonverbal communication, open- and closed-ended questions, reframing, focusing, exploration of logical consequences, use of confrontation, silence, self-disclosure and providing psychoeducation. Students are expected to transcribe their sessions verbatim and reflect on their verbalizations in the counseling sessions and reflect on the intentionality of the utterings.

The first video is a practice video, which is 10 minutes in length. In the first video, the students demonstrate that they can properly and efficiently explain confidentiality and the limits of confidentiality as well as review informed consent with the clients. These practice sessions also allow the students to test their technology to ensure that it is working properly. In addition, they are also testing the features of the Online Video Platform (OVP) in the virtual classroom.

Videos two through four are each 10 minutes in length and the fifth video is 20 minutes in length. The second video assesses the students' proficiency in attending behaviors, encouraging, paraphrasing and checkout and reflections of feeling. The third video assesses proxemics and/or haptics, nonverbal communication (client/counselor), open- and closed-ended questions, reframing, focusing and logical consequences. The fourth video assesses the student's skills in using confrontation, silence, information/psychoeducation and self-disclosure/feedback. The fifth video is the final capstone project, during which the student demonstrates a beginning, middle and end of a counseling session to include the use of the following stages: rapport or relationship, contract or story, focus or goal-setting, funnel or restory, closure and terminating the session.

The capstone video project is designed to demonstrate student counselor competence in all of the microskills, in what could be arguably the closest to a "real-world" counseling session. In the capstone video project, the students demonstrate micro-skills through a video recorded demonstration counseling session. The mock counseling session is expected

to be at least 20 minutes and all skills learned in the course are to be competently demonstrated.

Recording and transcribing the mock sessions allows students to self-critique and allows the faculty member to provide substantive feedback on the student's progress. Media, such as video, can help learners understand complex concepts and procedures that are difficult to explain simply with text and graphics (Hartsell & Yuen, 2006). In order to submit the videos, students use an online video platform (OVP). An OVP is a service that enables the computer to upload and store video content on the Internet. Formats vary according to the programs and operating systems employed by the students. There are many available formats for digital video including .avi (Microsoft), .mov (Quicktime), .wmv (Windows) and .flv (Flash video). There are many secure OVPs available on the Internet such as Panopto, 23video, Bright cove, Cisco and Share, Kaltura, Ooyala, Hightail, Mega and Voice Thread.

Faculty members complete formative and summative evaluations on each student and each evaluation is transmitted electronically to the technique course lead and the individual student. The evaluation rates each student on each of the assessed skills using the following scale: 0-3. A score of zero indicates skills are demonstrated inconsistently and the student does not adequately address the area of the client's concern. With a score of zero, the student will need continued review in this area before engaging in clinical work. A score of 1 indicates the student demonstrated skills somewhat inconsistently and the student minimally addresses the client's concern with faculty feedback. With a score of 1, the student will need continued review in this area before engaging in clinical work. A score of 2 indicates the student is mostly consistent in demonstrating skills and the student addresses the client's issue with faculty feedback, but the student will need some additional review before engaging in clinical work. A score of 3 indicates the student consistently demonstrated skills and there are no areas of concern for the student. Faculty members are instructed to include additional detailed comments for any student who receives a score of 0, 1, or 2.

Students are rated in the following areas: (a) the student relates to peers, professors, and others in a respectful and appropriate professional manner; (b) the student exhibits the spirit of advocacy and social change in her or his development as a professional counselor; (c) the student takes responsibility for compensating for her/his deficiencies; (d) the student is aware of her/his own belief systems, values and limitations and they do not actively affect his/her professional work; (e) the student demonstrates appropriate self-control (such as anger control, impulse control) in interpersonal relationships with faculty, peers and clients; (f) the student demonstrates the ability to receive, integrate and utilize feedback from peers, teachers and supervisors; (g) the student respects the fundamental rights, dignity and worth of all people, including respect for cultural, individual and role differences, including those due to age, gender, race, ethnicity, national origin, religion, sexual orientation, physical ability/disability, language and socioeconomic status; (h) the student behaves in accordance with the program's accepted code(s) of ethics/ standards of practice; and (i) the student demonstrates honesty and fairness, academically, personally and professionally.

Course 2

During this five-week introductory techniques course, students learn basic counseling skills and competencies essential to initiating and maintaining relationships with clients, regardless of specific theoretical orientation. This course offers a preliminary introduction to basic counseling skills. The course uses a revised version of the Counselor Competencies Scale (CCS; Swank, Lambie, & Witta, 2012), which assess the following competencies: nonverbal communication, accurate empathy, minimal encouragers, questions, paraphrasing, reflection of feeling and meaning, summarizing, challenging discrepancies and goal setting. By means of discussions, weekly structured practice assignments, two two-hour practical application sessions with the faculty member, journals and a transcript assessment of a practice 20-minute role-play session, students learn how to identify and conduct competent counselling interviews.

The platform for the online portion of the course is Moodle, which is a GPL open-source Learning Platform designed to provide educators, administrators and learners with a single robust, secure and integrated system to create personalized learning environments (Moodle, 2015). Moodle is built by the Moodle project, which is led and coordinated by Moodle HQ, an Australian company of 30 developers which is financially supported by a network of over 60 Moodle Partner service companies worldwide.

Students participate in an asynchronous discussion each week through Moodle. Discussion topics include conceptualizing helping, the impact of counselor/client differences, assessing clients, termination and integrating helping techniques into practice. Students are expected to spend approximately five hours per week in the asynchronous discussions, distributed throughout the week on three or more days and to be actively engaged in interactive discussion. The discussion posts reflect the degree to which the students have read, absorbed and then incorporated the assigned readings into the discussion.

Each week, students form groups and engage in learning activities designed to provide students with numerous ways of practicing, discussing, and processing the skills and competencies through interactive, synchronous, online group meetings. The weekly activities are critical to students' progress and directly tied to the competencies students must be able to demonstrate in order to be professional counselors. A Wiki signup sheet is available for students to form groups to complete these activities. Students utilize the OmniJoin (discussed in detail later) to meet as a group. In the past, students have also successfully used programs such as Skype, FaceTime, and Google Hangouts. Since the weekly activities do not include discussions of confidential information, these non-HIPAA compliant, video-conferencing technologies are allowed. Students submit a written summary and reflection on the activities via Moodle. Consistently, students note that the group interaction expands their perspective and enhances their understanding of the counseling skills being discussed.

Next, all students must participate in two two-hour Practical Application sessions via OmniJoin. OmniJoin web conferencing delivers highly secure voice and video collaboration through web meetings via a private cloud (Omnijoin, 2015). OmniJoin offers military-grade, end-to-end encryption; host authentication; SSL3/TLS/HTTPA transmission security; and multiple levels of meeting password controls. The program allows for secure sharing of media files, documents, and desktop screens. There is also a chat feature. One of OmniJoin's strengths is the immediate availability of support technicians who can join sessions to help problem solve technical difficulties.

During each two-hour Practical Application Session, students practice the skills being reviewed in class with up to three peers in an Omnijoin session with the instructor. Students have an active role during each Practical Application Session. The Practical Application Session opens with a brief discussion of the primary skills being practiced in the session. Then the instructor role-plays a counselor with one of the attending students. The last hour and a half of the Practical Application

Session consists of role plays in which students rotate through the roles of counselor, client and observer. Each role is active and has assigned tasks. Students provide a written reflective journal via Moodle after each Practical Application session. In their journals, students reflect on reactions, insights, skills acquisition and they set two or three SMART (Specific, Measureable, Achievable, Relevant, and Time-limited) goals related to the student's skill development as a counselor-in-training.

Finally, students work in small groups to conduct practice interview sessions of at least 20 minutes with an assigned classmate(s), taking turns being the counselor and the interviewee (the client). These sessions are recorded in OmniJoin. The "counselor" must ensure that his or her interviewee has signed an Informed Consent Form prior to recording the session. Each student completes a written portion of this assignment individually that has three components: role play context, transcription and analysis, and self-reflection. The written assignment and signed informed consent are submitted via Moodle. The recorded session is submitted as an OmniJoin link within the written assignment and is reviewed by the faculty member.

The faculty member reviews the role play via the OmniJoin recording and written transcription/analysis submitted via Moodle. Then, the faculty member provides quantitative and qualitative utilizing a revised version of the CCS (Swank, Lambie, & Witta, 2012). Students receive feedback via Moodle on the following competencies: nonverbal communication, accurate empathy, minimal encouragers, questions, paraphrasing, reflection of feeling and meaning, summarizing, challenging discrepancies and goal setting.

Training for Faculty and Students

When working with online technologies in the learning environment, the participants must receive training in order to make the learning environment as seamless as possible. In both courses, faculty members receive a minimum of one hour specific training on the technology prior to the start of the term. There is ongoing technical support available on demand for students and faculty for the technologies. Faculty members and students have access to online tutorials and 24-hour support. In addition, webinars are offered throughout the year to support basic and advanced uses of the technologies available.

In the second course, in addition to 24-hour technical support from the university, faculty and students can also contact Omni-Join technicians who are able to join sessions and problem solve issues immediately. Faculty members also receive an instructor's manual that provides detailed instructions on the use of the technology as well as the expectations for the course. Faculty members are encouraged to post prewritten bulletins in the course room throughout the term that provide helpful technological tips for using Omni-Join and Google Hangouts for assignments.

Challenges with Technology

Though there is training for the video platform that is consistently available on demand for all students, in the counseling techniques courses, there have been challenges with the technology. Primarily, students have reported difficulties uploading videos from their personal recording devices to the online video platform. Reasons for the difficulty in uploading assignments is as varied as the students themselves in the online learning environment. Depending on the original recording device settings (cell phone, lap top computer, video camera or digital video recorder), the recording settings may have been too large for the OVP to process. In such cases, students did not have the knowledge to change settings on their personal recording devices, and many chose to rerecord their sessions. Other

students contacted the technical support persons, also available on demand to students, who walked students through minimizing the size of the video so that it could be uploaded to the OVP.

Other challenges have been the time to upload videos and having the bandwidth to maintain video and audio conferencing. Some students have reported as many as 10 hours of uploading time. Likewise, students sometimes struggle to maintain a quality connection during the videoconferencing portion of the practical application sessions and role plays. Most often, these issues are due to slow wireless connections or even dial-up Internet connections. One solution that is now recommended to students with wireless only connections is a PowerLine adapter, which uses the student's home's electrical wiring as a wired data network.

CONCLUSION

Ultimately, technology has become an integral part of counselor education training for both on ground and online programs. Training programs who rely on technology have shown similar student progress to more traditional, less technology enhanced programs (Barnett, 2011; Coker & Schooley, 2012; Dubi, Ragg, & Reynolds, 2012; Karam, Clymer, Elias, & Calahan, 2014; Wilson, Brown, Wood, & Farkas, 2013). The challenge now is for programs to focus less on justifying the use of technology and moving more toward maximizing the use of technology for counselor educator training.

REFERENCES

Allen, I. E., & Seaman, J. (2013). *Changing courses: Ten years of tracking online education in the United States.* San Francisco: Babson Survey Research Group and Quahog Research Group, LLC.

Anthony, K. (2015). Training therapists to work effectively online and offline within digital culture. *British Journal of Guidance & Counselling, 43*(1), 36–42. doi: 10.1080/03069885.2014.924617.

Barnett, J. E. (2011). Utilizing technological innovations to enhance psychotherapy supervision, training, and outcomes. *Psychotherapy, 48*(2), 103–108. doi:10.1037/a0023381.

Blackboard. (2015). *About Blackboard*. Retrieved from http://www.blackboard.com/about-us/index.aspx.

CACREP. (2016). *2016 CACREP Standards*. Alexandria, VA: Author. Retrieved from http://www.cacrep.org/wp-content/uploads/2015/05/2016-CACREP-Standards.pdf.

Coker, J. K., & Schooley, A. L. (2012). Investigating the effectiveness of clinical supervision in a CACREP accredited on-line counseling program. In G. R. Walz, J. C. Bleur, & R. K. Yep (Eds.), *VISTAS 2012*. Alexandria, VA: American Counseling Association.

Dubi, M., Raggi, M., & Reynolds, J. (2012). *Distance supervision: The PIDIB Model*. Retrieved from http://www.counseling.org/docs/default-source/vistas/vistas_2012_article_82.pdf?sfvrsn=9.

Edwards, J. (2013). *Strengths-based supervision in clinical practice*. Thousand Oaks: Sage.

Goss, S., & Hooley, T. (2015) Symposium on online practice in counselling and guidance. *British Journal of Guidance and Counselling, 43*(1), 1–8.

Hartsell, T., & Yuen, S. C. (2006). Video streaming on inline learning. *Association for the Advancement of Computing in Education Journal, 13*(1), 31–43.

Karam, E. A., Clymer, S. R., Elias, C., & Calahan, C. (2014). Together face-to-face or alone at your own pace: Comparing traditional vs. blended learning formats in couple & family relationship coursework. *Journal of Instructional Psychology, 41*(1–4), 85–93.

Lyke, J., & Frank, M. (2012). Comparison of student learning outcomes in online and traditional classroom environments in a psychology course. *Journal of Instructional Psychology, 39*(3/4), 245–250.

Moodle. (2015). *About Moodle*. Retrieved from https://docs.moodle.org/28/en/About_Moodle.

Rapacki, T. M., & McBride, D. L. (2014). From awareness to practice: An online workshop on bringing culture into the counselling room. *Online Submission* [serial online], ERIC.

Rogers, C. R. (1942). The use of electronically recorded interviews in improving psychotherapeutic techniques. *American Journal of Orthopsychiatry, 12*, 429–434. doi: 10.1111/j.1939-0025.1942.tb05930.x.

Rousmaniere, T., Abbass, A., & Frederickson, J. (2014). New developments in technology-assisted supervision and training: A practical overview. *Journal of Clinical Psychology, 70*(11), 1082–1093. doi: 1-.1002/jclp.22129

Swank, J. M., Lambie, G. W., & Witta, E. L. (2012). An exploratory investigation of the Counseling Competencies Scale: A measure of counseling skills, dispositions, and behaviors. *Counselor Education & Supervision, 51*, 189–206. doi: 10.1002/j.1556-6978.2012.00014.x

U.S. Department of Education. (2014). *Enrollment in distance education courses, by state: Fall 2012 (NCES 2014-023)*. Washington, DC: Author.

Wilson, A. B., Brown, S., Wood, Z. B., & Farkas, K. J. (2013). Teaching direct practice skills using web-based simulations: Home visiting in the virtual world. *Journal of Teaching in Social Work, 33*(4–5), 421–437.

Chapter 37

THE ROLE OF ONLINE CAREERS WORK IN SUPPORTING MENTAL HEALTH

Tristram Hooley and Siobhan Neary

INTRODUCTION

There is a strongly documented relationship between positive career building and good mental health. Therapeutic counsellors and other kinds of mental health support workers have addressed this issue in one way, while career professionals have addressed this through a different set of paradigms and practices. In some places there have been interesting overlaps between the practices of these two groups but, in others, they have operated largely separately. However, the practices of both groups are shifting to take account of the affordances of the Internet (Goss & Hooley, 2015). This chapter will explore the relevance of the concept of career in supporting good mental health and consider how this can be translated into online practices which support individuals to improve their mental health and develop their careers.

The concept of career has a dialectical relationship with that of mental health. There is considerable evidence that mental health issues have a major impact on an individual's ability to work, work effectively and derive satisfaction from their work (Booth, Francis, & James, 2007; Royal College of Psychiatrists, 2008). People with mental health issues are disproportionately likely to be unemployed, in low-skilled employment and experience unmanaged breaks in their employment. On the other hand, the individual's experience of work is a strong influence on their mental health for both good and ill (Herr, 1989). A lack of employment or unsatisfactory employment impact on an individuals' self-esteem and can contribute to depression, addiction, disengagement from the workplace and other mental health issues (Vuori, Toppinen-Tanner & Mutanen, 2012; Waddell & Burton, 2006). Mental well-being and work are therefore both interrelated and interdependent.

The concept of career connects an individual's work with their learning and their wider life. Many of the interrelationships between work and mental health also hold true for participation in learning. Poor mental health can mitigate against participation in learning, while participation in learning can impact on mental health positively (Chandola & Jenkins, 2014) or lead to stress (Jayanthi, Thirunavukarasu & Rajkumar, 2015) and attendant mental health problems.

A career is not about the hierarchical progression through an organisation but is instead a key frame of reference for individuals in managing their own identity and aspirations. It provides a means by which individuals can access the good life while contributing to the world they live in. Consequently, good mental health impacts on individuals' capacity to manage their careers while effective career management maximises an individual's capacity to maintain good mental health (Walker & Peterson, 2012). This intersection is something that is appropriately of concern to counsellors, psychotherapists and other mental health workers as well as to career counsellors, careers educators and others involved in supporting career development.

Since the 1990s, the Internet has brought about a substantial shift in the way in which individuals' careers operate. This can be seen in the growth of online recruitment, e-learning and online career support. It can also be seen in the transformation of the lived experience of those in work and learning. For example, our increased capacity to work from home or to maintain numerous overseas contacts has the potential to improve our lives but also presents mental health challenges such as the observed relationship between email and workplace stress (Jerejian, Reid, & Rees, 2013; Reinke & Chamorro-Premuzic, 2014).

Hooley (2012) argues that the development of the Internet impacts on the concept of career in three main ways: firstly, it shifts in the context within which individuals live, learn, and work; secondly, it requires individuals to develop new kinds of career management skills to operate within this changed context; and finally, it opens up new opportunities for the giving and receiving of career support. Each of these shifts can impact on mental health, while the final one may open up new kinds of mental health support.

Careers Work and Mental Health

Career development is an interdisciplinary field which combines a range of different traditions including psychology, sociology, education and counselling. Watts and Kidd (2000) argue that while career development and counselling have distinct histories, by the 1960s, both were drawing on a common epistemology based in Rogerian counselling (Rodgers, 1965). However, since this point, despite frequent theoretical borrowings, the fields have developed along distinctive lines. Betz and Corning (1993) argue that this is a mistake and that career and personal counselling are "inseparable" due to both their theoretical similarities and the similarities in their processes. There is a strong tradition of careers work that builds on this shared heritage (e.g., Richardson, 2012; Westergaard, 2012) as well as traditions of careers work that draw from different epistemic basis, particularly those associated with education.

Within the work environment, there are a variety of processes such as restructuring, downsizing, and the requirement for increased flexibility which all place strains on people's mental health (Bamberger et al., 2012; Falkenberg et al., 2013) and require them to develop their career management competencies (Vuori et al., 2012). However, there is limited research that has explored the impacts of career guidance on mental health, although Robertson (2013) has identified this intersection as an area for further research and practice development.

Despite the limited evidence base in this field, it is possible to conceptualise four main ways in which careers work might support good mental health.

1. Increasing individuals' capacity to manage career and mental health challenges.
2. Supporting individuals through transitions
3. Contributing to the improvement of poor mental health.
4. Managing the impact of mental health conditions.

Increasing Individuals' Capacity to Manage

Some of the research on careers work and mental health has emphasised its capacity to prevent problems by enhancing individuals coping skills, adaptability and resilience (Akkermans et al., 2014; Bimrose & Hearne, 2012). Herr (1989) argues that most of the problems that are brought to career counsellors are not pathological or organic but are rather issues of personal competence. Consequently, the role of the careers worker becomes to help the individual to enhance their personal competence. This approach is strongly linked to the concept of career management skills (CMS). These skills can be defined as competencies that help individuals to identify their existing skills, develop career learning goals and to take actions to enhance their career (Gravina & Lovsin, 2012). These focus on providing individuals with the capacity to self-manage their career and to avoid crises that might lead to mental health problems. Brammer and Winter (2015) explore the use of Massive Open Online Course (MOOC) to deliver modules on career and employability skills to university students. The focus of the MOOC was to support participants to have greater control, clarity, confidence and courage in managing and progressing their career. Their research suggested that the MOOC supported people to improve their careers and their mental health concurrently. For example, the course helped participants to take risks, to step outside their comfort zone and to gain more control over their lives, which was particularly valuable to those reporting workplace stress.

Supporting Individuals through Transitions

The second area in which careers work seeks to intervene in ways that support positive mental health is in the provision of support for transitions. Life transitions, including those associated with career, place stresses on individual's mental health (Cleary, Walter, & Jackson, 2011; Wheaton, 1990). However, successful transitions can support well-being

and empower individuals (Robertson, 2013). In this role, career development seeks to providing individuals with the tools they need to ensure an effective transition.

Contributing to the Improvement of Poor Mental Health

Mental health issues commonly have a career component. While not all work is good for mental health, positive engagement with learning and work can support the enhancement of good mental health. As a consequence, it is possible to situate career interventions as part of an overall package to improve an individual's mental health (Vuori et al., 2002). Barker et al. (2005) explored the use of qualified career guidance practitioners working with hospital staff on an acute psychiatric unit and during the provision of post-discharge support. They identified that opportunities to consider the future contributed to recovery and encouraged individuals to continue with learning once they were discharged.

Barker et al. (2005) argue that a recovery model which focuses on supporting individuals to regain control over their life benefits from the inclusion of careers specialists. The inclusion of such specialists can help individuals to consider the multidimensional nature of their lives and to view themselves positively as a worker or potential worker as well as someone who is experiencing mental illness.

Managing the Impact of Mental Health Conditions

Finally, it is clear that for people with serious, complex and long-term mental health issues, there are considerable challenges to participating in the labour and learning markets. Where individuals are encouraged to focus on their treatments and therapies to the exclusion of considering how to participate in learning and work, there can be a detrimental effect which can increase levels of psychiatric illness (Centre for Mental Health, 2013). The Centre for Mental Health also notes that health professionals can contribute to creating barriers to employment by encouraging individuals with mental health issues to seek non-competitive employment opportunities such as voluntary or sheltered workplaces which do not allow individuals to progress. Contrary to this, the use of an individual placement and support model (IPS) provides a framework for counsellors which focuses on competitive jobs as an outcome. This provides in-depth support for individuals wanting to reenter the job market. This is currently being trialled broadly within the UK (Centre for Mental Health, 2013). Knaeps et al. (2015), in their study, explore counsellors' intentions in working with their clients. They argue that when working with people with mental illnesses, career professionals continue to focus first and foremost on competitive jobs unless it is felt to be detrimental to the individual. Such a focus can open up opportunities to progress for those with mental illness which can help them to access employment while achieving their recovery goals.

Careers Work Online

In recent years there has been a growing range of career guidance practice taking place in online spaces. Academics and practitioners have begun to explore the range of ways in which the online environment can support individuals to develop their careers in both blended and wholly online contexts. There is a tradition of research and practice on ICT and career development starting in the 1960s, which Watts (2002) recounts and argues moved through four phases: mainframe; microcomputer; web; and digital.

More recent work has examined the affordances of Watts' digital phase. Broadly, it is possible to characterise three distinct strands of practice which have developed (Hooley,

Hutchinson & Watts, 2010): (1) the use of the Internet to provide information and resources; (2) the use of various forms of online automated interactions to deliver career assessments, to replace aspects of what professionals would have done or to provide new kinds of automated experiences such as work simulations; and (3) the use of the Internet to provide online communication, networks and relationships.

Information

Information describes a range of online resources that can be utilised to support online career building. This includes conventional kinds of career information, e.g., job specifications and information about courses, but also allows for the development and utilisation of new types of information which make use of the interlinked and multimedia nature of the Internet. Since the mid-1990s, there has been a proliferation of career-related websites which have sought to provide careers information in a variety of forms. Included amongst this career information is a range of information which seeks to address mental health-related concerns. So, for example, *The Guardian* Careers site offers *top tips for dealing with stress at work* (Bird, 2012) while the university information site Top Universities offers advice on *how to stop feeling homesick at university* (Hunt, 2013). Mental health charities and government websites also provide a range of information online to support individuals with mental health concerns to manage their employment and their employers, much of this specifically focuses on how people can manage their return to work, for example, after sick leave (Mind, 2014). Online career information therefore regularly addresses mental health concerns, but there have so far been no studies that have sought to explore the reception or impact of such information.

Hooley (2012) argues that we need to be careful about viewing the Internet as a careers library and suggests that a better metaphor would be to see the Internet as a career marketplace in which traders with varying degrees of authority and integrity set out their wares. Elsewhere, Grubb (2002) has urged caution about celebrating the availability of online careers information without also recognising the skills and literacies that underpin the effective use of these. Empirical studies (Howieson et al., 2009; Howieson & Semple, 2013) have also questioned the usefulness of information-based careers websites without a strong supportive infrastructure for learning and development. In the context of mental health information, this raises further concerns about the challenges of self-diagnosis and the insensitivity of online information to the particular context that an individual might find themselves in. Reavley and Jorm (2011) raise concerns about the evidential base that underpins online mental health information.

Automated Interactions

The second strand to online careers practice is the use of automated interactions. Automated interactions seek to recognise the individual and to deliver a service that is, to varying extents, tailored to their needs without the direct use of a professional. Automated interactions can facilitate the initial exploration and diagnostic elements of a traditional advice and guidance service: for example, by offering psychometric, matching and reflective tools. Much online gaming can also be grouped under the heading of automated interactions. There is some emerged research that has identified career benefits that may accrue from participating in online gaming (e.g., Dugosija et al., 2008). Although this is of interest, there is not space within this chapter to explore this in detail.

There is considerable research that supports the idea that these kinds of automated interactions can be highly effective if administered appropriately (Dozier et al., 2014; Tirpak

& Schlosser, 2013). Gati and Auslin-Peretez (2011) highlight a number of features of effective design for such tools, noting, for example, the need to create tools that move beyond "diagnosing" and include resources that support individuals' understanding of the diagnosis and consider how best to act on this. They also highlight the way that such online resources can offer resources to counsellors as well as to individual career builders.

The challenges for online mental health assessments are even greater than with more traditional career assessments. For example, the Canadian Mental Health Association (2015) offers a range of self-assessment tools for Canadians. These includes a *Work/Life Balance Quiz*, which makes explicit reference to the intersection between career and mental health and an online *stress index* and *mental health meter*, which are both presented in sections of the site that discuss career and workplace issues. Within the UK, the Warwick Edinburgh mental well-being scale (Tennant et al., 2007) has become widely used to monitor mental well-being and to evaluate policies and project that aim to improve well-being. This instrument has been well validated and evaluated (Crawford et al., 2011) and is available as an on-line tool whereby individuals can take a *wellbeing self-assessment*. Respondents are encouraged to engage with five steps to mental well-being and to use other resources and to make use of other activities and resources such as *check your mood* (NHS, 2015). This site implements many of the recommendations of Gati and Auslin-Pertez, providing encouragement to make use of professional help, support in interpreting the conclusions, and encouraging reflection about context. However, it is worth noting that there is very little evidence that supports the effectiveness of these kinds of online assessments or theorising their use (Luxton et al., 2011).

The next generation of automated interactions frequently combines aspects of both assessment and gaming, delivering mental health interventions via mobile technologies. Such interventions are known as mHealth apps and may be used either as a stand-alone form of support or integrated into wider mental health support (Luxton et al., 2011). There is also an equivalent range of mCareer apps which provide career assessments and transition support such as helping with CV/resume creation. A minority of these tools also wrap forms of mental health support into the mCareer app; for example, the Mind Tools app[1] includes interactive assessments and resources on *stress, overcoming fear of failure, anger management* and a range of other mental health-related concerns within a suite of more conventional career management and employability skills such as *strategy, decision making, time management,* and *project management.* Again, the efficacy of such interventions has yet to be fully explored in the literature, nor has their use become well integrated into mainstream practice in either careers work or mental health support.

Communication

Finally, there are online tools that facilitate communication and interaction between people. In some cases, these online technologies have simply transferred offline practices (talking/writing etc.) online; in others, they have resituated other technologically mediated practices within the online arena (for example the move from telephone networks to video and audio online synchronous technologies). However, many types of online communication have created entirely new modes of communication. The many-to-many social networks of Facebook and Twitter with their conventions of short personal updates and the sharing of photos, weblinks, and resources have no direct offline equivalents.

The use of online communication tools opens up huge opportunities for online careers work. However, thinking about how to transfer career development online is unlikely to be simply a question of shifting existing practices into the online environment. Rather, it is likely to require a willingness to reimagine paradigms and to innovate. It is possible to classify communication tools into three categories: those that facilitate one-to-one, one-to-many and many-to-many forms of communication. These currently all exist in one form or another, but it would be useful to explore in more depth what these offer and to whom.

It is not possible within the scope of the current chapter to consider all of the different permutations of online communication that might serve to deliver career support. However, some brief examples can serve to open up some of the diversity. At one end, Haberstroh, Rowe, and Cisneros (2012) discuss the creation of a virtual counselling and advising service using chat software. Such a service translates many of the paradigms of face-to-face counselling into a text-based online interaction. Dowling and Rickwood (2013) argue that while such approaches have been extensively utilised, the evidence base for their efficacy in addressing mental health problems remains weak. Nonetheless, the virtual counselling and advising service remains as an interaction delivered by a professional trained in online counselling, operating within the context of an educational organisation and consequently open to quality assurance of various kinds.

At the other end of the spectrum, we might place something like the UK's mental health forum[2] where there is a specific forum dedicated to *education, employment, finances & debt, housing and legal issues,* which has over

---

[1] See http://www.mindtools.com/Apps/ for further information on the Mind Tools app.
[2] See http://www.mentalhealthforum.net/forum/.

2000 threads addressing topics such as *being run down because of the workplace* and *when you eventually go back to work what will you tell your employers.* This is a peer community managed by volunteers from which people can derive advice, support and information, but which offers little in the way of quality assurance. The evidence base for such resources is also emergent with a number of systematic literature reviews noting the need for higher quality studies in this area (e.g., Ali et al., 2015).

Conceptualising Online Careers Work and Mental Health

Individuals are accessing a range of online interventions to help support them with their careers and their mental health (sometimes both together). In many cases, these kinds of self-directed resources are being used without any direct reference to professionals. The unregulated and interdisciplinary nature of the Internet means that it is possible for boundaries between areas such as career development

and mental health support to be easily crossed and for hybrid practices to emerge. This chapter has identified a number of these hybrid practices and noted that in many of these cases, there is very limited research or theorisation that exists around them.

The task at hand is therefore to conceptualise what online careers work which address what mental health issues might look like. Figure 37.1 sets out a framework which may be useful in the further theorisation of this area. The categories suggested within each box are an attempt to begin this process of theorisation.

Figure 37.1 therefore suggests that it is possible to understand online mental health interventions in relation to two axes: firstly, the purpose to which the intervention is addressed (increasing individual capacity, supporting transition, improving mental health or managing mental health conditions) and secondly the kind of technology being used (information, automated interaction or communication). The use of this typology could aid the mapping

	Increasing individuals capacity	Supporting transitions	Improving mental health	Managing mental health conditions
Information	Information for CMS development e.g,. The Guardian Careers site	Transition information e.g., Top Universities	Career-related mental health information e.g., online advice about return to work following illness	Mental health relevant career information e.g., online advice about employment rights relating to mental health conditions
Automated interaction	Tools for CMS development e.g,. the Mind Tools app	Tools for transition e.g., C.V. builder apps	Tools for recovery e.g., the mental health meter.	Tools for managing e.g., mobile apps that reward you for maintaining work/life balance
Communication	Online career education e.g., MOOC	Online career support e.g., Linkedin	Online career counselling e.g., interviews delivered through video-link	Online career mentoring e.g., use of forums

Figure 37.1 Online career mental health support interventions.

and analysis of this emerging field. It would also provide both individuals and professionals working with them with a framework that could help diagnose the type of help required and the resources which may be available.

CONCLUSIONS AND A WAY FORWARD

This chapter has argued that there is a strong and appropriate overlap between careers work and mental health support. An individual's interaction with learning and work are both influenced by and can in turn influence their mental health. Consequently, there is an overlap in practice between careers workers and mental health workers, although there is considerable room for this overlap to be better developed and more clearly theorised.

Both careers workers and mental health workers are making increasing use of the Internet in their practice and there is an increasing amount of practice which addresses both career and mental health using online technologies. However, as this chapter has demonstrated, the development of such practice is rapidly outpacing evidence and research. This means that the efficacy and appropriate use of such technologies is often poorly understood. There is a clear need for a concerted research effort in this space in order to highlight the opportunities that new technologies offer, map their limitations and clarify where they are best employed in tandem with a professional. There is also need to ensure that the field of careers work is better engaged with the needs of those with mental health concerns and is able to provide specialist support and resources which will ensure greater inclusivity.

REFERENCES

Akkermans, J., Brenninkmeijer, V., Schaufeli, W. B., & Blonk, R. W. (2014). It's all about CareerSKILLS: Effectiveness of a career development intervention for young employees. *Human Resource Management.* Early view online prior to print publication.

Ali, K., Farrer, L., Gulliver, A., & Griffiths, K. M. (2015). Online peer-to-peer support for young people with mental health problems: A systematic review. *JMIR Mental Health, 2*(2), e19.

Bamberger, S. G., Vinding, A. L., Larsen, A., Nielsen, P., Fonager, K., Nielsen, R. N., Ryom, P., & Omland, O. (2012). Impact of organisational change on mental health: A systematic review. *Occupational and Environmental Medicine, 69*(8), 592–598.

Barker, V., Markby, P., Knowles, D., & Winbourne, R. (2005). Inclusion in work and learning: Providing information, advice and guidance to adults in acute psychiatric units. *Career Research and Development, 12*, 1–15.

Betz, N. E., & Corning, A. F. (1993). The inseparability of "career" and "personal" counseling. *The Career Development Quarterly, 42*(2), 137–142.

Bimrose, J., & Hearne, L. (2012). Resilience and career adaptability: Qualitative studies of adult career counseling. *Journal of Vocational Behavior, 81*(3), 338–344.

Bird, P. (2012). Top tips for dealing with stress at work. *The Guardian.* Available from http://www.theguardian.com/careers/stress-advice [Accessed 21st May 2015].

Booth, D., Francis, S., & James, R. (2007). Finding and keeping work: Issues, activities and support for those with mental health needs. *Journal of Occupational Psychology, Employment and Disability, 9*(2), 65–97.

Brammer, L., & Winter, D. (2015) 'I've been astounded by some of the insights gleaned from this course': Lessons learnt from the world's first careers abd employability MOOC by both instructors and participants. *Journal of the National Institute for Career Education and Counselling, 34*, 22–31.

Canadian Mental Health Association. (2015). Your mental health. Available from http://www.cmha.ca/mental-health/ [Accessed 21st May 2015].

Centre for Mental Health. (2013). *Barriers to employment* (Briefing 47). London: Centre for Mental Health.

Chandola, T., & Jenkins, A. (2014). The scope of adult and further education for reducing health inequalities. In British Academy, *If you could do one thing*. London: British Academy.

Cleary, M., Walter, G., & Jackson, D. (2011). "Not always smooth sailing": Mental health issues associated with the transition from high school to college. *Issues in Mental Health Nursing, 32*(4), 250–254.

Crawford, M., Robotham, D., Thana, L., Patterson, S., Weaver, T., Barber, R., Wykes, T., & Rose, D. (2011). Selecting outcomes measures in mental Health: The views of service users. *Journal of Mental Health, 20*(4), 336–346.

Dowling, M., & Rickwood, D. (2013). Online counseling and therapy for mental health problems: A systematic review of individual synchronous interventions using chat. *Journal of Technology in Human Services, 31*(1), 1–21.

Dozier, V. C., Sampson, J. P., Lenz, J. G., Peterson, G. W., & Reardon, R. C. (2014). The impact of the self-directed search form R internet version on counselor-free career exploration. *Journal of Career Assessment, 23*(2), 210–224.

Dugosija, D., Efe, V., Hackenbracht, S., Vaegs, T., & Glukhova, A. (2008). Online Gaming as Tool for Career Development, https://www.comsys.rwth-aachen.de /fileadmin/papers/2008/2008-steg-vaegs-gaming.pdf [Accessed 11 June 2012].

Falkenberg, H., Fransson, E. I., Westerlund, H., & Head, J. A. (2013). Short-and long-term effects of major organisational change on minor psychiatric disorder and self-rated health: Results from the Whitehall II study. *Occupational and Environmental Medicine, 70*(10), 688–696.

Gati, I., & Asulin-Peretz, L. (2011). Internet-based self-help career assessments and interventions: Challenges and implications for evidence-based career counseling. *Journal of Career Assessment, 19*(3), 259–273.

Goss, S., & Hooley, T. (2015). Symposium on online practice in counselling and guidance (Editorial). *British Journal of Guidance and Counselling, 43*(1), 1–7.

Gravina, D., & Lovsin, M. (2012). *Career management skills: Factors in implementing policy successfully*. ELGPN Concept Note No. 3. Jyväskylä: ELGPN.

Grubb, W. N. (2002) *Who am I: The inadequacy of career information in the information age*. Paris: OECD.

Haberstroh, S., Rowe, S., & Cisneros, S. (2012). Implementing virtual career counseling and advising at a major university. In R. Lupicini, *Cases on technologies for educational leadership and administration in higher education*. Hershey, PA: Information Science Reference. 174.

Herr, E. (1989). Career development and mental health. *Journal of Career Development, 16*(1).

Hooley, T. (2012). How the internet changed career: Framing the relationship between career development and online technologies. *Journal of the National Institute for Career Education and Counselling (NICEC), 29*, 3–12.

Hooley, T., Hutchinson, J., & Watts, A. G. (2010). *Careering through the web: The potential of web 2.0 and web 3.0 technologies for career development*. London: UKCES.

Howieson, C., & Semple, S. (2013). The impact of career websites: What's the evidence? *British Journal of Guidance and Counselling, 41*(3), 287–301.

Howieson, C., Semple, S., Hickman, S., & McKechnie (2009). *Self-help and career planning*. Glasgow: Skills Development Scotland.

Hunt, A. (2013). How to stop feeling home-sick at university. *Top Universities.* http://www.topuniversities.com/blog/how-stop-feeling-homesick-university [Accessed 21st May 2015].

Jayanthi, P., Thirunavukarasu, M., & Rajkumar, R. (2015). Academic stress and depression among adolescents: A cross-sectional study. *Indian Pediatrics, 52*(3), 217–219.

Jerejian, A. C., Reid, C., & Rees, C. S. (2013). The contribution of email volume, email management strategies and propensity to worry in predicting email stress among academics. *Computers in Human Behavior, 29*(3), 991–996.

Knaeps, J., Neyens, I., van Weeghel, J., & Van Audenhove, C. (2015). Counsellors' focus on competitive employment for people with severe mental illness: An application of the theory of planned behaviour in vocational rehabilitation programmes. *British Journal of Guidance & Counselling* (ahead-of-print), 1–15.

Luxton, D. D., McCann, R. A., Bush, N. E., Mishkind, M. C., & Reger, G. M. (2011). mHealth for mental health: Integrating smartphone technology in behavioral healthcare. *Professional Psychology Research and Practice,* (42), 505–512.

Mind (2014). We've Got Work to Do. Transforming Employment and Back to Work Support for People with Mental Health Problems. London: Mind.

National Health Service (2015). *Wellbeing self-assessment* http://www.nhs.uk/Tools/Pages/Wellbeing-self-assessment.aspx [Accessed 3rd June 2015].

Reavley, N. J., & Jorm, A. F. (2011). The quality of mental disorder information websites: A review. *Patient Education and Counseling, 85*(2), e16–e25.

Reinke, K., & Chamorro-Premuzic, T. (2014). When email use gets out of control: Understanding the relationship between personality and email overload and their impact on burnout and work engagement. *Computers in Human Behavior, 36,* 502–509.

Richardson, M. S. (2012). Counseling for work and relationship. *The Counseling Psychologist, 40*(2), 190–242.

Robertson, P. J. (2013). The wellbeing outcomes of careers guidance. *The British Journal of Guidance and Counselling, 41*(3), 254–266.

Rodgers, C. (1965). *Client-centered therapy.* Boston: Houghton-Mifflin.

Royal College of Psychiatrists. (2008). *Mental health and work.* Cross Government Health and Wellbeing programme, London: The Royal College of Psychiatrists and Health Work Wellbeing.

Tennant, R., Hiller, L., Fishwick, R., Platt, S., Joseph, S., Weich, S., Parkinson, J., Secker, J., & Stewart-Brown, S. (2007). The Warwick-Edinburgh mental well-being scale (WEMWBS): Development and UK validation. *Health and Quality Outcomes, 5*(1) 63.

Tirpak, D. M., & Schlosser, L. Z. (2013). Evaluating FOCUS-2's effectiveness in enhancing first-year college students' social cognitive career development. *The Career Development Quarterly, 61*(2), 110–123.

Vuori, J., Silvonen, J., Amiram, V. D., & Price, R. H. (2002). The Tyohon job search program in Finland: Benefits for the unemployed with the risk of depression or discouragement. *Journal of Occupational Health Psychology, 7*(1), 5–19.

Vuori, J., Toppenen-Tanner, S., & Mutanen, P. (2012). Effects of resource building group intervention on career management and mental health in work organizations: Randomised controlled field trials. *Journal of Applied Psychology, 97*(2), 273–286.

Waddell, G., & Burton, K. (2006). *Is work good for your health and well-being?* Department for Work and Pensions. Norwich: TSO.

Walker, J. V., & Peterson, G. W. (2012). Career thoughts, indecision, and depression: Implications for mental health assessment in career counseling. *Journal of Career Assessment, 20*(4), 497–506.

Watts, A. G., & Kidd, J. M. (2000). Guidance in the United Kingdom: Past, present and future. *British Journal of Guidance and Counselling, 24*(4), 485–502.

Watts, A. G. (2002). The role of information and communication technologies in integrated career information and guidance systems: A policy perspective. *International Journal for Educational and Vocational Guidance, 2*(3), 139–155.

Westergaard, J. (2012). Career guidance and therapeutic counselling: Sharing 'what works' in practice with young people. *British Journal of Guidance and Counselling, 40*(4), 327–339.

Wheaton, B. (1990). Life transitions, role histories, and mental health. *American Sociological Review, 55*(2), 209–23.

Chapter 38

USING TECHNOLOGY TO ENHANCE SUPERVISION AT THE UNIVERSITY OF SOUTHERN CALIFORNIA

Ginger Clark

INTRODUCTION

History

The Rossier School of Education at the University of Southern California (USC) had a doctoral program in Counseling Psychology for over four decades. Its commitment to the gold standard of supervision, at the time, was demonstrated through its allocation of resources to the program. When the school was smaller in size in the late 1980s and early 1990s, its building included a Counselor Training Center with counseling cubicles that had one-way glass and audio monitors that allowed supervisors and students to observe counseling sessions, live, in an unobtrusive way. Observing students were able to benefit from the supervising faculty's live feedback, and the counselor conducting the session would get a summary of the feedback at the session's conclusion.

However, keeping up with developments in supervision modalities, as well as advances in technology, is costly and, over time, the school had to reprioritize its resources. As the school grew, the counselor training space was needed for other programs and faculty, so the program partnered with a community mental health clinic in the city, and moved its training

and supervision operations there. One-way mirrors, along with audio monitors, were used at this facility and the one that followed. In trying to use the latest developments in technology to improve the quality of supervision, a USC faculty member, Joan Rosenberg, began to develop an approach that combined live supervision techniques with delayed, computer-mediated supervision strategies in her approach called "Real-Time Training" (see Rosenberg (2006) for a summary and evaluation of the approach). This method provided real-time written feedback visible on a monitor to students *observing* a session (not the counselor), so that observing counseling students were able to learn from the work of their colleague, who was conducting the therapy, and their professor, who was critiquing the therapy, at the same time. The benefit of using a computer to record the feedback, rather than dialogue in the observation room, was that the feedback was available later as subtitles superimposed on the video recording of the session, so that counselors who conducted the interview could view their session with the professor's real-time feedback scrolling under the video. This way the feedback did not interrupt the counselors' cognitive flow or emotional attunement during the session, but did allow them to experience the real-time feedback from an objective-observer vantage point.

Unfortunately, in 2000, the doctoral program was closed. The Master's Degree program in Marriage and Family Therapy (MFT) was retained, but many of the faculty associated with the doctoral program, and these community mental health partnerships, left the school for other Counseling Psychology doctoral programs, so these partnerships were lost. As a result, the MFT program had to rely on remote training placements, where faculty did not have supervision privileges on-site.

Loss of Resources Led to Less Effective Modes of Supervision

This shift in training arrangements, having students train off-site with supervision from site staff but no direct supervision from faculty, meant it was more difficult for faculty to directly evaluate students' clinical work. For a while, the MFT program relied on students' self-report and written conceptualization of clients during practicum and fieldwork supervision. This left many untapped opportunities to identify strengths or weaknesses, as the class and professor could only draw from the data presented from the perspective of the student. Any issues or critical moments that students missed because of their developmental stage, biases or countertransference were not visible in the supervision process. We found this to be unsatisfying for both students and faculty. Students felt they were not getting the oversight and feedback they needed, and faculty felt hamstrung by a lack of objective performance data. Worse, there were no direct checks and balances to ensure counselors were not somehow causing harm to their clients, so our ethical obligation to provide a gatekeeping function was compromised. Students were supervised at their site and were therefore held accountable to the training

site's therapeutic guidelines, but the MFT program did not have points of direct observation to ensure our own standard of care.

Reintroduction of Technology into Supervision

It soon became obvious that we needed to implement a requirement where students would have to bring samples of their work to their university fieldwork class, so that we could provide better supervision and fulfill our gatekeeping obligation to the public. We decided to require video recordings in most cases. The supervision literature historically has supported the use of video recording as a tool for the development of self-supervision skills, as well as the next best thing to live supervision (Binder, 1999; Huhra, Yamokoski-Maynhart, & Prieto, 2008; Kagan, 1980; Whiffen, 1982). There were a few rare sites that did not allow video recordings to be removed from the premises due to their own risk management policies, in which case we accepted either audio recordings or transcriptions of sessions.

We used Kagan's (1980) Interpersonal Process Recall model, where the counselor, supervisor and observers watch the video together, and anyone could request the video be paused to discuss what was happening in that moment of the recording. We found this approach brought counselors back into the session on a moment-by-moment basis, allowing for formative feedback, rather than only summative feedback at the end of the session. It forced students to re-enter the session from a supervisor role, and to examine their own work as an observer. This gave rise to far more conversations about therapeutic dynamics, such as countertransference, mirroring and attunement, as well as feedback on skills such as cultural competence, theory application, and "micro-counseling skills" (Ivey, Ivey, & Zalaquett, 2010).

The recordings initially came in on small

video cameras that were hooked up to computers, and projected onto a screen or monitor. Over time, however, as webcams became standard equipment in laptop computers, students moved to using their computers to directly record, and password protect, the sessions. This provided a bit more security than an average video camera, as both the operating system itself, as well as the video file can both be password protected. And the file can be easily deleted from the hard drive as soon as it has been viewed and evaluated.

In the past, we have discouraged students from using their mobile phones to record sessions. While the access to the phone's operating system can be password protected, the video file itself could not. Over the last couple of years, however, new mobile applications have allowed for this security function and hardware has evolved to allow the direct connection from the phone or tablet to the projector. We are beginning to see students move towards using their phones and tablets as their primary video recording device, though there are still some hard drive space concerns since 50 minutes of video recordings take up a lot of memory. Still, just as with their computers, they are able to delete the recordings after their use in supervision. An added security feature for phones, tablets, and computers is the ability to remotely wipe data should the device be lost or stolen. Something not possible with the old technology of videotapes, video discs or paper records. Obviously, this requires a back-up system to be in place so that records are not lost, but it still provides far greater mobility and security features when used correctly, abiding by the appropriate ethical guidelines outlined in the American Counseling Association's Code of Ethics (2005) and Stretch, Nagel, & Anthony (2012).

Use of Technology in Fieldwork Class

Aside from evaluating students' work via video recording, we have also begun to use technology as an immediate resource for information, tools, and communication in both clinical skills classes and fieldwork classes, where university-based supervision takes place.

Web-Based Information

The most obvious advancement in technology is immediate access to information. And not just textual information, but video demonstrations, news events and lists of books and articles on particular subjects germane to the client being served. We are able to pause in the middle of our review of a video recording of a session with a client who struggles with substance abuse, for instance, and use the same computer, phone, or tablet to find an online video of an expert doing Motivational Interviewing. Instead of the class hearing the professor recommend that they go buy William Miller's book "Motivational Interviewing: Preparing People for Change" (Miller & Rollnick, 2002), which they may or may not do at a later time, we are able to learn more about applying Motivational Interviewing by immediately calling up a video of Miller demonstrating an interview, then and there, and then discuss how that approach might have shifted the dynamic in the counseling session we are reviewing.

We will often refer to articles about recent news events, such as new policy related to mental health, or case examples of how issues of class, race, gender or sexual orientation are being portrayed in the media, so that students can see how these issues might be affecting the development and functioning of the client we are reviewing.

The web access also allows all of us (students and professors) to find books or articles we' have read or heard about that might be relevant to the case we are reviewing, so that all of the students can take note of the resource, or even buy it online during the discussion. We are able to access the webpages of leaders in the field of psychotherapy to look for book or article recommendations on particular subjects of interest. For example, Steven Hayes' website on Acceptance and Commitment Therapy (ACT) /Relationship Frame Theory (RFT) (Hayes, Pistorello, & Levin, 2012) contains a "State of the ACT Evidence" page (http://www.stevenchayes.com/the-association-for-contextual-behavioral-sciences/state-of-the-act-evidence/) that categorizes various studies that applied ACT to different clinical issues (e.g., depression, anxiety, psychosis, etc.). The site also offers multiple downloadable articles that evaluate ACT's effectiveness in randomized clinical trials.

This immediate access to information and resources has changed the face of the classroom. Our supervision groups have become much more agile and engaged, and the nature of the "era of access" has changed attitudes toward new information. I rarely see students who are resistant to new ideas or information anymore. The world is now a place where changing information is no longer only available to academics, scientists and wealthy corporations through print journals that are publishing information that is often a year or more old. It is now a place where anyone with an Internet connection can gain access to new information, sometimes as it emerges. Though many academic journals are still clinging to the old models of publication and pay to play usage agreements, given the forward momentum toward other models of monetization, and the expectation of free access to information, it is doubtful that these models will remain for long. Quick and easy access to verifiable information has become the expectation of our students, and they have developed the curious and critical minds necessary to filter through that information as a function of training in a program that utilizes it regularly.

Web-Based Tools

Another great advantage of having access to the web in supervision is the easy access to various tools, such as therapy assessments, diagnostic and treatment resource guides, activities that can be used in therapy, and referral sources. While our students receive training in measurement and assessment, once they begin to see clients, they are often overwhelmed by the anxiety that comes with the first time one is in a room with a client who expects them to know how to help. So we have to do a lot of reintroducing and reinforcement of training during this time, including helping students to remember how to evaluate their progress using outcome measures. One of the tools we like to have our students use in therapy is Scott D. Miller's "Session Rating Scale 3.0" and "The Outcome Rating Scale" (Miller, S. D., Duncan, B. L., Sorrell, R., & Brown, G. S., 2004). These measures are very simple to implement and students can chart the results over time with their clients. We will often refer to these measures as a way that students can evaluate their progress in developing the therapeutic relationship with their clients. Dr. Miller's website allows practitioners to download the measures and use them in their practice (http://scottdmiller.com). We are able to use the Web to gain access to various assessment tools that might be relevant to a students' work with their clients. As we discuss the evaluation of treatment, we are able to direct our students to these online assessments in class, which benefits all of the students in the supervision group, not just the student presenting their client.

We are also using our supervision time to reinforce the application of other aspects of classroom training, including diagnosis and treatment approaches. Diagnosis is one of the elements of therapy that is most anxiety provoking for students. They fear making the wrong diagnoses, and appropriately so. With the DSM 5 publication, they are even more unsure about how to navigate a changing diagnostic system. But, we can help them through this process in supervision by reviewing online resources like Psychcentral's "DSM-5 Resource Guide" (http://psychcentral.com/dsm-5/) to facilitate discussions around how diagnoses will be changing in the future, and how students can begin to incorporate those changes now (Grohol & Tartakovsky, 2013).

Blackboard (an online platform for classroom materials and interaction) has been a useful repository for materials that can be used in content classes, and accessed again during fieldwork classes. We have used it to upload videotaped demonstrations from students and professors on various skills, as well as publicly available treatment manuals and other reading materials. For example, John Briere and Cheryl Lanktree's (2013; 2011) "Integrative Treatment of Complex Trauma for Adolescents Treatment Guide" is a reference we regularly use in treating adults and adolescents with Complex Trauma. Our students receive training in this model during their first year, but we are able to refer back to the manual and its assessments on the fly in supervision by either accessing the Blackboard account for Child and Adolescent Psychotherapy course, or going straight to Briere's "USC Adolescent Trauma Training Center" (USC-ATTC) website (http://keck.usc.edu/Education/Academic_Department–and_Divisions/Departmentof_Psychiatry/Research_and_Training_Centers/USC_ATTC.aspx). Gaining quick access to this document helps us to apply evidence-based principles and strategies to real-life cases in front of an entire supervision group, enhancing the learning of every student.

Another use of technology that aids in supervision is suggesting and viewing various web-based activities for students' work with particular clients. For instance, Dan Siegel's free resources for teaching mindfulness come in very handy, particularly in trying to strengthen clients' resilience in the face of trauma and anxiety. "The Healthy Mind Platter" and "The Wheel of Awareness" have been useful tools in helping clients to recognize that the brain, like the body, requires a certain amount of self-care and "exercise." These can be easily accessed and discussed in class (http://drdansiegel.com/resources/). These activities are outlined in Siegel's books (Siegel & Hartzell, 2003; Siegel, 2010; Siegel & Payne Bryson, 2011), many of which are read by our students in other classes, but they have yet to apply these activities on actual clients. Having immediate access to them in supervision helps us to demonstrate when and how such activities might be appropriate to use, and with whom.

Finally, this Web gives us quick access to referral sources. For example, imagine a student is describing client who is a recent immigrant, whose citizenship is dependent on her marriage to her abusive spouse, and she feels she cannot leave him without threatening her residency in the US. We can quickly look online for legal aid, domestic violence shelters, and job training sites to help this student to collect the needed resources to have an informed discussion about the client's options. In doing the search in class, we are also demonstrating for students how to gain access to resources for their clients in the future.

Mobile and Computer Apps

A wonderful development that has taken place over the past five years is the advent of mobile applications to be used on computers, cell phones, or tablets. There have been many mental health-based applications that students have found useful in their work with clients. Some are very basic programs that help clients to keep track of the number of positive vs. negative thoughts throughout the day. Others are behavior modification programs for parents to use with children. There are meditation and hypnosis apps, as well as yoga and breathing applications. Psychoeducation applications around the symptomology of various disorders, such as PTSD or

Addiction, have been very useful in helping clients to understand their condition. In fact, the American Psychiatric Association has released an app for using the new DSM 5, purchased through the iTunes Store or the Android Market. And the California Board of Behavioral Sciences has also released a computer program called "TrackYourHours" that helps students to keep track of all of the different types of training hours they need to become licensed in the state (available at http://trackyourhours.com). Both students and faculty can recommend and demonstrate these applications during supervision to pool our knowledge of helpful resources in therapy.

Beginning counselors are looking for as many tools as they can acquire to help them to feel like they are "doing something" with their clients. We often have to consistently remind them that the vast majority of the help that comes from therapy lies in the development of a confidential, warm, empathic therapeutic relationship (Frank & Frank, 1993; Lambert & Barley, 2001). So we have to balance our willingness to support students' use of tools and gadgets in their clinical work, with our mandate that they learn "how to be in the room" with the client – how to be present. Still, these applications can be useful to counselors and clients, as long as they are not used as a crutch to circumvent the anxiety associated with the intensity and ambiguity of the therapeutic process for beginning counselors. As long as students are putting in the work to understand and validate the clients' experience, to set mutual goals, and to uncover resources and paths that facilitate those goals, these applications can be useful in helping students reinforce learning concepts and skills introduced in the classroom and are helpful to clients in reinforcing the concepts and skills learned in therapy.

Social Media

Social media is a primary source of communication in our program. Our Facebook site, for instance, is used to for announcements and job listings, training opportunities, important news articles, as well as a way for students and alumni to connect with each other for mentoring purposes. But, we also use this site as a consultation forum. All of our students and alumni are trained to use the site very carefully, never revealing identifying or confidential information about their clients. But, they are able to use it to ask for feedback, resources, or referrals for some of the therapeutic issues they are encountering in their training or practice. We often keep resource materials posted as files on this site, and will refer fieldwork students there for consultation with their colleagues or resources.

We've also used social media to create "secret groups" for our clinical training courses, where students role-play clinical scenarios as they practice their skills in a particular class, and then post those videos and information relevant to what we are learning in class, to the group. Because the groups are secret, only students enrolled in the class are invited to join, and no one who is not invited to join the group has access to the group or even knows of its existence (it is unsearchable in search engines and not visible to others on students' Timelines or their Group lists). Postings to the group only appear on group/class members' news feeds, and can only be viewed or commented on by group members. (Note: These are videos of student role-plays, not actual client sessions, so security breach concerns are not as much of an issue here.) The class members have access to the videos and notes posted to the group through their Facebook account, and are able to review each other's practice sessions, as well as the feedback sessions that follow. This allows them to review and comment on their own work outside of class, and the work of their classmates, and lets them review what the instructor and observers said about where they did well and where they can improve in their clinical practice. We find this centralized access to video review, outside of class, helps students to develop their skills in a much deeper way.

Communication

Probably, the least obvious change that has occurred in our program is the gradual evolution of modes of supervision-based communication, outside of class. We've slowly shifted from office-hours and landline phone calls, to the use of email, and then cell phones, texting, and now we are testing the usefulness of common video apps. Of course, once we left the world of secure landline telephone calls, we had to consider the security of these modes of communication, as none of them is immune to the threat of unauthorized interception of information. As we began to incorporate these technologies into our communication with students, we had to cultivate a culture of communicating in a new twenty-first century shorthand. This shorthand is predicated on the knowledge that almost no digital communication is completely secure. We discourage students from using any identifiable or confidential information in their emails or texts to us. In fact, we encourage them to use these forms of communication only to notify us of a need to talk on the phone or to provide us updates as to any changes in scheduling or administrative procedures. We will follow up with a phone call to discuss the particulars in a case, but even then, students are encouraged to not divulge identifiers if we are using cell phones. This allows us to consult anonymously, if students are not able to access their on-site supervisor, or if they need a second opinion. What has made this technology so useful to us is that students and supervising professors have much better access to one another, and response times are much shorter as a result. In the past, if I was not at my desk, I might miss an urgent phone call to my office line, and would sometimes not get back to my

student with support until the next day. Now, I carry my phone with me so that a text, email, or phone call reaches me much sooner, and I am able to respond within a timeframe that is useful for the student. Similarly, when something happens where I need to reach a student urgently, they also have access to their phone and can respond to my request for a phone call much sooner.

There has been much discussion around the use of video phone calls using applications like FaceTime and Skype. While this certainly makes more non-verbal information available to the supervising faculty, as to how a student in reacting to a situation, there are concerns about the security of the information being exchanged during these calls. And we haven't found it to provide significantly more benefits than the cost of its risks. Since we don't provide individual supervision for our students (that is provided by an on-site supervisor), and our communication outside of class is typically reserved for crisis consultations or second opinions, we are often not on a call long enough to benefit from the visual cues this medium might provide. Also, it requires more technology to be in place for it to work smoothly and without distracting glitches (such as a Wi-Fi connection) than a simple text or phone call. And there is no benefit in terms of students being able to count these calls as supervision time, as the state of California requires face-to-face, in-person supervision for all trainees in order for students to count a supervision hour. So for now, video phone calls are not something we are utilizing in the program for supervision.

However, we are using this technology extensively for admissions interviews. We believe it is important to level the playing field for all of our applicants during the admissions process, and we don't want to disadvantage applicants who cannot afford to fly out for an interview for the program. Historically, we've done phone interviews, but we have found those lacking in providing us the nonverbal information we are looking for as we evaluate an applicants' warmth, openness, confidence, humility, self reflection, etc. And in phone interviews, it is often tempting for applicants to read from prepared answers, which prevents us from getting a good sense of their interpersonal style. So we have found that video calls have helped us tremendously in providing equal opportunities for all of our applicants, while still allowing us to gather information from a more complete contextual picture of who they are and why they want to enter this field. In that way, video platforms have been invaluable to us.

CONCLUSION

As a program, we are cognizant of how we use technology. We are not interested in using it for its own sake, but are committed to using the technology when it supports the goals of our program. We want the technology to be a tool that helps us teach students to be critical thinkers who are able to access credible information and evidence to get their questions answered. We want it to be a mode of communication that keeps our students connected to us, and their colleagues, in a supportive way throughout their training, and in a way that follows them throughout their careers. Technology can allow us to keep close watch over the development of our students, even if they are not working in the same building as us. It allows us to easily use the expertise of leaders in the field to teach our students through the use of videos, activities, assessments, and other online resources. We believe technology has made our program more agile and has allowed us to more easily stay current and relevant as the field changes, because we have easy access to new information and tools.

REFERENCES

American Counseling Association. (2005). *ACA code of ethics.* Alexandria, VA: ACA.

Binder, J. L. (1999). Issues in teaching and learning time-limited psychodynamic psychotherapy. *Clinical Psychology Review, 19,* 705–719.

Briere, J., & Lanktree, C. (2013). *Integrative treatment of complex trauma for adolescents (ITCT-A) treatment guide* (2nd ed.). Retrieved from http://keck.usc .edu/Education/Academic_Department_and_Divisions/Department_of_Psychiatry/Research_and_Training_Centers/USC_ATTC.aspx.

Briere, J., & Lanktree, C. B. (2011). *Treating complex trauma in adolescents and young adults.* Thousand Oaks, CA: Sage.

Frank, J. D., & Frank, J. B. (1993). *Persuasion and healing: A comparative student of psychotherapy* (3rd ed.). Baltimore: The Johns Hopkins University Press.

Grohol, J. M., & Tartakovsky, M. (2013). *DSM-5 Resource guide.* PsychCentral. Retrieved from: http://psychcentral.com/dsm-5/.

Hayes, S. C., Pistorello, J., & Levin, M. E. (2012). Acceptance and commitment therapy as a unified model of behavior change. *The counseling psychologist, 40,* 976–1002.

Huhra, R. L., Yamokoski-Maynhart, C. A., & Prieto, L. R. (2008). Reviewing videotape in supervision: A developmental approach. *Journal of counseling and development, 86,* 412–418.

Ivey, A. E., Ivey, M. B., & Zalaquett, C. P. (2010). *Intentional interviewing and counseling: Facilitating client development in a multicultural society* (7th ed.). Belmont, CA: Brooks/Cole, Cengage Learning.

Kagan, N. (1980). Influencing human interaction – Eighteen years with IPR. In A. K. Hess (Ed.), *Psychotherapy supervision: Theory, research and practice* (pp. 232–283). New York: Wiley.

Lambert, M. J., & Barley, D. E. (2001). Research summary on the therapeutic relationship and psychotherapy outcome. *Theory, Research, Practice, Training, 38,* 357–361.

Miller, S. D., Duncan, B. L., Sorrell, R., & Brown, G. S. (2004). The partners for change outcome management system. *Journal of Clinical Psychology, 61,* 199–208.

Miller, W. R., & Rollnick, S. (2002) *Motivational interviewing: Preparing people for change.* New York: Guilford Press.

Rosenberg, J. I. (2006). Real-time training: Transfer of knowledge through computer-mediated, real-time feedback. *Professional Psychology: Research and Practice, 37,* 539–546.

Siegel, D. J., & Bryson, T. P. (2011). *The whole-brain child: 12 Revolutionary strategies to nurture your child's developing mind, survive everyday parenting struggles, and help your family thrive.* New York: Delacorte Press.

Siegel, D. J. (2010). *Mindsight: The new science of personal transformation.* New York: Bantam.

Siegel, D. J., & Hartzell, M. (2003). *Parenting from the inside out: How a deeper self-understanding can help you raise children who thrive.* New York: Penguin Putnam.

Stretch, L. S., Nagel, D. M., & Anthony, K. (2012). Ethical framework for the use of technology in supervision. *Therapeutic Innovations in Light of Technology, 3*(2), 37–45.

Whiffen, R. (1982). The use of videotape in supervision. In R. Whiffen & J. Byng-Hall (Eds.), *Family therapy supervision: Recent development in practice* (pp. 39–56). London: Academic Press.

Chapter 39

THE USE OF LIVE SUPERVISION IN A COMMUNITY-BASED TREATMENT PROGRAM

Glenn Duncan

Before implementing technology for the oversight of supervisees, one has to ask the following questions: (1) does clinical supervision have a beneficial effect on supervisees; and (2) does that beneficial effect translate into a positive impact on clients? Watkins (2011) stated that there is ample research showing clinical supervision's positive impact on supervisee development and stated "some of those positive effects include supervisee enhanced self-awareness, enhanced treatment knowledge, skill acquisition and utilization, enhanced self-efficacy (Kozina, Grabovari, De Stefano, & Drapeau, 2010) and strengthening of the supervisee–client relationship." Watkins stated that the research concerning the positive impact of clinical supervision on client care has much less empirical evidence. Proof of clinical supervision effectiveness for client outcome is overdue and needed in order to meet the same evidence-based challenge that clinical supervision's impact on supervisee development has met. In regards to clinical supervision, the assumption has been and continues to be, at the very least, the proven positive impact on the supervisee's professional growth will translate into better client care. However, Watkins' (2011) review of the literature posits that this assumption is conjecture as not enough studies have been done to make this an evidence-based statement. Thus we are only left with clear answers on the first question, that supervision has a positive impact on supervisees. Because of this clear evidence, we will focus on what are the best ways to ensure that clinical supervision will have the most effective impact on a supervisee.

The best way to ensure proper clinical oversight is to ensure that the supervisor is properly trained and competent. There is an abundance of evidence for the need to train clinical supervisors (Bernard & Goodyear, 2013; Falender & Shafranske, 2004; Milne, Sheikh, Pattison, & Wilkinson, 2011). In a review of 11 studies focused on training supervisors, Milne, Sheikh, Pattison, and Wilkinson (2011) stated the four most commonly used training methods of supervisors utilized were feedback, educational role-play, modeling through live and/or video demonstration and teaching. In academic and research settings training in clinical supervision occurs with many different types of training methods. However, the utilization of various methods in training supervisors has not translated to the community setting. There have been, and continue to be, wide variations regarding the requirement for clinical supervision training in the community setting. The source of clinical supervision training standards in community settings comes from the licensing standards of the various behavioral health professions. These varying standards in the community setting largely require much less intensive training standards than seen in academic and research settings. In a few instances, one may not need any additional training, or only need to attend a six hour workshop training in the community setting, to be considered a qualified supervisor.

During the last decade, many state regulating organizations have required that clinical supervisors demonstrate some level of competency before being considered qualified supervisors. The most common "proof" of supervisor competency is education in clinical supervision as demonstrated by either workshop attendance or a graduate-level course in clinical supervision. A small number of these regulatory bodies go further and require a national certification in clinical supervision. The requirements for a national certifications include education and supervision of one's own supervision. While more regulatory bodies have required some training in clinical supervision in the past 10 years, these requirements vary widely from region to region and can even vary widely within the same region, across different licensing standards. For example, in New Jersey the amount of training needed to be considered a qualified supervisor ranges from no training at all for certain licensures (i.e., Licensed Psychologists and Licensed Clinical Alcohol and Drug Counselors), only workshop attendance (i.e., Licensed Clinical Social Workers and Licensed Marriage and Family Therapists), to needing either a graduate-level course in clinical supervision or a national certification in supervision (i.e., Licensed Professional Counselors). This wide variation from region to region, or within the same region across different licensures, will have its impact on the effectiveness of clinical supervision given to supervisees.

The wide variation found in qualified clinical supervisor regulations narrows greatly when it comes to regulatory processes for supervisees just beginning in the field. For example, many state regulatory organizations in the United States have a two-tiered system of licensures; beginning licensures of professionals who require regular clinical supervision until they obtain their second tier, or end licensure. Given the wide variation in clinical supervisor training regulations, the implementation of clinical supervision in community settings is likely to reflect, in some instances, the adherence to only the minimum legal clinical supervision standards required by a particular license. While many licensure regulations define clinical supervision, define the number of supervisory hours that must be obtained per year, define how many supervisees a supervisor can have at one time, it is not common that the regulations define how the supervisor/supervisee interaction should occur. For example, out of 15 different licensures reviewed in over six different states, only one licensure required that a supervisee have some form of live (working as a co-counselor in a therapy session or live observation) or taped supervision oversight (video tape or audio tape). Thus while all the reviewed licensure regulations required clinical supervision, there was a lack of definition of how that clinical supervision should unfold with the supervisee.

The effectiveness of both individual and group supervision is well documented in both the training of supervisees (Bernard & Goodyear, 2013; Falender & Shafranske, 2004; Watkins, 2011) and supervisors (Bernard & Goodyear, 2013; Falender & Shafranske, 2004; Milne, Sheikh, Pattison, & Wilkinson, 2011). In a community-based treatment program setting, clinical supervision most often takes the form of feedback via self-report. Ellis (2011) stated there is a myth among supervisors that direct observation is unnecessary, either because it is too time consuming or seen as unnecessary. The data very clearly suggests otherwise; for example, supervisees often miss or are unaware, misinterpret or inaccurately recall that which transpires in the therapy session (Bernard & Goodyear, 2013).

Feedback via self-report has many problems attached to it. Without direct observation, you forfeit the opportunity for independent judgment regarding the client, and you forfeit the opportunity to illustrate directly from the case in question, how to draw inferences from the client and from the session. In an older piece of research, Wynne, Susman, Ries, Birringer, and Katz (1994) showed that experienced supervisees showed only a 42% recall rate for main ideas expressed in session, and 30% recall rate for supporting ideas expressed in session with a client.

The effectiveness of utilizing technology to train supervisees is also well documented (Bernard & Goodyear, 2013; Falender & Shafranske, 2004; Huhra, Yamokoski-Maynhart, & Prieto, 2008; Powell, 2004). The classic use of technology in live supervision has included the use of videotaping, which is an outdated name that never quite left our field's vernacular. Currently the word "videotaping" usually includes any type of recording of video and audio using digital and/or magnetic media. The use of audiotaping is another classic use of technology that has been used in our field for the purposes of recalling direct content from the therapy session.

The utilization of technology to incorporate live supervision has been occurring for a number of decades. There are many different ways to conduct live supervision. Live clinical supervision was initiated by Jay Haley and Salvador Minuchin in the late 1960s. Live clinical supervision combines direct observation of the session with some method that enables communication with the supervisee during the session. It is the highest safeguard of client welfare, but it can be time consuming for the clinical supervisor. Live supervision also allows for excellent and at times immediate feedback mechanism for the supervisee. Bernard and Goodyear (2013) cover many different aspects of live supervision which, on some level, incorporates technology. All of the live supervision methods listed below can occur utilizing video and audio equipment that allows a live feed of the session from the therapy room to the room where the supervisor is located. They can also occur by the supervisor being in an adjacent room behind a two-way mirror where the technology is an audio feed coming into the supervisor's room. These techniques include:

Bug in the Ear (BITE) is a wireless earphone worn by the supervisee that allows feedback from the clinical supervisor at any point in time, without the "interruption" of the therapy session. This requires higher levels of technology to have on hand, which may be something that a community organization, which is not a training institution, may not be able to incorporate. Bug in the ear is seen as having some major advantages: (1) it allows for minor adjustments in the therapy session without interruption; and (2) it protects the therapy relationship more fully because the client is unaware which interventions are coming from the supervisee and which ones are coming from the supervisor (Bernard & Goodyear, 2013).

An alternate of bug in the ear, is an interactional platform using of some type of video technology to serve the same purpose as the audio feed in the supervisees ear (sometimes referred to as bug in the eye). This can be utilized in many forms such as a television monitor placed behind the client, so it is out of sight of the client's vision but provides instant, ongoing feedback to the supervisee much in the same way as the audio feed in the ear would do. This feedback mechanism is done by the supervisor typing information into a keypad from the observation room which is then transmitted on screen to the supervisee to then incorporate in the therapy session. Supervisees can in theory be less distracted with video, than by having audio suggestions in their ear, and supervisees also have the control of when to read the feedback and incorporate it into the session.

Yu (as cited in Bernard & Goodyear, 2013) took this interactional platform and developed it using iPads and Google doc (or any other type of similar service or application). The supervisee has a tablet device such as an iPad on their lap and reads the feedback given by the supervisor. If the sessions are being recorded, the feedback is saved on the application to be reviewed later when the supervisee is watching the session recording. Yu (2013) has further developed this idea and has a website www.isupelive.com that bypasses Internet programs (such as Google doc) and applications by using a proprietary software to record these interactions. Using iSupe requires a computer or tablet device by the supervisor, a tablet device utilized by the supervisee, and requires an Internet connection. A supervisor license must be purchased ($50) and each supervisee requires a license ($5). iSupe is listed on their website as "a software package that allows supervisor and supervisee to communicate securely and in real-time across desktop, laptop, phone and tablet devices while the supervisee is meeting with a client." The software used is on a secured server, and while Yu's website states, "iSupe implements a number of industry-standard security measures to ensure the security of your communications," it is unclear as to whether or not this technology is HIPAA compliant as there was no statement found on their website regarding this issue. iSupe informs users to leave out client identifying information as a standard protocol when using their software.

Monitoring is another live supervision technique where the clinical supervisor observes the session and intervenes directly into the session, for example, if there is perceived difficulty within the therapy session. The clinical supervisor then takes over when coming into the session. The advantage of this process is the supervisor can experience the client/family dynamics while also allowing the supervisee to benefit from the modeling that the supervisor is doing when working directly with the client/family. The disadvantage of monitoring is when supervisors only intervene for client welfare issues. The argument here is the monitoring is not actually viewed as live supervision but rather is an intervention by the supervisor due to the urgency of the situation. Also, this method is not as sensitive to the supervisee-client dynamics as bug in the ear/eye (Bernard & Goodyear, 2013).

In Vivo is similar to monitoring, except the supervisor comes in and consults with the supervisee in front of the client(s), allowing the client(s) to have access to all information. This transparency of conversation between the supervisor and supervisee can heighten the client/family's awareness of the dynamics happening as long as they are phrased in a way that is understandable to the client. This transparency also allows the highest levels of openness by allowing clients a level of access to supervision content that is usually not available to them (Bernard & Goodyear, 2013).

Phone-ins, consultation breaks and walk-ins are interruption-based forms of live supervision implimented by breaking into the therapy session either by a phone call, a break of therapy session, or by the supervisor walking in, intervening and then walking back out. Although all these methods of interruption have documented training and supervision advantages, they also have the disadvantage of interruption, disrupting the flow of the therapy session (Bernard & Goodyear, 2013).

According to Bernard and Goodyear (2013) live supervision is especially popular in training programs. But the authors argue that live supervision is equally an important clinical supervision tool in community-based organizations as well. Along with live supervision protocols, such as the ones listed above, a modified "live supervision" protocol can be implemented also. This technique incorporates live direct observation, with feedback and discussion of that feedback provided at a later time. For example feedback and discussion of the case can occur either right after the therapy session or during the next regularly scheduled supervision time.

Tailoring a live supervision protocol, or modified live supervision protocol to a community mental health setting is not an arduous process. There are many issues that need to be addressed before implementing live supervision technology in a community-based setting. They include client confidentiality, informed consent and HIPAA compliance, administration support, policy and procedure development and the consideration of cost and logistics. Once all the issues are identified, researched and addressed, recommendations can be made to the administration/board of directors. Upon approval, the organization can then set upon the implementation of live supervision.

Hunterdon Drug Awareness Program, Inc. (www.hdap.org) is a small community-based, not-for-profit, substance abuse treatment program which works with clients who have primary substance use disorders and clients with co-occurring substance use and mental health disorders. Hunterdon Drug Awareness Program is an outpatient and intensive outpatient treatment program. Group supervision is provided weekly, as is individual supervision for all staff, as well as having live supervision and modified live supervision capacity. This is an organization, like many other community-based organizations, that supervises both staff and graduate student interns who are doing their field placement for their master's program.

Direct observation is done via technology that was incorporated into the organization in 2005, at a cost of just over $3,000. Since the initial start-up expenses, the organization has also purchased a tablet and iSupe licenses at an additional cost of $800. Fundraising monies were used to establish the technology

needed to perform live supervision. It is the core belief of the administration, with the support of the board of directors, that all supervisees require more than just feedback from self-report to grow clinically, and client welfare mandates a responsibility of the supervisor to have direct knowledge of the supervisee/client interaction.

The implementation of a live supervision protocol at Hunterdon Drug Awareness Program occurred by first hiring a local computer/networking organization. This company then gave the organization different options for video and audio. A high-definition color security camera was purchased and installed in one of the two large group rooms, along with an omnidirectional microphone. A low-tech solution to HIPAA HITECH privacy compliance was created, in that a closed-circuit transmission route was used from the television monitors (one located in the Executive Director's office and one located in the Clinical Director's office), to the camera and audio feed. The positioning of the camera allows for most of the seats in the room to be visible, though the static nature of the camera causes some seats to have better camera angles than others. The omnidirectional microphone was installed in the ceiling tile at the center of the room and is sensitive enough to pick up the sounds of people talking without having to directly mic individual participants.

All clients who enter into the program receive a complete explanation as to the use and purpose of this equipment and sign a video policy stating they fully understand the nature of the video/audio setup, the location, and the purpose it serves not only for the organization but the benefit it serves the client. When explained in the light of this service providing quality assurance for the client to ensure they are getting the best treatment possible, we have not had one client refuse to sign the consent to be on video. Clients are told this serves the purpose of clinical supervision monitoring and that it will not be used as any type of marketing tool. Clients are also told their image will not be reproduced for any purpose outside of the use for clinical supervision and that their image, if recorded, will always stay inside the physical building of the organization. While some graduate schools request that a student can tape a session to show in the classroom, this is not something that is allowed.

Initial installation of the video equipment, caused some anxiety among staff members who were going to be observed, but after the initial anxiety which was addressed in clinical supervision, the live supervision recording devices have been largely forgotten about by both supervisees and by clients. This technology setup allows a supervisor to turn on the monitor at any point and observe the supervisee in groups or family therapy sessions, without the supervisee knowing that they are being monitored at that moment. This allows for the most natural process of a supervisee running a group or family therapy session because they do not know they are being observed by their supervisor.

Upon the supervisor's request, the supervisee is asked to hold an individual therapy session in this group room instead of their office, for the purpose of direct observation. This allows for a less natural performance by the supervisee as they know they are being watched, which could change behaviors, interventions used and therapy dynamics compared to thos that existed when there was no observation.

The direct observation used by the supervisor can then take two different forms. It can be utilized in a modified live supervision format where the observation is viewed live, notes are taken by the supervisor and issues are discussed in a delayed format either after the therapy session or during the next regularly scheduled supervision session. The direct observation can also be utilized in a more traditional live supervision format. This

set-up allows the supervisor to engage in monitoring, walk-in, in-vivo or consultation break format. The live supervision format is utilized with the supervisee knowing that the supervisor will be monitoring the therapy activity and will engage in one the aforementioned live supervision methods. The modified live supervision format may or may not involve informing the supervisee that they will be observed.

The benefits that have been seen at Hunterdon Drug Awareness Program include the ability to monitor staff in more than just a self-report format. The utilization of the modified live supervision allows for direct clinical observation that captures the most natural counseling style due to the counselor not knowing if the supervisor will have the monitor on at any given time. The live supervision also provides the direct and immediate feedback needed that allows the supervisee to implement feedback and see its effects immediately. In summary, it is the belief that live supervision is not only good for treatment effectiveness and supervisee growth, but it can also be a cost effective alternative for community-based treatment programs. The live supervision system that has been incorporated in our community-based treatment organization also provides the clinical supervisor flexibility to utilize a variety of live supervision or modified live supervision techniques. This enhances their functioning as a supervisor while helping to deliver the best array of services to the client and maintain an ethical fidelity to consumer protection.

REFERENCES

Bernard, J. M., & Goodyear, R. K. (2013). *Fundamentals of clinical supervision* (5th ed.). Boston: Pearson.

Ellis, M. V. (2010). Bridging the science and practice of clinical supervision: Some discoveries, some misconceptions. *The Clinical Supervisor, 29*:1, 95–116.

Falender, C. A., & Shafranske, E. P. (2004). *Clinical supervision: A competency-based approach.* Washington, DC: American Psychological Association.

Huhra, R. L., Yamokoski-Maynhart, C. A., & Prieto, L. R. (2008). Reviewing videotape in supervision: A developmental approach. *Journal of Counseling & Development, 86*, 412–418.

Kozina, K., Grabovari, N., De Stefano, J., & Drapeau, M. (2010). Measuring changes in counselor self-efficacy: Further validation and implications for training and supervision. *The Clinical Supervisor, 29*:2, 117–127.

Milne, D. L., Sheikh, A. I., Pattison, S., &

Wilkinson, A. (2011): Evidence-based training for clinical supervisors: A systematic review of 11 controlled studies. *The Clinical Supervisor, 30*:1, 53–71.

Powell, D. J., & Brodsky, A. (2004). *Clinical supervision in alcohol and drug abuse counseling.* San Francisco: Jossey-Bass.

Wynne, M. E., Susman, M., Ries, S., Birringer, J., & Katz, L. (1994). A method for assessing therapists' recall of in-session events. *Journal of Consulting Psychology, 41*:53–57.

Yu, A. (2013). www.iSupeLive.com: "The Future of Live Supervision." [online: Accessed May 30, 2013]. Retrieved from http://www.isupelive.com/?page_id=272.

Conclusion

FUTURE DIRECTIONS OF TECHNOLOGY IN MENTAL HEALTH

LoriAnn Sykes Stretch, Kate Anthony, and Stephen Goss

Technology in mental health practice, training and supervision is here to stay. As demonstrated in this text by the multitude of experts in the field utilizing technology in the delivery of mental health, technology is a vital tool in the practice, training and supervision of mental healthcare. The goal of this conclusion is to highlight the themes that cross the uses of technology and discuss future directions for the use of technology in the mental health field. Finally, we will acknowledge the challenges related to technology in mental health practice, training, and supervision.

THEMES OF TECHNOLOGY IN MENTAL HEALTH

Technology offers a variety of promising approaches to mental health practice, training and supervision. Whether email (Recupero & Harms, Chapter 1), telephone and mobile communication (Groman, Chapter 27; Huggins, Chapter 3; Saunders & Osborn, Chapter 9), web-based information (Grohol, Chapter 7), social networking (Thompson, Chapter 4), online support groups (Boniel-Nissim, Chapter 5), podcasting (Quinones, Chapter 17), film (Sutherland, Chapter 22), or gaming (Matthews & Coyle, Chapter 13), quite apart from all the other matters dealt with in this book, these technologies have become modalities that increase access to mental health services and training. Bennett and Glasgow (2009) noted the common reasons used to justify using technology in mental health include (a) decreasing cost, (b) reducing time constraints and transportation barriers, (c) overcoming problems in the availability of care, (d) increasing the efficiency of care, (e) reducing discomfort associated with traditional face-to-face services and (f) allowing practitioners and clients to express themselves in a broader variety of ways, some of which particularly suit some peoples' preferences or are particularly useful in addressing certain conditions, like using virtual reality to expose people to known fears or problematic situations (Riva & Repetto, Chapter 11).

In this text, authors from around the world have shared a wide variety of ways technology can be used in practice, training and supervision. Each author noted the ways in which technology is selected, utilized and evaluated. In all the approaches, the authors noted the importance of informed consent, staying current and protecting confidentiality. Another common theme was ensuring that all users of the technology have training on how to use the technology and that a backup plan exists for when technology fails.

FUTURE DIRECTIONS AND CHALLENGES

Staying Current

Practitioners, educators and supervisors will need to stay current in the rapidly developing world of technology. Kazdin (2015) noted that as we evaluate the future of technology in mental health, we need to consider the following aspects: reach (who can we connect with services), scalability (typically larger than individual therapy), affordability (lower costs than traditional therapy), convenience (for clients, counselors and supervisors), expansion of settings where services are provided and acceptability to consumers (clients and practitioners) and effectiveness. Evaluating technology will require far more than simply looking at the approach's efficacy with a specific population. Ben-Zeev, Davis, Kaiser, Krzsos, and Drake (2012) noted that researchers, administrators and practitioners will need to come together to create technologies that are responsive to mental health needs and evidence-based. This has been carried out by a now increasing number of service providers such as PlusGuidance, which offers an exemplar of what can be achieved (see www.plusguidance.com). The added challenge for practitioners is that each technology itself will need to be evaluated for usability and accessibility as well as efficacy, and they must ensure their competence with each technology they wish to add to the range of ways in which they connect with their clients.

Additional challenges include that research is relatively slow to be published while technologies continue to change rapidly. This combined effect makes staying current a major challenge for most practitioners unless they commit to specific training and skills development for each one. Traditional methods of program evaluation will result in validation long after the technology being evaluated is obsolete (Mohr, Burns, Schueller, Clarke, & Klinkman, 2013). In addition to peer reviewed journals, practitioners will also have to utilize resources such as technology usability and feasibility reports to determine appropriateness of technologies for use with specific populations. Price et al. (2014) pointed out that future research on technologies must incorporate assessments of usability and adherence in addition to their incremental benefit to treatment. For example, as Luxton, McCann, Bush, Mishkind, and Reger (2011) noted, there is no current oversight or quality control of applications related to behavioral health. Instead, practitioners need to consider the developer of the technology, the recommended use for the technology and must evaluate potential benefits and risks. Learning how to critically analyze technology and ascertain potential risks is a skill set of its own and many practitioners utilizing technologies are also likely to need additional training in these areas.

The existing research regarding technology and mental health is growing but, for some technologies more than others, still has some important gaps. For example, Computer-aided Cognitive Behavioral Therapy (CCBT; Cavanagh & Grist, Chapter 12) has a promising evidence-based practice and, in the UK, the National Institute for Health and Clinical Excellence has issued a wide approval for its use in the UK National Health Service. On the other hand, each variant of a technology, like new virtual reality environments or specific online therapy platforms, still require to be tested each time.

As Luxton et al. (2011) and Wilson, Onorati, Mishkind, Reger and Gahm (2008) noted, while there are promising technological approaches, many still need further research to determine acceptability for use. Some of the key challenges in the existing research needing to be addressed are small sample sizes, restricted populations, and a limited scope of mental health disorder types and severity (Boydell et al., 2014). Similarly, Boydell, Volpe, and Pignatiello

(2010) noted that many studies were brief and more longitudinal studies were needed, though they are relatively costly.

Nonetheless, while research in some areas or for some specific platforms or technologies is limited, much more research is underway and the evidence base is growing at a rate that promises much greater, more accurate and reliable information for practitioners. Mohr et al. (2013), for example, found that in the existing research on technology in mental health: (a) videoconferencing and standard telephone technologies have been well validated; (b) web-based interventions have shown efficacy across a broad range of mental health outcomes; (c) social media, such as online support groups, have produced disappointing outcomes when used alone; (d) mobile technologies and gaming have received limited attention for mental health outcomes; and (e) virtual reality has shown good efficacy for anxiety and pediatric disorders.

Educating the Public

Technology can also be used to educate the general public regarding mental health as well. For example, Ebert et al. (2015) found that a simple informational video was helpful in educating clients about the use of technology in the treatment of depressive symptoms. Likewise, technologies, such as virtual reality, can offer education and practice for clients in a safe, accepting environment (Riva & Repetto, Chapter 11; Tan, Chapter 16). While technology has the potential for making mental health services accessible and efficient, mental health providers will need to practice due diligence in training the public about reasonable expectations regarding the use, benefits and risks involved in using each given technology. Future technological approaches must incorporate training of both the practitioner and client, student or supervisee as the case may be.

Most advocacy organizations utilize social media and the Internet to promote the organization's mission. In fact, frequently, technologies have been cited as one way to overcome stigma and access barriers to mental health care (Wilson et al., 2008). Online assessment is one way practitioners can reach populations who might be skeptical or hesitant to access services. As Klion (Chapter 14) and Dombeck (Chapter 18) noted, there is great potential for online assessments, though the development of these needs to move to creating assessments specific to an online delivery and less on converting paper-and-pencil assessments to online usage.

An additional caution is that clients may assume with the speed at which technologies such as email and text messages transmit that they can expect an immediate response from a clinician. In addition, the lack of formality of entering a professional office may lead to a blurring of the therapeutic boundaries that an office setting can help create and maintain. Therefore, as a profession, we will need to continue to fine tune the process of informed consent for mental health services integrating technology. Fortunately, more and more of our professional organizations, such as the American Counseling Association (ACA, 2014), the American Psychological Association (2010a; American Psychological Association Practice Organization, 2010b), the British Association for Counselling and Psychotherapy (Anthony & Goss, 2009, 2015; Hill & Roth, 2015), Canadian Psychological Association (2015), the National Board of Certified Counselors (NBCC, 1997, 2009, 2012), and the Center for Credentialing and Education (CCE, 2011) and a growing number of other professional associations around the world are recognizing the need for ethical guidance – some issuing repeated guidance on the topic to keep up with developments as they emerge (see Goss & Anthony, 2012, for a more detailed account).

Another area of concern is safety for

high-risk clients. Technology is unreliable at times and interrupted connections, intercepted communication and/or miscommunications could potentially put clients at greater harm. In fact, Luxton, Sirotin, and Mishkind (2010) pointed out that safety and usability need to be the first steps in utilizing technology within a standard of care. Practitioners will need to continue to establish broad networks for additional support in the local areas in which clients live and solidify crisis plans with clients well before they become needed. Educating the clients about what to do in cases of technology failure and establishing support networks local to the client will require practitioners to establish and maintain large collegial networks. Developing collegial support may occur at conferences, annual meetings of professional organizations, or via listservs and other networking tools.

Educating the Profession

Practitioner training programs need to be equipped to train students in how to effectively ethically and legally utilize technology in clinical practice, administratively and in supervision. Technology is a necessity in this day and age and not including technology as part of mainstream practitioner training poorly prepares graduates for the realities of our technological world. Fortunately, in an increasing number of countries, bodies responsible for accreditation standards, such as the Council for the Accreditation of Counseling Related Educational Programs (CACREP, 2016), are beginning to recognize the importance of training practitioners about technology in mental health. Specifically, the 2016 CACREP Standards require graduate programs to train students in the following areas: "technology's impact on the counseling profession" (Sec. 2.F.j.), "ethical and culturally relevant strategies for establishing and maintaining in-person and technology-assisted relationships" (Sec.2,

F.5.d.), "the impact of technology on the counseling process" (Sec.2, F.5.e.), and "modalities of clinical supervision and the use of technology" (Sec.6, B.2.g.). In contrast, the 2009 CACREP Standards only mentioned that programs needed to demonstrate "the use and infusion of technology in program delivery and technology's impact on the counseling profession" (Sec II.F.).

In addition, professionals in the field must seek out ongoing training and supervision regarding technology (see the Online Therapy Institute – www.onlinetherapyinstitute.com for a range of affordable and high quality exemplars). All counselors use some form of technology in their work, whether email, telephone, videoconferencing, etc. Technology is part of our professional lives. Moreover, even the most technologically-resistant practitioners must recognize that the vast majority of their clients live and communicate, at least in part, in a technologically mediated world so it is incumbent upon them – at *minimum* – to be able to understand how technology affects their experiences, relationships and ways of communicating.

Technologies are already being used successfully in clinical supervision for EAP (Mani & Vader, Chapter 31; Practica/Internship (Lent, Burck, & Stretch, Chapter 35), public health (Buxton & Devaney, Chapter 32), private practice (Stokes, Chapter 33), play therapy (Stretch & Vincenzes, Chapter 34), and career counseling (Hooley & Neary, Chapter 37). Multiple authors noted the importance of ethical guidelines that are responsive to the advances in technology (Stretch, Nagel, & Anthony, Chapter 30) and research to identify best practices in distance supervision and training (Coursel, Lewis, & Seymour, Chapter 28; Nagel & Anthony, Chapter 24; Speyer & Yaphe, Chapter 23).

Public Policy

Additionally, there are challenges for

public policy. In many countries, laws and regulations vary, often inhibiting counselors from serving clients across jurisdictions either because of the complexity for practitioners in maintaining an adequate working knowledge of numerous regulatory or legal frameworks or because services across borders may even be prohibited, as is the case in some US states. Considering the increased mobility and access of both practitioners and clients, laws may be more limiting than technology. Professional associations have an opportunity to advocate for laws and regulations that allow qualified practitioners to provide services beyond political boundaries.

Another potential barrier to use of technology in mental health services is accessibility due to costs. Ben-Zeev et al. (2012) found that many clients identified costs as the main barrier to owning a mobile phone, for example, and these same clients were not aware of governmental programs to assist with access. Practitioners will need to be aware of – and stay current with – programs that can assist clients with accessing technologies, such as mobile phones, Internet access and videoconferencing.

CONCLUSION

The question is no longer, as it once was, whether we should use technology in the delivery of mental health services, counselor training or clinical supervision. Instead the question now is *how* to best use technology, *with whom*, and *when* as noted in several chapters including Carey and Stretch (Chapter 26); Kaltenthaler, Cavanagh, and McCrone (Chapter 21); and Simpson, Richardson, and Reid (Chapter 10). Integrating technology into mental health is far more than adapted face-to-face techniques and interventions. Klion (Chapter 14) noted that we need to shift from adapting non-technical tools to developing tools specifically for Internet-based delivery.

Hooley and Neary (Chapter 37) noted that

in the world of technology and mental health "the development of . . . practice is rapidly outpacing evidence and research." The more we research current distance technology in the mental health field, the more opportunities we will have to understand the specific components that most impact our clients, students and supervisees. As Matthews and Coyle (Chapter 13) noted, further research into efficacy will eventually lead to more purposeful design. Hooley and Dodd (Chapter 20) stressed that as a profession we have to research the "psycho-socio-technical phenomenon" to truly understand how and when technology is best utilized in mental health delivery and training.

The future is certainly bright for increasing use and quality of technological means of extending mental health care well beyond the four walls of the consulting room. Futurology is an inexact science, at best, and the history of the development of information and communication technologies is replete with examples of products that, once hailed as The Next Big Thing, failed to deliver their hoped-for potential. Some became obsolete simply because a new, previously unimagined option removed the need they had sought to fulfill – digital cameras are one example, now that most mobile phones include one as standard. Others struggled to find a place in the socially sophisticated world of technologically mediated living. It would be foolhardy, therefore, to attempt to predict the future of technologies in mental health care with great precision. We may not have robots fitted with the Genuine People Personalities envisioned in the science fiction of books like *The Hitch Hikers' Guide to the Galaxy* (Adams, 1978), but we *do* know that there will be innovations that are equally amazing and, perhaps, even more useful. After all, many of us really do carry devices that give us instant access to everyone we know (and many people we don't) along with pretty much the sum total of all human learning and history.

To an ever-increasing degree, we are being enabled to be who we want to be online and, what is more, to express that in an ever-increasing variety of ways that we can choose for a given purpose or simply because they suit our need at the time.

What is already certain is that existing technologies can provide far greater possibilities for accessing mental health services and care than would otherwise be the case. It is also certain that these technologies will continue to be refined by their developers and, we hope, the input of mental health practitioners and their clients. If the history of technology in mental health care shows anything, it is that new opportunities will continue to emerge. Some will extend previous options into new areas or will use them in new ways. Others will be innovations on a greater scale and take us in directions we have not yet had the chance to think through. Their development and implementation will need to be carried out thoughtfully and with appropriate care and research. Practitioners, clients, the public, policy makers and professional associations will all need to be enabled to use them well through training and dissemination of high quality, unbiased and reliable information. However, if this is done, there is every reason to expect that mental health care as a whole will continue to be improved enhanced, perhaps especially by those nascent technologies yet to come to the fore.

REFERENCES

Adams, D. (1978). *The hitchhikers' guide to the galaxy.* [radio broadcast]. United Kingdom: British Broadcasting Corporation.

American Counseling Association. (2014). *Code of ethics and standards of practice.* Alexandria, VA: Author.

American Psychological Association. (2010). American Psychological Association ethical principles of psychologists and code of conduct. Retrieved from http://www.apa.org/ethics/code.

American Psychological Association Practice Organization. (2010). Telehealth: Legal basics for psychologists. *Good Practice.* Summer Issue, 2–7

Anthony, K., & Goss, S. (2009). *Guidelines for online counseling and psychotherapy. Including guidelines for online supervision.* (3rd ed.) Lutterworth, UK: British Association for Counselling & Psychotherapy.

Anthony, K., & Goss, S. (2015). *Good practice in action 27 and 28.* Lutterworth, UK: British Association for Counselling and Psychotherapy.

Ben-Zeev, D., Davis, K. E., Kaiser, S., Krzsos, I., & Drake, R. E. (2012). Mobile technologies among people with serious mental illness: Opportunities for future services. *Administration and Policy in Mental Health Services Research. 40*(4), 340-343.

Bennett, G. G., & Glasgow, R. E. (2009). The delivery of public health interventions via the Internet: Actualizing their potential. *Annual Review of Public Health, 30,* 273–292. doi: 10.1146/annurev.publhealth.031308.100235.

Boydell, K. M., Hodgins, M., Pignatiello, A., Teshima, J., Edwards, H., & Willis, D. (2014). Using technology to deliver mental health services to children and youth: A scoping review. *Journal of the Canadian Academy of Child and Adolescent Psychiatry, 23*(2), 87–99.

Boydell, K. M., Volpe, T., & Pignatiello, A. (2010). A qualitative a study of young people's perspectives on receiving psychiatric services via televideo. *Journal of the Canadian Academy of Child and Adolescent Psychiatry, 19*(1), 5–11.

Canadian Psychological Association. (2015). *Providing psychological services via electronic media.* Ottawa, ON: Author.

Center for the Credentialing and Education. (2011). *Distance credentialed counselor (DCC).* Greensboro, NC: Author.

Council for the Accreditation of Counseling Related Educational Programs. (2016). *2016 CACREP standards.* Alexandria, VA: Author. Retrieved from http://www .cacrep .org/wp-content/uploads/2013/12/2009-Standards.pdf.

Council for the Accreditation of Counseling Related Educational Programs. (2016). *2016 CACREP standards.* Alexandria, VA: Author. Retrieved from http://www .cacrep.org/wp-content/uploads/2015/ 05/2016-CACREP-Standards.pdf.

Ebert, D. D., Berking, M., Cuijpers, P., Lehr, D., Pörtner, M., & Baumeister, H. (2015). Increasing the acceptance of internet-based mental health interventions in primary care patients with depressive symptoms. A randomized controlled trial. *Journal of Affective Disorders, 176,* 9–17. doi. org/10.1016/j.jad.2015.01.056.

Goss, S. P., & Anthony, K. E. (2012). The evolution of guidelines for online counselling and psychotherapy – the development of ethical practice. In B. Popoola & O. Adebowale (Eds.), *Online guidance and counselling: Towards effectively applying technology.* New York: IGI Global.

Hill, A., & Roth, A. (2015). The competences required to deliver psychological therapies "at a distance." Retrieved from http:// www.bacp.co.uk/admin/structure/files/ pdf/13919_background_document.pdf.

Kazdin, A. E. (2015). Technology-based interventions and reducing the burdens of mental illness: Perspectives and comments on the special series. *Cognitive and Behavioral Practice, 22*(3), 359–366. doi. org/10.1016/j.cbpra.2015.04.004.

Luxton, D. D., McCann, R. A., Bush, N. E., Mishkind, M. C., & Reger, G. M. (2011). mHealth for mental health: Integrating smartphone technology in behavioral healthcare. *Professional Psychology: Research and Practice, 42*(6), 505–512. http://dx.doi .org/10.1037/a0024485.

Luxton, D. D., Sirotin, A. P., & Mishkind, M. C. (2010). Safety of telemental healthcare delivered to clinically unsupervised settings: A systematic review. *Telemedicine and e-Health, 16,* 705–711. doi: 10.1089/tmj.2009.0179.

Mohr, D. C., Burns, M. N., Schueller, S. M., Clarke, G., & Klinkman, M. (2013). Behavioral intervention technologies: Evidence review and recommendations for future research in mental health. *General Psychiatry, 35,* 332–338. doi:10.1016/j. genhosppsych.2013.03.008.

National Board of Certified Counselors. (1997). *Standards for the ethical practice of webcounseling.* Greensboro, NC: Author.

National Board of Certified Counselors. (2009). *The practice of internet counseling.* Retrieved from http://www.nbcc.org/ Assets/Ethics/internetCounseling.pdf.

National Board of Certified Counselors. (2012). *NBCC policy regarding the provision of distance professional services.* Retrieved from http://www.nbcc.org/Assets/Ethics/ NBCC Policy Regarding the Practice of Distance Counseling - Board - Adopted Version - July 2012- PDF.

Price, M., Yuen, E. K., Goetter, E. W., Herbert, J. D., Forman, E. M., Acierno, R., & Ruggiero, K. J. (2014). mHealth: A mechanism to deliver more accessible, more effective mental health care. *Clinical Psychology & Psychotherapy, 21*(5), 427–436. doi: 10.1002/cpp.1855.

Wilson, J. A. B., Onorati, K., Mishkind, M., Reger, M. A., & Gahm, G. A. (2008). Soldier attitudes and technology-based approaches to mental health care. *CyberPsychology & Behavior, 11*(6), 767–769. doi: 10.1089/cpb.2008.0071.

INDEX

E-Health Law, 161, 166
Ekselius, L., 13
Elford, D., 163, 165
Elford, R., 164, 166
Elhai, J., 99, 114, 310, 321
Elliot, R., 112
Elliott, J., 346
Elliott, R., 112
Elveling, E., 135
e-mail, 5, 10, 14–15, 215, 217, 333, 343–44, 347
email
   communications, 6–9, 12–13
   contacts, 7, 294
   exchanges, 206, 232, 295–97, 299–300, 332–33
   therapist-client, 8
   therapy, 11–12, 14–15, 128
   therapy-related, 10
Email and chat supervision, 315
emojis, 16, 33–34
emoticons, 11, 16, 33–34, 54, 66
emotions, 11, 48, 57, 97, 111, 122, 125, 209, 225, 263, 267, 317
Employee and Family Assistance Programs. *See* EFAP
Employee Assistance Programs. *See* EAPs
encryption, 8–9, 35, 39–41, 94–95, 112, 191, 244, 284, 286, 300, 306
Enhance Client Peer Support, 53, 55, 57, 59, 61
Enrich Counselor Training, 242, 321
environment, therapeutic, 104, 110, 288
Epley, N., 14, 10
equipment, 29, 37–38, 108–9, 266, 381
Erdman, H., 186
Eriksson, M., 241
Eriksson, S., 137
Eriksson, T., 15, 222
Ertelt, T., 100, 102, 112
Essock, S., 210
e-supervision, 240, 343, 348
E-supervisor, 235–40
e-therapy, 11, 93, 98, 168, 302
Ethical and practical dimensions of online therapy, 302
Ethical framework, 14, 34–35, 42, 90, 179, 302, 321, 338, 376
ethics, 6–7, 34–35, 41–46, 48–50, 133–34, 148–49, 204–5, 207–10, 247–48,

262–63, 286–89, 299–300, 321–22, 341–42, 346–48
   code of, 35, 44–45, 88, 94, 186, 287, 289
Etienne, J., 137
Ett, T., 97
European Eating Disorders Review, 14–15, 60, 114–15, 124
Excerpt of Asynchronous Email Supervision, 334
exchanges, 16, 37, 40–41, 57, 68–69, 150, 234, 236, 238, 240, 300, 316, 318, 332, 334
   therapeutic, 30, 37, 86
Exergames, 145
Eysenbach, G., 213, 215, 220

F

Fabregat, B., 179
Facebook, 43, 45–47, 49–50, 59, 61, 79, 88, 90, 177, 202, 205–6, 292–93, 362, 373
Facebook Messenger, 29–30
face-to-face supervision, 246, 275, 280, 308, 321, 328–29, 344, 348
face-to-face supervision sessions, 286, 341
face-to-face therapy, 18–19, 33, 132–33, 135, 144, 219
Fairley, M., 166
Falender, C., 261, 270, 377-379, 383
Falicov, C., 261, 270
Falkenberg, H., 358, 365
Family Brief Therapy, 23–24
Family Therapists, 243, 247, 287, 341, 378
family therapy, 114, 264, 269–71, 327, 382
Family therapy supervision, 269–71, 376
Farrand, P., 132, 136
Farren, C., 72
Faulkner, L., 158, 166
Fearfighter, 131–32, 134, 192, 216
Fedak, T., 346
feedback, 78, 88, 142–43, 183–85, 189, 215–17, 250–52, 256–57, 261, 264–65, 267–68, 293–95, 353–54, 368–69, 377–82
   faculty, 352
   supervisor's, 268
Feltey, K., xi, 224, 227, 228
Feltham, C., 302
Fenichel, M., 243, 246
Ferguson, J., 100, 103, 113, 115, 171
Ferguson, D., 264, 271
Ferlin, G., 124

CHARLES C THOMAS • PUBLISHER, LTD.

INTEGRATED HEALTH CARE FOR PEOPLE WITH AUTISM SPECTRUM DISORDER
By Ellen Giarelli & Kathleen Fisher
2016, 420 pp. (7 x 10), 19 il., 14 tables.
$65.95 (paper), $65.95 (ebook)

BEHAVIORAL GUIDE TO PERSONALITY DISORDERS (DSM-5)
By Douglas H. Ruben
2015, 272 pp. (7 x 10), 31 il., 1 table.
$42.95 (paper), $42.95 (ebook)

HAIR AND JUSTICE
By Carmen M. Cusack
2015, 224 pp. (7 x 10)
$35.95 (paper), $35.95 (ebook)

THE PROFESSIONAL HELPER (2nd Ed.)
By Willie V. Bryan
2015, 354 pp. (7 x 10)
$53.95 (paper), $53.95 (ebook)

SOLVING THE PUZZLE OF YOUR ADD/ADHD CHILD
By Laura J. Stevens
2015, 266 pp. (7 x 10), 7 il., 13 tables.
$35.95 (spiral), $35.95 (ebook)

THE USE OF CREATIVE THERAPIES IN TREATING DEPRESSION
By Stephanie L. Brooke & Charles Edwin Myers
2015, 368 pp. (7 x 10), 38 il.
$69.95 (hard), $69.95 (ebook)

THE SOCIOLOGY OF DEVIANCE (2nd Ed.)
By Robert J. Franzese
2015, 398 pp. (7 x 10), 21 il., 6 tables.
$64.95 (paper), $64.95 (ebook)

HYPNOSIS, DISSOCIATION, AND ABSORPTION (2nd Ed.)
By Marty Sapp
2015, 238 pp. (7 x 10), 4 tables.
$34.95 (paper), $34.95 (ebook)

DEALING WITH THE MENTALLY ILL PERSON ON THE STREET
By Daniel M. Rudofossi
2015, 252 pp. (7 x 10)
$51.95 (paper), $51.95 (ebook)

POSITIVE BEHAVIOR SUPPORTS FOR ADULTS WITH DISABILITIES IN EMPLOYMENT, COMMUNITY, AND RESIDENTIAL SETTINGS
By Keith Storey & Michal Post
2015, 196 pp. (7 x 10), 9 il., 27 tables.
$34.95 (paper), $34.95 (ebook)

HELPING SKILLS FOR HUMAN SERVICE WORKERS (3rd Ed.)
By Kenneth France & Kim Weikel
2014, 384 pp. (7 x 10), 6 il.
$59.95 (paper), $59.95 (ebook)

MULTICULTURAL ASPECTS OF HUMAN BEHAVIOR (3rd Ed.)
By Willie V. Bryan
2014, 278 pp. (7 x 10)
$45.95 (paper), $45.95 (ebook)

PERSONAL COUNSELING SKILLS (Rev. 1st Ed.)
By Kathryn Geldard & David Geldard
2012, 340 pp. (7 x 10), 20 il., 3 tables.
$45.95 (paper), $45.95 (ebook)

FOUNDATIONS OF MENTAL HEALTH COUNSELING (4th Ed.)
By Artis J. Palmo, William J. Weikel & David P. Borsos
2011, 508 pp. (7 x 10), 6 il., 3 tables.
$87.95 (hard), $64.95 (paper), $64.95 (ebook)

RESEARCH IN REHABILITATION COUNSELING (2nd Ed.)
By James L. Bellini & Phillip D. Rumrill, Jr.
2009, 320 pp. (7 x 10), 3 il., 5 tables.
$49.95 (paper), $49.95 (ebook)

PRINCIPLES AND PRACTICES OF CASE MANAGEMENT IN REHABILITATION COUNSELING (2nd Ed.)
By E. Davis Martin, Jr.
2007, 380 pp. (7 x 10), 7 il., 2 tables.
$54.95 (paper), $54.95 (ebook)

IDEOMOTOR SIGNALS FOR RAPID HYPNOANALYSIS
By Dabney M. Ewin & Bruce N. Eimer
2006, 296 pp. (7 x 10), 15 il.
$67.95 (hard), $47.95 (paper), $47.95 (ebook)

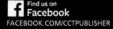
Find us on
Facebook
FACEBOOK.COM/CCTPUBLISHER

TO ORDER: 1-800-258-8980 • books@ccthomas.com • www.ccthomas.com